T0314257

A CATALOG OF BENEVOLENT ITEMS

A CATALOG OF BENEVOLENT ITEMS

Li Shizhen's Compendium of Classical Chinese Knowledge

Selected Entries from the *Ben Cao Gang Mu*

Translated, Edited, and Introduced
by Paul U. Unschuld

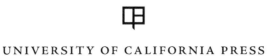

UNIVERSITY OF CALIFORNIA PRESS

University of California Press
Oakland, California

© 2024 by Paul U. Unschuld

Library of Congress Cataloging-in-Publication Data

Names: Li, Shizhen, 1518–1593, author. | Unschuld, Paul U. (Paul Ulrich), 1943– translator, editor, writer of introduction.
Title: A catalog of benevolent items : Li Shizhen's Compendium of classical Chinese knowledge / translated, edited, and introduced by Paul U. Unschuld.
Other titles: Ben cao gang mu. Selections. English
Description: Oakland, California : University of California Press, [2024] | Includes bibliographical references.
Identifiers: LCCN 2024013162 | ISBN 9780520404236 (hardback) | ISBN 9780520404243 (paperback) | ISBN 9780520404250 (ebook)
Subjects: LCSH: Li, Shizhen, 1518–1593. Ben cao gang mu. | Materia medica—China—Early works to 1800. | Medicine, Chinese—Formulae, receipts, prescriptions—Early works to 1800. | Natural history—China—Pre-Linnean works.
Classification: LCC RS180.C5 L4513 2024 | DDC 615.3/210951—dc23/eng/20240416
LC record available at https://lccn.loc.gov/2024013162

33   32   31   30   29   28   27   26   25   24
10   9   8   7   6   5   4   3   2   1

publication supported by a grant from

The Community Foundation for Greater New Haven

as part of the **Urban Haven Project**

The *Ben Cao Gang Mu* Series

The complete Chinese text
translated and annotated by Paul U. Unschuld

Tools

The *Dictionary of the Ben Cao Gang Mu*

Contents

4

Preface

This book opens the view to a unique encyclopedia that was first printed under the title *Ben cao gang mu* in China in 1593 and which, in its time, found no comparable counterpart on the entire Eurasian continent.

Li Shizhen (1518 - 1593) created a work which, at first glance, seems to be dedicated solely to healing with natural and also artificially produced substances. On closer inspection, however, the *Ben cao gang mu* proves to be an almost inexhaustible source of data, not only on historical Chinese natural science as a whole, but also on countless facets of Chinese historical culture.

Since the opening of the country in the 1970s, China has shown an exceedingly impressive capacity to become a world leader technologically and scientifically, and often in a very short time. To understand China, it is essential that we recognize the historical foundations of this success. In the middle of the 19th century, the encroachment first of Western European powers, then Russia, the USA and finally Japan, forced an independent knowledge dynamic, until then only sporadically enriched by foreign influences, to come to a virtual standstill. It was only after more than a century of the struggle to find a suitable place for the country in a changed world order that it once again came to fruition.

In the *Ben cao gang mu* we encounter the culmination of the pre-modern development of natural and medical knowledge in China. We recognize the seriousness of the search to explain natural processes. We observe an ancient culture of discussion with an openness to dissenting opinions that is without parallel in the documented history of knowledge in Europe. Through the testimonies of hundreds of authors of the past two millennia, we gain unprecedented access to all kinds of health hazards and suffering to which the population was exposed, and we learn, as nowhere else, about the manifold efforts to work for human welfare with the help of substances from nature and on the basis of varying theoretical approaches and practical interventions. To this end, we are also confronted with innumerable details of historical Chinese everyday culture, which are not brought before us in this density in any other pre-modern work. There are many reasons to study the historical foundations of Chinese culture and civilization in great depth today and in the future; the *Ben cao gang mu* offers what was hitherto largely inaccessible.

After many years of studying the history of ancient Chinese medical literature and translating the classics of Chinese medical theory from antiquity, I began a translation of the *Ben cao gang mu* almost two decades ago now. My aim was to produce for the first time an English version of the text based on European philological methodology and to render the views of Chinese authors of the past two millennia in their own understanding, rather than reinterpreting them according to contemporary knowledge. I was able to complete the translation in August 2022; the total of ten volumes of original Chinese text and English translation will be available in print from University of California Press by January 2024. [1]

Finally, the time had come to conclude the project with an anthology. No one can be expected to read all of the nearly 10,000 pages of the English version, but it is possible to recognize the value of *Ben cao gang mu* and become aware of its place in the history of the literature of human knowledge. This selection of about 500 text excerpts presented here conveys, not least, a completely new picture of traditional Chinese medicine. And above all, it may act as a first incentive to deal with the many facets of this work.

The *Ben cao gang mu* offers untold data and unique information on the culture of China that needs to be further explored. Studies by Chinese and Japanese authors already fill many volumes. It is hoped that the book presented here, as a narrow but stimulating reference to the full translation, will initiate outside of East Asia a similarly intensive study of this encyclopedia.

Paul U. Unschuld

Berlin, 2023

---

[1]   *Ben cao gang mu*, Vols. I through IX. *16th Century Chinese Encyclopedia of Materia Medica and Natural History*. The complete Chinese text translated and annotated by Paul U. Unschuld University of California Press, Oakland California 2021 – 2024.

Prolegomena

The disappointment resulting from Li Shizhen's failure to meet the expectations of his family may have been traumatic. Here was a young man who had been educated since childhood to raise the family from the status of socially rather disrespected physicians to the nobility of Ming society, that is, to being a Confucian scholar and official. The young man, 14 years old, had passed the first, not really challenging level of government exams. But that was it. He failed in all subsequent attempts to successfully pass higher level exams and eventually had no choice but to learn what his father and forefathers had practiced for a living, that is, medicine.

Medicine in China since its earliest appearance in historical documents had been depicted as a means to earn a livelihood not regarded worth a gentleman's attention. Zhu Xi (1120 – 1200), the eminent Song philosopher and driving force behind a revival of Confucius' teachings as Song-Neo-Confucians, had delivered a final deathblow to numerous attempts made by practicing physicians in their appeals to the public at reaching appropriate social recognition for what they termed a most humanitarian occupation. In an ongoing debate on what were "petty teachings," Zhu Xi listed "agriculture, horticulture, medicine, prophecy and all the other types of specialized work." It was only beginning with the Yuan dynasty, when learned Confucian scholars no longer easily found a government job, that some of them turned to medicine as the only alternative realm of knowledge based on a large literary corpus. Although their voices increased in number and quality in their demands for recognition as contributing to society as much humanitarian service as Confucian scholars claimed to monopolize, their status remained as low as ever. Some became renowned practitioners, some wrote texts reprinted for many centuries, and some became rich. But the status of Confucian scholar official remained the one and only longed-for status in the highest echelon of society.

Li Shizhen sat the provincial exams for a third time at the age of 23, when he joined the large number of unsuccessful candidates. He made the best of the alternative path in life that he was forced to take, eventually leaving behind a monument of literacy and scholarship that was to survive the writings produced by his more successful contemporaries. Li Shizhen studied and practiced medicine, he occupied several positions in medical offices, and he eventually set out to demonstrate that he was not simply a practitioner of some specialized work, who got his hands dirty like a gardener, but a scholar commanding a wide range of knowledge, and a scholar author capable of offering information at least as valuable for society as the contents of the well-respected works of Confucian scholar literati. He chose for the work he was going to give mankind the title *Ben cao gang mu*.

Ben cao was an established term for *materia medica* ever since the Han dynasty. With the addition *gang mu*, Li Shizhen combined two messages. The terms *gang* and *mu* were to signal that he planned to provide data in a consistently structured manner, offering a division into major, *gang*, and more specific, *mu*, sections. But there may have been more behind this. We cannot look into Li Shizhen's mind, but when he chose a title for his encyclopedia, he may have been thinking of the only major and widely known work published as a *gang mu* before, the *Tong jian gang mu* edited by Zhu Xi as a condensation of the famous Song historian Sima Guang's *Comprehensive mirror to aid in government.*

Sima Guang (1019 – 1086) was repelled by the cumbersome and un- wieldy conventional writings dominating historiography. He adopted the annalistic style in which Confucius around 1500 years earlier had written his *Spring and Autumn Analects*. By combining the terms and concepts of *ben cao* and *gang mu*, Li Shizhen went right to the heart of Confucianism. He positioned himself next to Zhu Xi's *Gang mu,* and at the same time with his own *Gang mu* he demanded the highest respect for a knowledge belittled by the great Song philosopher. The *Ben cao gang mu* in a way is annalistic. Never before had an author given as much space to history and tradition in the field of natural science and health care as did Li Shizhen in his encyclopedia. Never before had an author brought together as many diverse sources of information as had Li Shizhen. He signaled a digression from what he, too, must have perceived as the cumbersome and unwieldy structure of earlier comprehensive *materia medica* works. At the same time, he linked his work, intentionally or somewhat unconsciously, with the are- na of social and scholarly life in which his education made him a player, that is, Confucianism as modified by the so-called Cheng-Zhu school.

Zhang Zai (1020 – 1077) had initiated this new interpretation of Con- fucius's teachings when pressure increased to save them from being pushed into oblivion by Buddhism and Daoism. Zhang Zai emphasized the reality and materiality of all things by pointing at *qi* as the finest vapor of matter in permanent aggregation and dissolution. His nephews Cheng Hao (1032 – 1085) and Cheng Yi (1033 – 1107) saw a basic principle, *li*, underlying all workings of *qi*. All three of them, Zhang Zai and the two Cheng brothers, urged scholars to study real objects so as to eventually grasp the workings of *qi* and the underlying principle *li*. Zhu Xi forged this into a system that, beginning with the Ming era, was accepted as orthodox Confucian doctrine. *Li*, he taught, constitutes the immaterial organizational principle controlling all genesis, existence, and decay, and *qi* are the vapors of matter that bring genesis, existence, and decay to fruition. A hands-on study of nature had so far been the domain of Daoism, regarded by Confucian scholars as "off-limits." Competence in natural processes and the crafts transforming them into items of daily use was more or less required now to prove real scholarship. In recognizing *qi* as a matter uniting all dead things and all living beings, an ethical obligation was created to focus not only on a connection between humans and their affairs but including all phenomena alike. This served to offer a secular ethics contrasting with the charity required by Buddhism with its denial of reality.

The contents of the *Ben cao gang mu* are the results of Li Shizhen's search for and collection of mostly down-to-earth information on nature and how nature could be employed to assist humans in times of need. Li Shizhen carried out his project with unique ambition. He evaluated a vast number of available sources with great care. He read texts and talked to informants from all social classes. Evidently, all scholarly arrogance was alien to him. He did not shy away from gathering data from all levels of society. Historians have found numerous "firsts" in his substance monographs, previously hidden in some obscure sources.

One example is his account of a disease called "red bayberry sores," identified now as syphilis, in the monograph on the herb glabrous greenbrier (18-27), the first of such detail in *materia medica* literature: "Red bayberry sores are not recorded in ancient recipes; and there were no patients affected by them. In recent times, they emerged in Lingbiao and from there spread into all directions. The fact is, Lingbiao is a region with inferior natural conditions and extreme heat, and with stifling vapors and miasma. People drink and eat acrid, hot items. Males and females engage in licentious behavior. When the evil qi of moisture and heat have accumulated to an extreme, they will effuse as poisonous sores. This, then, is transmitted from one to another, from the South to the North, extending everywhere. Still, only people committed to the evil of licentiousness get this disease. It may appear in numerous varieties, but there is only one way to cure them."

Li Shizhen was the first to accept sweet potato and corn as *materia medica*; they had reached China, imported from the Philippines, only during his own lifetime. Joseph Needham, always in search of insights, conclusions, and methods apparently recorded much earlier in China than in Europe, was successful in the *Ben cao gang mu* several times: "Li Shizhen tells us, too, of hygienic practices such as the fumigation of sick-rooms and the steam sterilization of patients' clothes in epidemics, ... But perhaps the most outstanding example of Li Shizhen's insight and intelligence in iatro-chemical matters is his detailed account of the making of steroid hormone preparations from large quantities of urine, and their use in suitable endocrinological disorders."[2] It is often overlooked, though, that, unlike in Europe, such spectacular finds appeared as isolated notes and remained unnoticed rather than becoming practices widely accepted and practiced by Chinese physicians.

In many ways, the completion and publication of the *Ben cao gang mu* should not be viewed merely as the extraordinary achievement of a uniquely gifted and dedicated individual. Li Shizhen was also a child of his time. The Ming dynasty had fostered a social environment that had a direct bearing on Li Shizhen and his encyclopedia. One is tempted to compare Li Shizhen's achievement with that of Song Yingxing (1587 – 1666?); their lifetimes overlapped for seven years. Song Yingxing, a minor official living in southern China, compiled the *Tian gong kai wu*, published in 1637, four decades after the appearance of the *Ben cao gang mu*. Dagmar Schäfer in her *The Crafting of 10,000 Things* offers a biography of Song Yingxing and locates his work in his time.[3] Apparently, *Works of Heaven and the Inception of Things*, as she translated *Tian gong kai wu*, was compiled out of a late Ming scholar's frustration over the progressive violation and decay of a social order that a Confucian felt was essential.

Song Yingxing had a family background of scholars that stretched back over several generations; one of his ancestors was remembered as a local eminence. The claim to occupy such a high rung on the social ladder had remained alive in the family for generations. Song Yingxing noted enough signs that he and others interpreted as portents of imminent social disintegration, with dire consequences not only for his own and his family's future, but also for the dynasty and the country as a whole. He sat down and put his concerns to paper. He published several smaller pieces; the *Works of Heaven and the Inception of Things* was his most important work. For historians of today it is a source of almost unlimited information – on the author and on his time, on Chinese culture in general and on the situation of artisans and their crafts in particular.

---

2   Joseph Needham, *Science and Civilisation in China*. Vol. VI: 1. Biology and Biological Technology. Cambridge University Press, Cambridge. 1956: 320. See there for more.

3   Dagmar Schäfer, *The Crafting of the 10,000 Things. Knowledge and Technology in Seventeenth-Century China*. The University of Chicago Press. Chicago and London. 2011.

A comparison of Song Yingxing's *Tian gong kai wu* with Li Shizhen's *Ben cao gang mu* should cast additional light on Li Shizhen and his encyclopedia. However, the two sides of such a comparison are not yet equally visible. Schäfer's meticulous analysis of Song's personality, his motivation and his written work as influenced by his environment, cannot yet be matched with a similarly informed study of Li Shizhen's. This is all the more true because Song Yingxing has left behind several additional texts reflecting on his personal views and reflecting on the ideal role of scholars in Ming society.

Li Shizhen has left us no such evidence of his intellectual orientation. There is only one line in the Introductory Notes to the *Ben cao gang mu* where he abandons his reluctance to talk about his motives and identifies himself as a Ming era Confucian: "I, Li Shizhen have added another 374 items. They may be called 'pharmaceutical items' by medical experts, but the way I have studied and explained their nature and the principles underlying it is in fact part of the investigation of things, pursued by us Confucians/scholars, to fill the gaps in the *Examples of Refined Usage*,[4] and the commentaries on the *Classic of Songs*."[5] Any further clues as to stimuli and concerns that may have prompted Li Shizhen to realize his unprecedented program are to be sought in notes scattered far apart in his *Ben cao gang mu*.

Song Yingxing wrote a thoughtful piece on *qi*, the finest vapors of matter, so important to Neo-Confucian philosophy. Li Shizhen simply used the term and concept in a context strictly defined by morphological, physiological and pathological argumentation. *Qi* vapors and blood had been identified as the two essential foundations of life in antiquity. Li Shizhen quoted earlier authors who had written of *qi* congealing, accumulating and aggregating, causing blockage and disease. *Qi* move in the human organism with different functions. They may enter the organism hidden in food and beverages or with the air through inhalation. They may leave the body through any of the various orifices, including the pores of the skin. The body's *qi* can be manipulated based on the expert's knowledge of the *qi* transmission through an ingestion of natural substances, and also through fumigation. Li Shizhen left such information alone; he did not join the philosophical discussion on the wider, universal significance of *qi*.

Li Shizhen's handling of *li* is not much different. He used the term *li* to connote a concept comprising underlying principle, innate order, and also

---

4   The *Er ya*, an authoritative lexicographic guide to Chinese classic texts ca. 200 BCE.

5   The *Shi jing*, allegedly compiled by Confucius.

structure. Every now and then he comments on a more or less noteworthy, if not spectacular, relationship between natural substances as an example of "the principle of things mutually affecting each other." He speaks of "the wondrous principles underlying things that nobody can imagine." And he acknowledges man's ignorance in comments such as "the principles underlying the activities of objects are that strange" and "that walnuts check the poison of copper is one of those enigmatic principles in the nature of things."

And yet, the requirement imposed by Cheng-Zhu-Confucianism on scholars is also mirrored in such statements as "the land to produce tree fruits and melons may be normal or unusual, their nature and flavor may be good or poisonous. How could one simply long for and indulge in them without being familiar with their underlying principles?" Possibly, Li Shizhen thought here of an inherent cosmic order to be revealed by the "investigation of things." Two or three similar lines, hidden in the vast amount of information gathered in the *Ben cao gang mu*, hit the same note: "The Sages paid greatest attention to even these small creatures. How could scholars of today not do research on these creatures and their underlying principles, and check whether they are good or have poison?" "The structure of things assumes myriad appearances like that. Is this not something a learned person must know?" And: "To carefully read the texts requires first to approach their underlying principles and not to cling strictly to the written words."

Unlike Song Yingxing, Li Shizhen did not see it as his task to give new impetus to the philosophical debate, or even to explicitly express thoughts on it. He had not been accepted into the higher ranks of recognized scholarship. Practicing medicine and writing on herbal, mineral and animal substances and how they were processed to become valuable pharmaceutical drugs, he remained down to earth while still fulfilling the basic role of a Cheng-Zhu Confucian scholar: he investigated things and wrote about them to expand knowledge. With his sober attitude he created an encyclopedia informed by his time, but not limited to his time.

Song Yingxing, if we follow Schäfer's conclusions, wrote on the "crafting of things" to demonstrate the control held by his class, the scholars, over a field as indispensible for daily life as craftsmanship and the artisans involved in it. Li Shizhen wrote on objects found in nature and processed for the benefit of man as a field of knowledge to which he himself applied his own hands. Song Yingxing is praised for the intellectual reflections that he brought to fruition in his *Works of Heaven and the Inception of Things*. His name and his writings are still known and valued by the highly educated in China and by a few sinologist experts in the world. Li Shizhen's *Ben cao gang mu* is known to virtually everybody with a basic education in China. He is remembered with postal stamps, children's books and TV series. In 2011, the United Nations Educational, Scientific and Cultural Organization (UNESCO), following a suggestion submitted by this author, certified the inscription of the *Ben cao gang mu* on the Memory of the World International Register.

Historical background

The *Ben cao gang mu* is the most comprehensive and most innovative and therefore most informative encyclopedia of natural science compiled and published throughout the Eurasian continent prior to the 19th century. It is also the culmination of a 1600-year history of Chinese *materia medica* literature, including information from the realms of botany, zoology and mineralogy, in addition to countless data on their cultural context. This history began at some time during the Han dynasties when, between the 2nd century BCE and the 2nd century CE, two in China hitherto undocumented genres of medical-therapeutic works appeared in Chinese bibliographies.

Stimulated by impulses whose origin and nature remain enigmatic today, the new therapeutic approach of needling 365 "holes" spread over the human body, on the one hand; and a first detailed description of 365 individual pharmaceutical substances on the other, marked the onset of two traditions of health care. They remained conceptually separate for one thousand years. Why 365, the number of days in a solar year, – rather unusual in the history of Chinese categorization of natural phenomena – was chosen as the starting point for both traditions is unclear.

Needling therapy, or so-called acupuncture, remained an isolated facet of Chinese medical culture until the 11th/12th century. Its seminal texts, the Yellow Thearch classics,[6] were either lost during the first millennium or survived only through a somewhat tenuous tradition, supported by a few members of the social elite. Apparently, the yin yang and Five Phases

6   Including the *Huang Di nei jing su wen* 黃帝內經素問, *Huang di nei jing ling shu* 黃帝內經靈樞, and a late sequel, the *Nan jing* 難經. For philological translations of these classics, see Paul U. Unschuld and Hermann Tessenow, *Huang Di Nei Jing Su Wen. An Annotated Translation of Huang Di's Inner Classic*, 2 vols. University of California Press, Berkeley and Los Angeles, 2011. Paul U. Unschuld, *Huang Di Nei Jing Ling Shu. The Ancient Classic on Needle Therapy*. University of California Press, Oakland, 2016. Paul U. Unschuld, *Nan jing. The Classic of Difficult Issues*. Oakland 2016.

doctrines of systematic correspondences, which legitimated and guided needle therapy from its beginning, failed to achieve the status of a world view widely acknowledged by the elite and broad segments of the population. In contrast, pharmaceutical therapy, as evidenced by published recipe collections and works focusing on the description of individual substances, have constituted the mainstay of medical practice in China from the first millennium to the present day.

Since the early 1970s, recipe manuscripts with data on the therapeutic properties of combinations of herbal, mineral, and animal substances have been recovered from late Zhou and early Han era tombs.[7] The list of therapeutic indications and the highly developed pharmaceutical technology outlined in these texts evidence the lengthy development of knowledge on the therapeutic value of herbs, minerals, and animals, as well as some man-made substances, prior to the compilation of works with descriptions of the properties of individual substances. The earliest of these works known is *Shen nong's materia medica*. Historians agree that it was written at some time between the 1st century BCE and the 1st century CE.[8]

Even though at that time Chinese civilization recognized and documented in bibliographies and catalogues the individual authorship of literary works, the authors of the seminal texts of both the needling and the pharmaceutical traditions remained anonymous. Their origins were traced to legendary culture heros, that is, to Huang Di, the Yellow Thearch, and Shen Nong, the Divine Husbandman. Shen Nong, also known as the Fiery Thearch, was said in the *The Master of Huainan* to have pitied the suffering of mankind. Hence, he tasted all kinds of herbs and "discovered 100 with poison per day." From the very beginning, for a natural substance "to have poison" or "to be nonpoisonous" was seen as an important criterion for assessing its acute or long-term therapeutic potential.

Tao Hongjing (452 – 536), a Daoist naturalist, was the first author to revise and expand the *Original Classic*, as he called *Shen nong's materia medica*. In a first work, titled *Shen nong's classic on materia medica*, he retained the original division into three chapters, but added 365 "additional records on pharmaceutical substances recorded earlier by renowned physicians." In a second work shortly thereafter, the *Various annotations to Shen nong's classic on materia medica*, Tao Hongjing significantly expanded

7   Donald Harper, *Early Chinese Medical Literature. The Mawangdui Medical Manuscripts.* Kegan Paul International, London and New York, 1997.

8   For details on the *Sheng nong ben cao* and the subsequent history of Chinese *materia medica* literature, see Paul U. Unschuld, *Medicine in China. A History of Pharmaceutics.* Berkeley, Los Angeles, London, 1986.

his annotations to the 730 substances listed and also divided the text into seven chapters.

Tao Hongjing initiated a "main tradition" of material medica works, which would be continued by subsequent authors until the early 13th century. This tradition was characterized by an expansion of the *Original Classic* with ever more data on the nature, origin, therapeutic effects and pharmaceutical processing of natural and man-made substances. This data was often adopted from an increasing number of *materia medica* works published outside of the main tradition whose authors did not feel committed to the structure and contents of the *Original Classic*. They focused on regional knowledge, their own experience, substances used as both medication and food, substances enabling survival in times of famine, pharmaceutical processing, and other such special aspects of pharmaceutical lore. In the middle of the 7th century, an official named Su Jing (fl. 657) suggested that the emperor support a new edition of the *Original Classic* to correct older data since regarded as erroneous, and include more recent knowledge of the therapeutic potential of natural substances. The result, the *Newly revised materia medica* of 659, combining 850 substance entries in 54 chapters, was the first government-sponsored and illustrated *materia medica* work in China.

The main tradition came to a halt in the 13th century for at least two reasons. The lengthy title of one of the final works of this tradition, published in 1249 and describing 1746 substances in 30 chapters, offers a clear indication of one of these reasons: *Newly revised materia medica of the reign period "uprightness and harmony," based on data from the classics and historical annals, based on evidence and ordered on the basis of groups, prepared for clinical application.* The main tradition was stifled by the abundance of its data and the perpetuation of its claim to be merely extending the original classic. The last works were extremely unwieldy. More recent data were added to previous statements, without comments on contradictions or earlier errors. Readers were left abandoned with ever longer sequences of quotes from a wide range of sources of varying quality.

We see a second reason for the end of the main tradition in a completely new genre of *materia medica* texts initiated by Kou Zongshi's *Extended ideas on materia medica* in 1119 and exemplified by Wang Haogu's *Materia medica of decoctions* in the mid-13th century. With the rise of Song Neo-Confucianism, the more than one-millennium-old schism was bridged between the therapeutic approaches of needling and pharmaceutical therapy. Needling, i.e. acupuncture, was based on the yin yang and Five

Phases doctrines of systematic correspondences. *Materia medica* literature and recipe collections until now had completely bypassed the doctrines of systematic correspondences. Rather, they were based on ever increasing empirical knowledge and a continued belief in pre-historic magical correspondences.

The convergence of these two separate approaches resulted in a first genuine pharmacology of systematic correspondences, i.e., a theory of the effects of medicinal substances in the human organism based on the yin yang and Five Phases teachings. Authors committed to this new perspective categorized each pharmaceutical substance according to its presumed association with certain kinds of flavor (sour, acrid, bland, sweet, salty) and thermo-quality (hot, warm, cool, cold). As these flavors and thermo-qualities were associated, in turn, with certain yin and yang qualities, as well as with the Five Phases, a link appeared possible to pathologies also defined in terms of yin and yang and the Five Phases.[9]

The main tradition was unable to integrate the ideas published by the various authors of the so-called Song-Jin-Yuan epoch of *materia medica* literature. As a result, the publication of comprehensive *materia medica* texts ended. Each of these works claimed to offer all available pharmaceutical knowledge, old and new. It was only three centuries later, in the 16th century, that two authors introduced a new structure to the contents of comprehensive *materia medica* works, leading to a brief revival of the tradition. The first result was the *Materia medica written on imperial order, containing essential data arranged in systematic order* in 1505. The second and more successful of these newer *materia medica* works was the *Ben cao gang mu* of 1593 compiled by a team led by Li Shizhen (1518 – 1593).

Biographical sketch of Li Shizhen (1518 – 1593)

Li Shizhen, style Dongbi, "ceremonial jade disc of the east," assumed name Binhu, "on the shore of the lake," was born in Qi zhou, today's Qi chun county, province Hu bei, to a family of physicians. His grandfather is known to have practiced as an itinerant healer. The earliest known biography of a professional Chinese medical healer, published by Sima Qian (fl. 90 BCE) in his historical account *Shi ji*, is devoted to an itinerant healer, Chunyu Yi. To this day, itinerant healers have played an important role in the medical care of large segments of the population. At the same time,

---

9   Ulrike Unschuld, Traditional Chinese Pharmacology: An Analysis of its Development in the Thirteenth Century. *Isis* 68, no. 2 (June 1977): 224-248.

they were and still are commonly denounced as fraudsters by resident physicians. Li Shizhen's father, Li Yanwen, rose to a more respected class of physicians and was engaged for a while as Medical Secretary in the Imperial Medical Office. For his therapeutic skills he was praised as Immortal Li. He is remembered as the author of monographs on ginseng root and mugwort, a plant used for moxibustion. He also wrote texts on smallpox and pulse diagnosis.

Li Shizhen was supposed to rise even higher on the social scale. He was introduced to Confucian learning by Gu Wen, grandfather of the renowned Gu Jingxing (1621 – 1687), who was the first to write an account of Li Shizhen's life. At the age of 14, Li Shizhen passed the county level exams. However, even though he continued his studies for several years, he failed to pass exams on the next higher level and eventually turned to the occupation of his father and grandfather. Over time, based on experience and knowledge acquired from his father as well as on his own literate knowledge and dedication to understanding the principles underlying natural processes, Li Shizhen became widely known as a competent practitioner. He was invited to noble and other high-ranking families, and his successful cures in 1543 led to an invitation from the King of Chu, Zhu Xianrong (1506 – 1545), a regional prince, to manage his palace medical office. Details of the following years are unclear. We know that Li Shizhen was offered and accepted a position in the Imperial Medical Office but returned to his hometown after only a year. The exact date and circumstances of this journey to Beijing and the reasons why he left so soon are not known. From the contents of the *Ben cao gang mu*, though, it is obvious that he returned from the north having accumulated much new knowledge.

In Beijing he also encountered practices he considered highly objectionable. Among the elite, a widespread practice was to "cure human ills with human substances." Based on a notion that a reverse flow of menstrual blood left the body as breast milk, practitioners advocated kneading the breasts of girls until they released some liquid. This liquid was termed "flat peach wine," allegedly an elixir granting immortality. Li Shizhen recorded this practice in chapter 52, entry 15, on "human milk," clearly condemning it as "deceitful rhetoric to make a profit, aimed at those who are ignorant. It is voiced by fraudulent persons, and punished by royal law. The gentleman is to denounce it." In Beijing he also learned of the use of opium as an aphrodisiac and considered this a therapy that ought not be applied by a proper healer.

Back home in 1552, at the age of 34, Li Shizhen began to compile the *Ben cao gang mu*. It was only 27 years later, in 1578, that he concluded his manuscript. To compile a work of 1.6 million characters, based not only on extensive reading of earlier literature but also on the results of repeated short and long-distance travelling, is an enormous achievement. Li Shizhen mentions family members and disciples as assistants, but the size of his team is not known. His achievement is even more astonishing given that during these 27 years he wrote and published several books as well. Two of these, *Binhu's study of vessel movements*, a book on pulse diagnosis, and the *Studies of the eight extraordinary conduit vessels*, survive to this day. Others, like a collection of medical cases in which he himself had achieved successful outcomes, a *Collection on Li Binhu's easy to use recipes*, and an *Illustrated study of the five long-term depots*, have been lost as individual texts.

None of these books became as influential as the *Ben cao gang mu*. Nor, initially, was the completed manuscript of the *Ben cao gang mu* received with much enthusiasm. It took Li Shizhen ten years, knocking at doors here and there, until eventually Hu Chenglong in Jinling, today's Nanjing, agreed to print the text. It was published in 1593 with a preface by the famous scholar Wang Shizhen (1526 – 1590) and supplemented by two chapters with 1109 illustrations rather hastily made by his sons Li Jianyuan and Li Jianmu. Whether Li Shizhen ever saw this "Jinling edition" is not known. He died that same year.

Today eight complete copies of the first edition and four fragments are known to exist in China, in Japan, and in the USA. A second edition, supported by a local government office, was published by Xia Liangxin and Zhang Dingsi in neighboring Jiangxi province in 1603. Even though some errors crept into the text, the print and the illustrations were excellently executed. The widespread dissemination and the fame of the *Ben cao gang mu* began with this Jiangxi edition.

Structure and contents of the *Ben cao gang mu*

A major challenge met by an author compiling an encyclopedia with descriptions of individual substances from the realms of mineralogy, botany, and zoology is the classification and arrangement of the entries. Li Shizhen conceptualized a new order. The Han era *Original Classic*, within the three groups of upper, middle, and lower rank, had listed substances following their identification as mineral, herbal, and animal-human – i.e. proceeding from dead and immobile to living and immobile, and then on to living and mobile substances. A fourth and final group consisted of victuals. Later works of the main tradition omitted the upper, middle, and lower rank divisions, but retained the mineral, herbal, and animal-human classifications.

Li Shizhen introduced a different order. Based on the sequence of the Five Phases, after four introductory chapters he began the subsequent 48 chapters with a list of waters, followed by fires, soils, and metals, including salts and minerals (chapters 5-11), and then herbal substances (chapters 12 through 37). Separated by chapter 38 listing "fabrics and utensils," he then devoted chapters 39 through 50 to animals, ranging from "tiny" to "large," that is, from worms/bugs through fowl to four-legged creatures. Again, separated by a chapter on "strange items," he eventually reached the pinnacle of his scale, human substances suitable for a medicinal application. In all, Li Shizhen wrote down ca. 1.6 million characters to describe 1,892 pharmaceutical substances.

The entries in chapters 5 through 52 were divided into 16 sections, for 13 of which Li Shizhen identified subsections. These serve to identify related items within broader groups such as waters, herbs, and worms/bugs. The section on worms/bugs, for example, is subdivided into those born from eggs, those generated through transformation, and those originating from moisture. Each section is introduced by a general statement explicating the special nature of the substances grouped in it. These statements are cited in full length in 01 of the present anthology.

Each individual substance is given a heading stating its earliest name as documented in pharmaceutical literature and, if this was the "original classic," the upper, middle, or lower rank to which it had been assigned. Given the different names by which natural things had come to be known over the millennia and in different regions, Li Shizhen often went to great lengths to explain the origins and meanings of mineral, plant, and animal names. Examples are offered here in 16 of the anthology.

Where required, Li Shizhen began an entry by pointing out a formerly erroneous listing of the substance in question. Whenever he found identical substances listed twice in previous *materia medica* works under different names, he justified the combination of these names in one entry.

Li Shizhen offered what he may have considered comprehensive lists of therapeutic indications associated with individual items. The quotes on the ability of substances to "control" disease are taken from sources spanning more than 1,500 years. The *Ben cao gang mu* includes more than 4,500 key disease terms; by the time of Li Shizhen perhaps most of them were still self-explanatory or could be understood by experts from their context.

In today's China, many of the disease names referred to in these quotes are no longer easily understood. Similarly, for readers of the *Ben cao gang mu* outside China, the therapeutic indications are often given with rather enigmatic disease names written in single, unfamiliar characters or using metaphors that are no longer easily grasped. As an essential tool required for a meaningful reading and translation of the *Ben cao gang mu* we have prepared in collaboration with Zhang Zhibin the first volume of the *Dictionary of the Ben cao gang mu*, and published it through University of California Press. It traces each of the 4,500 disease terms to its earliest appearance; it identifies their meaning in that early context and, where applicable, at the time of Li Shizhen. [10]

Another central feature of the descriptions of pharmaceutical substances is their place of origin. From early on it was known among Chinese experts that one and the same herb was endowed with different therapeutic powers depending on where it grew in the country. The climate and the nature of the soil varied from North to South and from East to West, and so did the *qi* a plant was exposed to. Hence, where considered necessary, substance entries in the *Ben cao gang mu* include related information. This is mostly comparative: that is, Li Shizhen provided a ranking of the substances from different regions in accordance with the presumed strength of their therapeutic effects. Again and again, the *Ben cao gang mu* emphasizes the effects of local climate on local *qi* and how local soil transmits the therapeutic effects of these *qi* onto the objects originating from there. All the dynasties that followed each other during the imperial age regularly rearranged administrative structures. Consequently, place names and the names of administrative structures were assigned new designations. As a result, hardly any location kept one and the same name throughout history. In his time, Li Shizhen regularly explained the location of places mentioned in an ancient quote under a name no longer in use. Today, however, the current location of even more places can no longer be easily identified by their ancient names.

In collaboration with Hua Linfu and Paul D. Buell we have therefore prepared and published the second volume of the *Dictionary of the Ben cao gang mu*. It traces each of the place names and those of administrative structures mentioned in the *Ben cao gang mu* to their current location.

---

10 See Zhang Zhibin and Paul U. Unschuld, *Dictionary of the Ben cao gang mu*. Vol. I: *Chinese Historical Illness Terminology*. University of California Press, Oakland, 2015.

More importantly, the *Dictionary* offers the history of each name and each administrative structure so that a quote from a specific time period may be compared to the existence of a name and administrative structure at that time. This is of particular relevance if one identical name was given to different locations in the course of history, or if the borders of an administrative structure were altered to such a degree that it may have had a significant impact on the climate or nature of soil suggested by its name.[11]

No *materia medica* text prior to the *Ben cao gang mu* was based on a comparable range of literary and non-literary material. It should come as no surprise that Li Shizhen exploited the *Materia medica of the reign period "uprightness and harmony"* of 1249, the final work of the former main tradition of *materia medica* works, as his major source. Apparently, Li Shizhen intended to continue this tradition, but he went far beyond it. In a bibliography at the very beginning of the *Ben cao gang mu*, he listed more than 868 titles he had consulted. The exact number of titles quoted or mentioned in passing in the main text exceeds by far these 868 texts. To be sure, Li Shizhen may not have held all of them in his hands as original editions. Many texts were quoted second- or third-hand from quotes in later encyclopedias.

In addition to drawing his data from all kinds of literary genres, Li Shizhen personally travelled to places all over the country where he expected to access data available nowhere else. In this way, he was also able to record valuable data on substances not mentioned in *materia medica* literature or publicly documented previously elsewhere. For example, *san qi* 三七, identified today as *Panax notoginseng* (Burk.) F. H. Chen, is one of the herbs most commonly resorted to in Chinese medicine. Li Shizhen was the first to learn of its therapeutic potential from "locals," and he introduced it with the following lines:

"This medication was discovered for the first time only recently. The people in the South use it in their military as an important medication for wounds caused by metal objects/weapons. It is said to have an extraordinary therapeutic potential. It is also said: For all injuries resulting from flogging and blows, when stagnant blood is set free, it should be chewed until it is pulpy. Once this is applied to the affected region, the bleeding ends. Greenish swelling is dissolved. If one is to be flogged, let him ingest beforehand one or two maces, and his blood will not rush to his heart. Af-

---

11 See Hua Linfu, Paul D. Buell and Paul U. Unschuld, *Dictionary of the Ben cao gang mu*. Vol. II: *Geographical and Administrative Designations*. University of California Press, Oakland, 2017.

ter a flogging it is even more advisable to ingest it. To ingest it after a birth is good, too. Generally speaking, this medication has warm qi and a sweet and slightly bitter flavor. Hence it is a medication for the blood section on the yang brilliance and ceasing yin conduits and can serve to cure all kinds of blood diseases, similar to dragon blood (*Daemonorops draco* Bl.) and shellac."[12]

In this manner, the *Ben cao gang mu* refers to hundreds of texts and their authors, in addition to individuals (including Li Shizhen's own father Li Yanwen) unassociated with any literary genre.

Many of the persons quoted or referred to as authors, patients, healers or actors in some anecdote have remained nameless to posterity. In bibliographical and biographical reference works today's readers of the *Ben cao gang mu* may easily find the more prominent book titles, authors and historical personalities encountered in the *Ben cao gang mu*. But an identification of numerous titles and many more persons requires extensive research. It is here that one wonders how many collaborators Li Shizhen may have had.

Wang Shizhen, the author of a preface to the first edition of the *Ben cao gang mu*, quotes Li Shizhen verbatim as stating that he had rewritten the entire manuscript three times. A question arising here is whether he had failed to notice numerous inconsistencies in the references to book titles and authors quoted. Not infrequently, one book is quoted with either its complete title or several different abbreviations. Similarly, one identical author is quoted by his full name, by his first or last name, by his style, or by using other possible designations. Such diversity appears plausible if one imagines a larger team around Li Shizhen supplying him with data without prior agreement on how to quote a text or refer to a person. If this diversity makes it difficult enough for readers to immediately identify a text or author quoted, the hardship is further aggravated by numerous quotes misleadingly ascribed to source texts they were never part of.

Not much later, Zhao Xuemin (ca. 1730 – 1805), author of the book *Addition of Data Omitted in the Ben cao gang mu*, suggested with the title of his book that he not only intended to list pharmaceutically useful substances Li Shizhen had failed to include. He was also the first to identify 30 substantial errors in the description of substances recorded. In recent years, with a steep rise in *Ben cao gang mu* research, many more such errors and misleading

---

12 *Ben cao gang mu*, chapter 09, entry 09. See also, Zheng Jinsheng 郑金生 and Zhang Zhibin 张志斌, *Ben cao gang mu dao du* 本草綱目导读, 2016, 175 - 177.

data have been identified, as for instance in Mei Quanxi's (1962 –) *Supplementing omissions and correcting errors of the Ben cao gang mu.*

A comparison of numerous quotes in the *Ben cao gang mu* with their original sources often enough shows significant divergence. It is not always clear whether these are intentional modifications, perhaps adapting an ancient wording to usages preferred at the time of Li Shizhen, or errors due to careless copying.

In collaboration with Zheng Jinsheng, Nalini Kirk and Paul D. Buell we have prepared and published the third volume of the *Dictionary of the Ben cao gang mu,* devoted to "Persons and Literary Sources." It offers biographical and bibliographical data on all the texts and persons encountered in Li Shizhen's encyclopedia, with a few exceptions for sources and people that appear undocumented elsewhere. This volume of the *Dictionary* includes the various versions of titles and names assigned by Li Shizhen or his collaborators to quotes and anecdotes. It also indicates where quotes ascribed in the *Ben cao gang mu* to a specific text or author, in fact, originated elsewhere. [13]

Ever since Tao Hongjing's *materia medica* book of 500 CE and throughout the history of the main tradition, authors introduced their *materia medica* works not simply with a single preface to inform readers of their motives, aims and (where relevant) the history of their texts. They also offered more general information associated with the origin, gathering, pharmaceutical processing, contra-indications, synergies, and applications of pharmaceutical substances. Here, too, Li Shizhen extended the introductory sections to four voluminous chapters occupying one-eighth of the entire text.

Li Shizhen was fully aware of and explicitly acknowledged the information he was offered by previous authors and their works. In chapter one, before he set out to manage received information and combine it with new data in often innovative ways, he enumerated 40 earlier *materia medica* works with brief commentaries by other authors and himself. This list is followed by another, already mentioned above, of all the literary sources he had taken into account, divided into two groups: 277 older and more recently published medical and pharmaceutical works, and 591 classics, historical annals and others. Next, Li Shizhen went into more detail, informing readers of all the earlier *materia medica* works he had taken sub-

---

13 Zheng Jinsheng, Nalini Kirk, Paul D. Buell and Paul U. Unschuld, *Dictionary of the Ben cao gang mu,* Vol. III: *Persons and Literary Sources,* University of California Press, Oakland, 2018.

stance descriptions from. Li Shizhen paid homage to the beginning of the main tradition by quoting the preliminary sections of the *Original Classic*, including commentaries by Tao Hongjing and others.

He eventually switched to the Song-Jin-Yuan understanding of health and pharmaceutical therapy by first quoting a passage from the *Yellow Thearch's Inner Classic, Plain Questions* concerning the effects of climatic factors on drugs. This is followed by a section on "The seven ways of compiling a recipe," with commentaries by the legendary Qi Bo, the 8th century commentator of the *Basic Questions,* Wang Bing, and various Song-Jin-Yuan authors. Next is a section on "The effects of the ten kinds of recipes," with commentaries by Xu Zhicai (ca. 510 – 590), several Song-Jin-Yuan authors again, and Li Shizhen himself. The first chapter ends with ten treatises on the medical-theoretical teachings of the Song-Jin-Yuan period.

Chapter 2 begins with an enumeration of pharmaceutical substances known by up to five alternative names. It continues with an enumeration of pharmaceutical substances according to their reciprocal, synergistic effects when ingested together, an enumeration of foods whose consumption is forbidden during an ingestion of specific pharmaceutical substances, an enumeration of substances that must not be taken by pregnant women, and an enumeration of beverages and foods that must not be consumed together. Also in chapter 2, Li Shizhen quotes a section on how to treat illness without engaging in theoretical considerations. This is from Li Gao (1180 – 1251), one of the main authors and theoreticians of the Song-Jin-Yuan era, whose treatise acknowledges that the treatment of certain illnesses escapes theorization. Hence, he simply lists certain pathological signs and the pharmaceutical substances suitable for their treatment – without reference to the yin yang and Five Phases doctrines of systematic correspondences.

Similarly, the next treatise is an "enumeration of all pharmaceutical substances that, according to Chen Cangqi (8th century), are used in the treatment of depletions." From another core theoretician of the Song-Jin-Yuan era, Zhang Zihe (1156 – 1228), Li Shizhen adopts the treatise "The three processes of sweating, vomiting and purging." Chapter 2 ends with a section from a work known as *Pharmaceutical Drugs matched up*, a text allegedly predating the *Original Classic*, and the tables of contents of the *Original Classic* and the *Materia medica based on data from the classics and historical annals, based on evidence and ordered on the basis of groups, prepared for clinical application* by Tang Shenwei (fl.1082), one of the final works of the main tradition, written between 1080 and 1107.

Chapters 3 and 4 of the *Ben cao gang mu* include lists of all diseases, and where necessary a detailed description of their pathological conditions, with the appropriate pharmaceutical substances and more or less abbreviated information concerning their pharmacological function, preparation and administration. The full text of these recipes can often be found in the Added Recipes sections of their main ingredient entries. Perhaps, chapters 3 and 4 were meant to save practitioners consulted far from home from having to deal with all 52 chapters. The abbreviated recipes in chapters 3 and 4 included enough information to remind a well-trained practitioner of a full recipe that he may have seen in a later chapter and studied earlier in his career.

Li Shizhen was the first author in the tradition of comprehensive works to combine the genres of *materia medica* and recipe literature. With very few exceptions, he added to every substance a list of recipes with the information he may have considered essential for their application in actual clinical practice. One or more therapeutic indications, mostly down-to-earth without theoretical embellishment or legitimation, are followed by the recipe's ingredients with brief data on their raw or processed states. The recipes further include concise data on their preparation, on the external or internal mode of their application, and on the number and required time span of their applications. A source is given for each recipe. For each list of recipes added to the entry on a specific substance, Li Shizhen also specifies how many of them were recorded in previous recipe collections and how many he has recorded for the first time.

It is here that we should address a question that might at first seem trivial. For whom did Li Shizhen write this encyclopedia? With its title's first two characters, "materia medica," the answer may seem obvious. His audience comprised all those healers interested in a pharmaceutical therapy based on herbal, animal, and mineral substances. In fact, for the first four chapters Li Shizhen introduces an ingenious structure. Chapters 2 and 3 offer practioners a fairly comprehensive survey of theoretical and practical foundations for their applied, clinical work. Chapters 3 and 4 offer virtually all the diseases, illnesses, complaints, side-effects, and more that one might think of as a healer. We learn of the detrimental side-effects, not only of mineral drugs but also of moxibustion. We learn of the health problems of eunuchs resulting from castration and of women who have had an abortion, of battle wounds that fail to close, of injuries resulting from sexual intercourse, and of the means for preventing bruises resulting from flogging.

For modern historians this is a unique panoramic account of two millennia of health problems recorded in a comprehensiveness and detail unlike any other Chinese pre-modern text, and also in no other region of the Eurasian continent. The list of health problems is completely systematic. From general diseases/illnesses, often with numerous variations in different age groups, males and females, married and unmarried females and others, it proceeds to an enumeration of pathologies, of body parts affected, and, with women and children marking the end, of groups of patients deserving special attention.

For each health problem, no matter how specific, different substances are attached, often with a brief hint at the pharmaceutical processing required and dosage forms recommended. The individual paragraphs are further divided by lists of therapies to be applied internally and externally, and by the origin of the substances advocated for therapies as to their grouping as herbs, vegetables, minerals, animals with or without scales and shell, etc. Chapters 5 through 52 turn the information around. Here the focus is on the individual substances, their detailed description, and their application in "attached recipes."

In other words, a practitioner may approach the information offered from two angles. Presumably, a healer is confronted with a client's health problem and needs to know more about those variations requiring differential diagnosis. He then is led to the substances he should use for a therapy. The many different substances listed permit a choice also based on local availability. Once a choice is made, a healer may then turn to the monograph of a substance and select a suitable recipe. He may, of course, be familiar with the ailment to be treated and start his quest for a suitable recipe from the monograph of a substance he was thinking of right away.

Obviously, Li Shizhen certainly had the needs of healers in his mind when he set up the structure of his work. But there must have been more to this, and the question, for whom he compiled the encyclopedia, is not yet answered. At least it suggests that there are further questions to be answered. It is difficult to define a clientele of practitioners and patients who may have had access to the many substances required for the recipes recommended. Many herbal, animal, and mineral constituents of the recipes may have been ubiquitously available. But many presumably were not. Who could afford herbal and mineral substances imported from overseas? Who stored and sold mercury and other chemical substances recommended so often in the *Ben cao gang mu*? And who was supposed to process the individual constituents of a recipe into the recommended dosage forms?

When Li Shizhen selected all this information, did he have – in addition to clinical practitioners – another agenda in mind? Was he convinced that his readers were interested in all the information presented that goes beyond the arena of illness and therapies? All these questions cannot be answered right away. The *Ben cao gang mu* is not only a most informative source for the history of medicine in China. It will also become an area of multi-directional research.

Notes on the translation

The translation of the *Ben cao gang mu* which has resulted in the nine-volume series published by University of California Press since 2021 and, hence, underlying the anthology in the present volume is based on a most remarkable critical edition of the text prepared and published by two Chinese scholars Zheng Jinsheng and Zhang Zhibin. I have had the privilege of collaborating with them since 1986, first in the translation of the *Yellow Thearch's Inner Classic, Plain Questions, Huang Di nei jing su wen*, and then in the translation of the *Ben cao gang mu*.

Zheng Jinsheng and Zhang Zhibin have traced all the quotes encountered in the *Ben cao gang mu* to their original source text. Wherever the first 1593 Jinling print of the *Ben cao gang mu* differed from the original texts because of intentional abbreviations, they have added a note with the original wording. Divergences interpreted as unintended errors, such as omissions or mistakenly written single characters, as well as erroneous ascriptions of quotes to original texts and authors, have been corrected in the main text with a note added to explain such modifications. The complete text presented in my nine-volume edition together with its translation includes these corrections. Readers interested in all the details, both of the errors corrected and the original wordings that were abbreviated or otherwise modified by Li Shizhen and his collaborators, are advised to consult the critical text edition by Zheng Jinsheng and Zhang Zhibin.[14]

I am most grateful to both of these scholars for supplying me with a pre-publication version of their work. I wish to especially express my thanks to Prof. Zheng Jinsheng for helping me to understand passages and single characters my own research had been unable to clarify. Almost

---

14 Zheng Jinsheng 郑金生 and Zhang Zhibin 张志斌, *Ben cao gang mu su yuan* 本草綱目溯源, "Tracing the quotations in the *Ben cao gang mu* to their sources." A volume of the *Ben cao gang mu yan jiu ji cheng* 本草綱目研究集成, "Collection on research on the *Ben cao gang mu*," edited by Zhang Zhibin and Zheng Jinsheng, Ke xue chu ban she 科学出版社, Beijing, 2019.

all philological notes accompanying my translation are based on the text edition prepared by Zheng Jinsheng and Zhang Zhibin. I have also greatly benefitted from consulting the Japanese translation of the *Ben cao gang mu* published in 1965.[15] In particular, secondary quotes within primary quotes have been marked in my translation based on the Japanese edition.

In 2003, the Foreign Language Press in Beijing published a first English version of the *Ben cao gang mu*. It was not suitable for publicizing the value of the *Ben cao gang mu* outside East Asia. Mistranslations of entire passages, omissions, the absence of the Chinese original text, as well as a lack of notes identifying persons, unfamiliar place names, and cryptic references to literature cited prevented the Foreign Language Press edition from becoming a starting point for the vast range of research projects on numerous issues related to the history of culture in general and various areas of science in particular in China. The approach that was chosen to translate medical terminology differed significantly from the one adopted in my translations of ancient Chinese classics. In the Foreign Language Press edition as many as possible of the diseases, ailments, and signs of illness encountered in the *Ben cao gang mu* are rendered in terms of modern Western medical concepts.[16]

The *Ben cao gang mu* is an encyclopedia compiled in the 16th century, based on literary and non-literary data of the preceding 1,800 years. It quotes authors of varying expertise and offers today's readers an incomparable view of almost two millennia of the development of pharmaceutical science and related realms of knowledge and more general aspects of culture.

The translation of the Chinese text offered in the nine-volume edition of University of California Press, and, hence, in the present anthology, honors the authors of bygone days by illuminating as clearly as possible their thoughts and their wisdom as formed by the conceptual, social, economic, and natural environment of their time. I do not consider it meaningful to tell the ancient authors what they should have said if they had had the knowledge of the 20th and 21st century, thereby dispossessing them, as it were, from their own level of knowledge.

---

15 Kimura Kouichi 木村康 (ed.), Suzuki Shinkai 鈴木真海 (transl.), *Shinchu Koutei Kokuyaku Honzou Koumoku* 新註校定國本草綱目譯, , "A translation of the *Ben cao gang mu*. Newly annotated and checked against the original text." Shunyoudou Shoten 春陽堂書店, Tokyo 1965.

16 *Compendium of Materia Medica.* (*Bencao Gangmu*). Compiled by Li Shizhen. Translated and Annotated by Luo Xiwen. Foreign Language Press, Beijing, 2003.

The translation offered here has resisted a temptation to make ancient views appear modern and agreeable with today's biomedical reality. Such an approach, not infrequently met in recent renderings of ancient Chinese medical texts in Western languages, is not only a sign of disrespect for the intellectual integrity of ancient experts. It is also an obstacle blocking a recognition and appreciation of the never-ending historical process of understanding nature and the management of human life as part of nature, which has been pursued in China since antiquity.

Authors from previous centuries and millennia relied on metaphors and allegories to elucidate their understandings of human physiology and pathology. Modern pathology and physiology are no different. Such fields of science need to draw on metaphors and allegories to illustrate their findings.[17]

Disease names are a case in point. The *Ben cao gang mu* includes quotes with about 4,500 core terms to specify all kinds of pathological conditions. The translation offered in the nine-volume series and in the present anthology provides, where appropriate, the literal meaning of disease terms. Occasionally, ancient single characters keep their meaning secret; in such cases, they are given in pinyin transcription. Notes are added to all occurrences of historical disease terms that are not self-explanatory, and readers are led to the relevant pages of Vol. I of the *Dictionary*.

Place names, designations of administrative structures, names of persons, and book titles appear in the translation without additional notes. Readers interested in further details should consult volumes II and III of the *Dictionary of the Ben cao gang mu*, which provide information both on the geographic and adminstrative designations and on the persons and literary sources mentioned.

A challenging feature of translating an ancient text on *materia medica* is the identification of natural substances recommended for medicinal use. Since the 17th century European scientists have been eager to identify herbal and mineral substances they have encountered in China. From the beginning, this has turned out to be a difficult endeavor. Different names were used for identical substances in different parts of the country; different pronunciations of an identical name in the dialects of different regions led to different writing. One and the same substance has been recorded with varying names in the course of history.

17 Cynthia Taylor and Bryan M. Dewsbury, On the Problem and Promise of Metaphor Use in Science and Science Communication. *J Microbiol Biol Educ*. 2018; 19(1): 19.1.46.

An herb listed in an 8th century *materia medica* text might not have been available at a later time and was replaced by another herb sold under the same name. The marketing of fakes as substitutes was so widespread that Li Shizhen cautions his readers about fakes in the first chapter of the *Ben cao gang mu*. In his descriptions of individual substances, he devotes much space to such issues. The fact is that, despite all the many attempts published over the past three centuries, uncertainty remains as to the true identity of numerous herbs and minerals recorded in historical Chinese *materia medica* works. This translation offers – with a caveat – identifications of the substances recorded in the *Ben cao gang mu* based on the most reliable reference works available today. Wherever a commonly known English name was available, such as "ginger" and "ginseng root," it was used in the translation. All other translations refer to the Latin name of a substance.

My desire in compiling the following anthology has been, by means of a selection of suitable passages, to show that the *Ben cao gang mu* can be regarded as a rich source not only of medical knowledge in ancient China. In 17 chapters, references to generally valid cultural aspects of ancient China are also given prominence. Readers who wish to find the quoted text excerpts in their original context are referred to the volumes of the complete edition published by University of California Press.

1. Division of items: 16 sections

In his "Introductory Notes" Li Shizhen addresses one of the major challenges he was confronted with. Almost two millennia of literary evidence lay before him. A quantity of historical data which had never been evaluated in as much variety as he intended to provide was to be examined for its usability in the realm of *materia medica*. We imagine a young man, aged 35, in a region not really close to the centers where well-stocked libraries gave access to the many works of the past. To this day it is an unsolved mystery how he could manage to acquire and read all the many texts he quoted. He did not see all the books as separate editions; often he used earlier collections of past texts. Still, it was for him to identify all the sources he wished to excerpt, and to locate them somewhere not too far away. How many assistants could he send out? How much of his time did he spend on reading and how much on pondering how to manage the data he considered worth excerpting and commenting on?

Li Shizhen's approach to knowledge management, resulting in information that he assumed would be useful to his readership, was aptly characterized by Georges Métailié in his volume on *Traditional Botany: An Ethnobotanical Approach*, in volume 6 of Joseph Needham's epochal *Science and Civilisation in China*: "His concern is ... simply correctly to identify the medicinal products that the natural products produce and to verify the information that he has gleaned about them in his reading. He therefore takes as his starting point primarily and above all the writings of his predecessors. If he innovates at all, it is in the uses of those products. .... His originality consists in adding to the *materia medica* products already known that he judges to be interesting from what others have written about them or even from hearsay. Li Shizhen is first and foremost a doctor writing about plant, animal and mineral *materia medica*. ... When he records observations about plants, animals or even minerals, he is neither a botanist, a zoologist nor a mineralogist, but simply a member of the Confucian literature elite practicing what he calls a 'study of the investigation of things.'"

Métailié has laid out in great detail Li Shizhen's adoption of earlier categorizations of natural items, and his decisions about departing from past formats and rearranging an unsuited order. For almost two millennia, astute observers of plants, animals, and minerals had thought about groupings and differences. The writings of previous authors were often detailed enough to allow a fairly exact identification today, and this in turn shows that quite a few objects that modern botany, for example, considers closely related were already seen as such in ancient China. It was claimed that such relationships existed because of agreements in their therapeutic effects, flavor, appearance, and habitat. Detailed differences in the shape of leaves despite an agreement in the shapes of an herb's or tree's stem were noted and considered criteria for classification into various suborders. The growth of a root vertically or horizontally, as a single extension or as multiple tubers, the color of petals, and virtually all other characteristics perceptible to the human senses had led to naming and classification in the course of the centuries.

This is not the place to recall all the details of Métailié's subtle penetration of all the factors he identified as leading to Li Shizhen's final arrangement of what are now identified as natural botanical substances. Li Shizhen addressed a similar problem in his arrangement of minerals and metals, with the additional task of integrating and distinguishing between natural and man-made substances. As in the area of plants, so also in the area of minerals and metals, many previous authors had described things, products, and processes. The same was true for the vast realm of living beings, including man. Insects, worms, snakes, birds, and quadrupeds; some animals found only in the wild, others not even in China, others domesticated as livestock; and so many creatures more – Li Shizhen faced a gigantic range of subjects requiring a careful overview, a meaningful classification and a description that was to offer only the most useful and reliable information. Did he attribute a hidden link connecting all natural things? He realized that their relations with each other were led by "underlying or innate principles." He urged scholars to discover these principles, and at the same time he agreed that many of them were strange and enigmatic, beyond human understanding. He acknowledged the pervasion of all things by *qi*, finest vapors of matter. The omnipresence of *qi* was a fact; Li Shizhen saw no need to say a word about them. The anthology presented below consists of the explanatory introductions that Li Shizhen placed at the beginning of all the 16 sections into which he had divided the heterogenous realm of natural phenomena.

Li Shizhen was a man of the 16th century, raised, educated, and writing in a cultural environment often seen as very distant and differing in many ways not only from today's China, but even more so from the so-called Western world and its civilization. A close look at the 16 sections in the *Ben cao gang mu* and its many subsections reveals almost immediately that there are no fundamental, perhaps insurmountable, cultural barriers that substantially hinder or even prevent an understanding of Li Shizhen's cate-gorizations. Indeed, his criteria were not those of modern science, but they were self-explanatory. If we were to meet him today, a discussion among peers could begin immediately.

The following references to Vol. and ch. refer to the volumes of the translation of the *Ben cao gang mu*, published by University of California Press, 2021 – 2024, and the chapters in the original text.

Section Waters. Vol. II, ch. 5

Li Shizhen: Water is the visible realization of the trigram *kan* in the *Classic of Changes*. In a horizontal representation, the arrangement of the lines is ☵. The vertical arrangement is ☵. The body is pure yin; its function is pure yang. Above, water takes form as rain, dew, frost, and snow. Below, it takes form in lakes, rivers, springs, and fountains. Water can flow or rest. It can be cold or warm. All of these are different concentrations of qi. Water can be sweet, tasteless, salty, or bitter. That is, the taste qi that entered the water is not the same. This was also the reason why ancient people distin-guished between the waters and earths in the nine regions of China, so that they could also distinguish between the good and bad endowments of people and find confirmation that they enjoy a long life or die early.

The fact is, water is the origin of the myriads of changes; the earth is the mother of the myriads of things. The natural endowment that comes to man through drinking is that of water. The natural endowment that he takes in through eating is that of the earth. Eating and drinking are man's lifelines. His storage qi and his protective qi depend on them. Therefore, it is said: as soon as there is no more water, the storage qi are exhausted; as soon as the grain is consumed, the protection qi are lost.

The fact is, for the prevention of sickness and the maintenance of life, the peculiarities and tastes of waters must be taken into account. Now here are united 43 kinds of waters, which have a meaning for the preparation of medicines and food. They are divided into two groups, the waters of heaven and those of earth. In earlier materia medica texts, the waters included 32 species and they were scattered in the sections "Jade" and "Rocks/Minerals."

Section Fires. Vol. II, ch. 6

Li Shizhen: The people are nourished by water and fire, and the people's life depends on them. Still, all the medical recipes recorded in *materia medica* works distinguish between different types of water, but fail to distinguish between different types of fire. This is truly a significant omission! Fires rage in the South. The character *huo* 火, "fire" when written horizontally is the trigram ☲; when written vertically is 火 to reflect rising flames. The qi of fire move toward heaven; they are deposited in the earth; they are made use of by humans.

In High Antiquity, a Mr. Tinder Mirror Man observed heaven above and the earth below. He drilled wood to obtain fire and he taught the people to cook food, so as to avoid abdominal illness. Among the officials of the Zhou, a Mr. Sunlight resorted to a tinder mirror to obtain brilliance fire from the sun, and by means of a tinder mirror he obtained brilliance water from the moon for sacrificial usages. A Mr. Sacrificial Fire Manager handled the administration of the various types of fire. The fires in the country in accordance with their changing nature in the course of the four seasons were used to protect the people from seasonal illness.

The *Record of Rites* states: The Sage Kings of the past used waters, fires, metals, and wood, and they saw to it that the preparation of beverages and food corresponded to the seasons. That is, the ancient Sage Kings were very careful to handle the various types of fire in accordance with the changing relationship between heaven and man. Why did later generations fail to pay such respect? Here now altogether 11 kinds of fire as resorted to in daily life and for cauterization have been selected to form a section on fires.

Section Soils. Vol. II, ch. 7

Li Shizhen: Soil is the chief of the Five Phases; it is the physical embodiment of the trigram representing latency. It appears in all the five colors, but yellow is the proper color of soil. It appears with all the five flavors, but sweet is the proper flavor of soil. Hence in the chapter "The Tribute of Yu" in the *Documents of the Elder* the colors of the soil of the nine divisions of our country are distinguished, and the *Offices of Zhou*, i.e., *Rites of Zhou* distinguishes among the natural dispositions of the soil of the 12 regions. The fact is, soil is endowed with utmost softness and hardness, as well as utmost calmness as its regular feature. It is linked to the Five Phases' engendering of the myriad items, but this does not exhaust its potential. It exemplifies the utmost endowment of feminity as reflected by the trigram representing latency. In man, the spleen and the stomach correspond to it. Hence, whenever soil is added to medication, this serves always to assist the activities of the long-term depot and short-term repository associated with the 5th and the 6th of the ten celestial stems. Here now 61 kinds of soil are brought together to form the section on soils. In older versions of materia medica works 39 kinds had been listed scattered in the section on jades and minerals/stones.

Section Metals and Stones/Minerals. Vol. II, ch. 8

Li Shizhen: Stones/minerals are qi turned to kernels; they are soil turned to bones. Large ones form cliffs and rocks; fine ones form sand and dust. Their essence manifests itself in gold and jade. Their poison manifests itself in *yu* and arsenic. When qi coagulate, they conglomerate and appear as red and greenish coloring. When qi transform, they turn into liquids and appear as alum and mercury. As a result of changes, what was soft becomes hard, such as when stalactites and brine turn into stones/minerals. What has moved becomes sedentary, such as when herbs and trees turn into stones/minerals. When what once has flown and what once has run with a numinous nature turns into stones/minerals, this is a change from what has feelings to something that has no feelings. When thunderbolts and meteorites turn into stones/minerals, this is a change from something without physical appearance into something with physical appearance.

Nature has provided us with metals and minerals. They may be dull items but by means of the pans and bellows of the pharmaceutical experts they can be transformed to be useful in innumerable ways. Individuals and their households rely on them for protecting and maintaining their existence. This is why the *Yu gong* and the *Offices of Zhou,* i.e., *Rites of Zhou* listed their places of origin, and why the *The Farmer's Classic* and the *Xuan's Canon* specified in detail their nature and functions, as these are data to be taken into account by good statesmen and by good physicians.

In the following sections are gathered 160 kinds that are of benefit to the country and that serve to eliminate disease; they form the "section on metals and stones/minerals," divided into four groups, namely metals, jade, stones/minerals, and salty items. Old versions of *materia medica* literature distinguished in the section on jade and stones/minerals among three ranks, including altogether 253 kinds. Here now 28 kinds are newly included. Thirty-two kinds are removed to the section on waters. Thirty-nine kinds are removed to the section on soils. Three kinds are integrated into the section on garments and utensils. One variation is integrated into the section on shells. One variation is integrated into the section on man.

Section Herbs. Vol. III, ch. 12

Li Shizhen: Heaven creates, the earth transforms, and herbs and trees grow. When hardness interacts with softness, roots form. When softness interacts with hardness, twigs and branches form. Leaves and the calyxes of flowers are associated with yang; blossoms and fruits are associated with yin. Hence, there are trees among herbs, and herbs among trees. Those herbs that receive pure qi are good. Those that receive violent qi, they are poisonous. Herbs may appear in five physical variations, i.e., metal, wood, water, fire, and soil. They have five qi, i.e., fragrant, malodorous, foul, fishy, and rank qi. They appear in five colors, i.e., greenish, red, yellow, white, and black. They have five flavors, i.e., sour, bitter, sweet, acrid, and salty. They have five natures, i.e., cold, hot, warm, cool, balanced. They have five functions, i.e., rising, descending, floating, sinking, and remaining in the center.

The Fiery Thearch, Shen nong, tasted and distinguished them. Xuanyuan and Qi Bo told the respective knowledge by writing it down. Throughout the Han, the Wei, the Tang, and the Song dynasties, enlightened sages and good physicians added new writings and boosted the knowledge. However, even though a division into three ranks existed, when the rivers Zi and Sheng have joined they are no longer discernible. All sorts of entries appeared doubled. The rivers Jing and Wei were no longer separated.

When subtleties are not examined, when good and malign are not known, how can one make use of the seven kinds of recipes and weigh the ten kinds of dosage forms to bring the dead back to life? Hence here we have cut out redundancies and eliminated repetitions. We have corrected errors and supplemented what was missing. We have formed classes and distinguished groups. We have ordered the herbs in accordance with basic principles and we have further divided the entries in accordance with individual topics.

Apart from grain and vegetables, the herbs that can be supplied to physicians as medicinal substances amount to 610 kinds. They are divided into ten groups, namely mountain herbs, fragrant herbs, marshy land herbs, poisonous herbs, creeping herbs, water herbs, rocky land herbs, mosses, miscellaneous herbs, and those that are known by name but are out of use. In old *materia medica* works, herbs were listed in three sections, upper, middle, and lower rank, 447 kinds in all.

Here now, 31 kinds have been joined with other substances. Twenty-three kinds have been introduced into the section on vegetables. Three kinds have been introduced into the section on grain. Four kinds have been introduced into the section on fruits. Two kinds have been introduced into the section on trees. Fourteen kinds were taken from the section on trees and introduced into the section on herbs. Twenty-nine kinds from the creeping herbs section and 13 kinds from the vegetables section were removed to be included in the herbs section. Four kinds from the fruit section were removed to be included in the herbs section. Two hundred forty-seven kinds are known by name but are out of use.

Section Cereals. Vol. V, ch. 22

Li Shizhen: In ancient times, people had no cereals to eat. They consumed hairy animals and drank their blood. Then came the Venerable Shen nong, and he was the first to taste herbs and differentiate those that can be consumed as grains. He taught the people the art of working the land. Also, he tasted herbs and differentiated those that can be ingested as pharmaceutical drugs. He saved the people from illness and premature death. Then the Venerable Xuanyuan appeared. He taught them how to cook and how to design recipes and make medicinal preparations. People in later time acquired the DAO of how to nourish their life.

The *Offices of Zhou*, i.e., *Rites of Zhou* lists the names of five cereals, six cereals, and nine cereals. Poets recited songs naming eight cereals and one hundred cereals. That is, the number of grains is huge. The *Basic Questions* states: "The five types of cereals provide nourishment." Sesame seeds, wheat/barley, non-glutinous rice, glutinous panicled millet, beans are associated with the liver, the heart, the spleen, the lung, and the kidneys. An official named Overseer of Feudatories distinguished the cereals of the nine *zhou*. An Office of the Land distinguished the Nine Provinces in terms of their being suitable for cultivating the different kinds of rice. When they taught the people the art of farming, all of this showed their appreciation of the people.

The qi of the five cardinal directions, the products of the Nine Provinces, and the hundred cereals, their nature differs. How could one eat them every day without knowing the harmful and beneficial properties of their qi and flavor? Now, herbs and fruits that are edible are combined here in the section "cereals." It includes 73 kinds, divided into four groups. They are first, sesame, wheat/barley and rice, second, millet, third, legumes/beans, and fourth, prepared and brewed items. In former editions of *materia medica* works the section on rice/cereals comprised three ranks with altogether 59 kinds. Here now nine kinds are added. One kind is moved to the section on vegetables. One kind is moved here from the section on herbs.

Section Vegetables. Vol. VI, ch. 26

Li Shizhen: All herbs and woods that can be eaten are called "vegetables." Leeks, Chinese chives, mallows, onions, and bean leaves are the "five vegetables." The *Basic Questions* states: "The five cereals provide nourishment. … The five vegetables provide filling." They assist the qi of the cereals and help them to dredge obstructing and stagnating qi. In antiquity, the three husbandmen grew the nine types of cereals; on fields and in gardens they cultivated herbs and woods/trees to be prepared for times of famine because of crop failure.

For sure, the vegetables were not limited to the five just mentioned. At the beginning of the present dynasty of our country, Prince Zhou Xian wang surveyed more than 400 kinds of herbs and trees able to offer relief and he compiled the *Materia Medica for Famine Relief*. It serves as a directive.

Now, the growth of yin items depends on the five flavors. Harm caused to the Five Mansions (i.e., the five long-term depots) is caused by the five flavors. When the five flavors eaten are carefully harmonized, the passage through the long-term depots and short-term repositories is open and the flow of qi and blood is free. The bones will be properly firm and the sinews will be soft. The interstitial structures in the skin will be firmly closed, and life can last for a long time.

For this reason, the "Pattern of the Family" section in the *Record of Rites* includes relevant instructions, and dietetic medicine is based on relevant recipes. The benefits to humans granted by vegetables are by no means insignificant! However, whether their five qi are good or poisonous may differ and where the five flavors enter is based in their preferences. People use them every day but are unaware of these characteristics nevertheless.

Here now, a total of 105 types of edible vegetables are summarized in one section, divided into five groups. They include fragrant-acrid items, softing and smoothing items, melons, water items, and mushrooms-fungi. The vegetable section in former editions of *materia medica* works included three ranks, with a total of 65 kinds. Here now five kinds are added. Thirteen kinds are removed from here to the herbs section. Six kinds are added to the fruit section. Twenty-three kinds are removed from the herbs section to be included here. One kind is removed here from the cereals section. One kind is removed here from the fruit section. Three kinds are removed here from the Additional Items group, items known by name but not in use.

Section Fruits. Vol. VI, ch. 29

Li Shizhen: The fruits of wood are called *guo* 果; the fruits of herbs are called *luo* 蓏. When they are ripe they can be eaten; dried they can be made to preserved fruit. When they are available in abundance, they can be stored to be of help in times of need. In the case of illness and suffering, they can serve as medication. They support cereals and cooked meals and nourish the people. Therefore the *Basic Questions* states: "The five fruits provide support." The five fruits with their five flavors and their five colors correspond to the five long-term depots. They are plum, apricot, peach, chestnut, and Chinese date.

Ancient books advise for predicting a good or bad harvest of the five cereals to simply observe the increase or decrease of the five fruits. Plums control the amount harvested of mung beans. Apricots control the amount harvested of barley. Peaches control the amount harvested of wheat. Chestnuts control the amount harvested of rice. Dates control the amount harvested of millet. In the *Record of Rites*, section "Internal Rules," the following fruits are listed: water chestnut, fruit of the oriental raisin tree, fruit of the hazelnut tree, and melon.

Among the officials of the Zhou a Mr. Fang was responsible for distinguishing the items to be planted on one of the five types of land. Mountain forests were considered suitable for black items, such as *xylosma* tree fruits and chestnuts. Rivers and marshland were considered suitable for pasty items, such as water chestnuts and foxnut fruits. Hills were considered suitable for items with kernels, such as dark plums and ordinary plums. A Master of the Crops was in charge of wild tree fruits and melons. A "field person" planted precious tree fruits and melons to store them when it was their season.

Seen from this, the land to produce tree fruits and melons may be normal or unusual, their nature and flavor may be good or poisonous. How could one just long for and indulge in them without being familiar with their inherent cosmic order? Here now the fruits of herbs and woods are collected as "fruits of woods," and "fruits of herbs" in the section "fruits." They include 127 kinds, divided into six groups, as are the five fruits: mountain fruits, fruits of non-Chinese origin, spices, herbal fruits/melons, and fruits in waters.

Section Woods. Vol. VII, ch. 34

Li Shizhen: Wood is a plant item; it is one of the Five Phases. Its nature is endowed with the benefits of soil; woods grow in mountain valleys, on the plains and in marshland. Beginning with a transformation of qi they acquire a material shape as tall trees, boughs, densely growing woods, and shrubs, with roots and leaves, flowers and fruits. They may be hard or brittle, beautiful or unsightly, all reaching their extremes. They are distinguished on the basis of color, fragrance, qi and flavor. They may produce edible fruits and vegetables, timber, pharmaceutical substances, and vessels. They may be cold or warm, poisonous or good. All this needs to be considered and recorded.

If many of their names are known, why should it be just the result of reading poetry? Their wide-spread familiarity is increasingly guaranteed by *materia medica* works. They have gathered relevant data and grouped the woods accordingly. This is the section "woods." In all, it comprises 180 kinds, divided into six groups. They are the fragrant woods group, tree-size woods group, shrub group, epiphyte woods group, densely growing woods group and miscellaneous woods group.

In ancient *materia medica* editions the section "woods" included three ranks, with altogether 263 kinds. Here now, 25 kinds have been included from other groups. Fourteen kinds were removed into the section herbs. Twenty-nine kinds were removed into the section creepers. Thirty-one kinds were removed into the section fruits. Three kinds were removed into the section vegetables. Sixteen kinds were removed into the section utensils. Two kinds were removed into the section worms/bugs. Two kinds were removed from the section herbs to be included here. Eleven kinds were removed from the group of additional items, known by name but not in use, to be included here.

Section Clothes and Utensils. Vol. IX, ch. 38

Li Shizhen: Worn-out curtains and covers were not overlooked by the sages. Wooden scraps and bamboo tips were paid attention to by the virtuous. Nothing was neglected. A kettle floating in a stream may save a drowning person. The felt used to cover snow in a pit might rescue someone in a critical situation. Nothing is to be considered despicable. Clothes, silk, and utensils, as petty and trivial as they are, in situations of unexpected turmoil they may be of good use and offer extraordinary results. So, why should they be looked down upon instead of being appreciated!

In the old *materia medica* editions, they appeared scattered among herbs, trees, jade and stones/minerals, worms/bugs, fish, and human substances. Here now 79 varietes are gathered together in a "clothes and utensils section" to make them available for medicinal use. This section is further divided in two sections again, namely clothes and silk, and utensils and further items. Sixteen kinds are grouped as herbs. Nineteen kinds are grouped as woods/trees. Two kinds are grouped as jade and stones/minerals. Five kinds are grouped as worms/bugs and fish. One kind is a human substance. Together these are 43 kinds.

Section Worms/Bugs. Vol. VIII, ch. 39

Li Shizhen: Worms/bugs are small creatures; there are very many kinds of them. Hence the character *chong* 蟲 is based on the idea of "three worms/bugs, *chong* 虫." According to the *Records of the Investigation of Crafts*, those with their bones outside, those with their bones inside, those moving backward, those moving sideways, those moving one linked to another, those moving in curves, those chirping from their neck, those chirping from their beak, those chirping from their side, those chirping from their wings, those chirping from their abdomen, and those chirping from their chest, they are said to belong to the small worms/bugs.

Even though these are small creatures and cannot be grouped together with creatures such as *lin*, phoenix, tortoise, and dragon, and even though their physical appearance may have wings, hair, scales, or armors, or they may be naked, and they differ in that they are born from the womb, from eggs, from wind, from dampness, or through transformations of other creatures, still all these wrigglers have some numinous potential; each has its specific nature and qi.

The ancients recorded their respective abilities, and they knew their poisons, and distinguished them accordingly. Also, that the cicada, the bees, the ants, and the eggs of ants could be offered as royal dishes, this is recorded in the *Record of Rites*. That centipedes, silkworms, toads, and scorpions may serve to prepare medications, this is recorded in the recipe literature.

Among the Zhou officials were a Mr. Shu, responsible for eliminating poisonous *gu*, a Mr. Jian, responsible for eliminating moth-like creatures, a Mr. Guo, responsible for eliminating frogs and toads, a Mr. Chi fu, responsible for removing worms/bugs such as earwigs from the walls, and a Mr. Hu zhuo responsible for removing water worms/bugs, these are fox-toads. That is, the Sages paid greatest attention to even these small creatures. How could scholars of today not do research on these creatures and their underlying principles, and check whether they are good or have poison?

Here now of those small worms/bugs that have a positive effect and of those that may be detrimental, a section on worms/bugs is recorded, with altogether 106 kinds, distinguished in three groups. These are those born from eggs, those born from transformation, and those born from moisture. In the old texts, the section on worms/bugs and fish comprised three ranks with altogether 236 kinds. Here now, the two sections of scaly and armored creatures are deleted, while six kinds are newly introduced. Eight kinds are moved into the sections of fowl and four-legged animals, as well as garments and utensils. Six kinds are moved here from the section on those that are known by name but are out of use, and two kinds are moved here from the section on woods.

Section Animals with Scales. Vol. VIII, ch. 43

Li Shizhen: There are two groups of bugs with scales: those living in the waters, and those living on land. These groups may not be identical, but they all alike have scales. Hence, numinous items such as dragons and snakes, and animals living in the waters, like fish, even though they are different kinds, they are interrelated through their changes and transformations. The fact is, their substance differs while their feelings are identical.

All animals with scales are born from eggs, with the exception of the pit vipers that are born from a womb. Those living in waters have eyes that never close; the globefish can blink with its. The tail of a blue snake serves to resolve the poison of its head. The skin of sharks serves to dissolve accumulations of minced fish. If nobody knew of this, who could carry out pertinent investigations?

In the *materia medica* literature of the Tang and Song era, bugs and fish were not separated. Here, now, a section "animals with scales" is introduced with altogether 94 kinds, separated into four groups: dragons, snakes, fish, and fishes without scales.

Section Animals with a Shell. Vol. VIII, ch. 45

Li Shizhen: There are 360 worms/bugs with a shell, and tortoises are the most outstanding among them. The fact is, tortoises are the spiritual leaders of worms/bugs with shells. Among the officials of the Zhou, "the tortoise men were responsible for collecting, during their season and by pulling them out of mud, items with two shells above and below fitting each other. In spring, they submitted tortoises and clams. In autumn, they submitted tortoises and fishes. For sacrifices, they supplied mussels, wasps, and the eggs of ants to hand them over to those officials responsible for preparing minced fish." That is, during the time of the Sages, animals with shells were given out as delicious food because they were not considered useless. So, there is even more reason to serve them as medication. The *materia medica* works of the Tang and Song indiscriminately subsumed them under worms/bugs and fishes. Here now they are treated separately in a "section animals with shells." It includes 46 kinds, divided into two groups, namely tortoises and clams.

Section Fowl. Vol. IX, ch. 47

Li Shizhen: Creatures with two legs and feathers are called fowl. Shi Kuang in his *Bird Classic* states: There are 360 creatures with feathers. Their fur corresponds to the four seasons; their colors correspond to the five cardinal directions. Mountain fowl live in rock caves. Fowl of the open country live on the ground. Forest fowl sing in the morning; water fowl cry at night. Mountain fowl have a short trunk and a long tail. Water birds have a long trunk and a short tail. When they mate, some do so by shaking their tails, some do so by glancing at each other, and some do so by making sounds. Some mate with other kinds of animals. For example, pheasants and peacocks mate with snakes. When fowl reproduce, some may hatch their eggs under their wings. Or their qi, because they are identical, undergo a change, such as when a goshawk transforms into a turtledove. It may also be that some other type of animal transforms into a bird, such as when a field mouse transforms into a quail. It may also be that a bird transforms into some being without feelings, such as when a sparrow enters water and becomes a clam.

Wow! The structure of things assumes a myriad appearances like that. Is this not something a learned person must know? Five kinds of turtledoves and nine kinds of button-quails were used by Shao Hao to designate official ranks. Male pheasants and owls have inspired poets. This is so subtle! There were requirements not to molest the young of certain birds, not to overturn a nest of certain birds, not to break open the eggs of certain birds. On the other hand, a cook may offer six birds for food. The *chi* 翟, read *chi* 翅, officials of Zhou times were ordered to attack ferocious birds. And the official designated as "collector of nests" overturned the nests of those birds that indicated early death. That is, the attitude of the Sages toward things was to use them and to leave them, to keep them alive and to kill them - how could all this be meaningless!

It is recorded: What heaven brings forth is yang. Feathered kinds of animals, then, are yang in yang. That is, they basically serve to nourish the yang. Here now are collected data that must be known no matter whether the birds are offered to the cook or for medical use, or whether they are poisonous and malign. This is the section on fowl, including 77 items, divided in four groups: water fowl, open country fowl, forest fowl, mountain fowl. In the *materia medica* volumes of former times, the section on fowl included three ranks with altogether 56 items. Here now one item was added. One item was moved here from the section on wild animals. One item was moved here from the section on worms/bugs. One item was moved here from the section on those that are known but are not in use.

Section Four Legged Animals. Vol. IX, ch. 50

Li Shizhen: *Shou* 獸, animal, is a general designation of living beings with four legs and body hair/fur. They reproduce on land. Those raised as livestock are called *chu* 畜. When the *Basic Questions* states: "The five domestic animals provide enrichment," it correctly refers to these animals. The administrative structure of the Zhou included a cook who supplied the Court with meals prepared from six domestic animals, i.e., horse, cattle, chicken, sheep, dog, and pig, and six wild animals, including Pére David's deer, deer, wolf, river deer, hare/rabbit, and wild boar. He distinguished between items delivered dead and alive, fresh and preserved.

Persons in charge of four legged animals distinguished them according to their names. Dead or living animals were supplied for sacrifices and to host visitors. Their skin, fur, sinews, and bones were stored in the Jade Palace treasury. A Mr. Darkness was responsible for catching ferocious four legged animals. A Mr. Cave was responsible for catching hibernating animals.

Alas! The WAY how the sages raised living and handled dead animals, how they distinguished items and how they made use of them, this can be said to have been cautious and well prepared. In later times, animals like the yellow sheep and the yellow rodent, nowadays they are supplied to the Court. The tail of the yak-ox and the skin of the marten are widely used.

The exotic nature of the mountain otter, and the effects of the dogs' bladder stones, are all required for life-prolonging ingestion. But there are no records of them in ancient texts. When asked about the spirit goats/sheep found deep in the earth, it was only Xuan fu who knew their identity. When confronted with a *zhong* rodent, Zhong Jun knew how to examine it. The sheep living on land, and the meat of the *peng hou*, is there anyone apart from widely learned scholars who knew how to distinguish them?

Also, the nature and the underlying principles of things/beings appear in a myriad variations. When one makes use of them, this should be with caution. It is simply not enough to know their many names. In the following section, devoted to the group of four legged animals, descriptions of all animals are gathered that may be supplied to prepare dietetics and ordinary meals, medication, garments and utensils. In all, these are 86 kinds, divided into five groups, i.e., domestic animals, wild animals, rodents, residential animals, and strange animals. The *Examples of Refined Usage*, section "Explanation of animals" has "those belonging to rodents" and "those belonging to residential animals." Xing Bing commented: "Monkeys to a certain degree resemble humans. They reside in the mountain forests. Hence, they are said to be "those belonging to residential animals."

In older versions of *materia medica* texts, the section "animals" was divided into three ranks, including 58 kinds. Today, five kinds are added. One kind was removed to the section "animals with scales." One kind was removed to the section on domestic animals. Three kinds are moved here from the section "worms/bugs."

Section Human Substances. Vol. IX, ch. 52

Li Shizhen: *The Divine Farmer's Materia Medica* includes only hair as one item from the realm of human substances. The reason is, humans are different from all other substances. In later times, the experts of the recipe arts extended their understanding of pharmaceutical substances to include human bones, flesh, muscles, and blood. That was extremely inhumane. In the present section, not one of all those parts of the human body that are in use by humans is to be omitted. But only those that are not harmful to righteousness will be discussed in detail. Those that show cruelty and are evil and filthy will be left out from a detailed description. However, they are briefly mentioned at the end of the respective entries. In all, these are 37 items. They are not subdivided any further.

2. Widespread culture, local customs, personal interventions

When Li Shizhen set out to compile a major work on health care utilizing pharmaceutical drugs prepared from items both found in nature as well as manmade, he must have had in mind from the very beginning an encyclopedia exceeding by far the contents of conventional similar texts. He was the first to offer not only data on the origin, nature, pharmaceutical preparation, therapeutic indications, dosage forms, and methods of administration. He also presented data on much of the cultural environment of drug use, offering insights into aspects of 16th century Chinese civilization that are difficult to learn of from other sources.

Certainly, no *materia medica* work prior to the *Ben cao gang mu* had depicted the social setting of pharmaceutical therapy with such a wide lense. For example, he repeatedly felt obliged to inform readers of the widespread practice of preparing fakes of expensive or difficult to obtain items. He focussed his critique for the most part on merchants in general and market traders in particular. He accused them of running after profit and being deeply involved in murder and robbery. However, when he spoke of "people" producing fakes, he suggested that this practice was not limited to those whom one might think of first. Interestingly, he contrasts the majority with those people in one region where chances of obtaining the genuine commodity are good because the people there "are not much interested in producing fakes." Warnings concerning fraudulent pharmaceutical substances are regularly combined with detailed explanations of how fakes are made and how to test a substance to gain clarity, as well as with statements on the consequences of their use. They may be harmful or simply be a waste of money because they have, in contrast to genuine goods, no therapeutic effects at all.

Similar to references to regionally distinct hotspots of faking, notes on other local practices show an awareness, present at least throughout the upper echelons of Chinese society, of a multi-cultural reality in their country. Li Shizhen refers to the Liao people, to the people in Guangnan, to the people in Lingbiao, the Hu and Man people, and the girls of Yao, but also to "people in the north" and "people in the south." The use of brick beds with their negative effects on health, or the application of certain substances to poison others are regionally specific.

A notion of cultural diversity is closely linked to social behavior, especially to the degree of social connectedness, or the absence of it. The people in Guangnan, the *Ben cao gang mu* informs its readers, use a certain substance to poison others, and so do the Hu and the Man people, or the people in the south in general. Cultural diversity means that ethnic groups can pursue different interests and be guided by different values. This in turn is accompanied by an inevitable lack of trust in people who do not belong to one's own family, clan, or social network. This again results in only a weak motivation to treat "the others" as equals and facilitates cheating and deception.

Still, quite a few customs are depicted in the *Ben cao gang mu* as common facets of social life. Softening of little girls' bones to prepare them for foot binding is described as a normal procedure, not condemned. The practice of *gu*-poisoning is referred to as a fact that is severely punished once a culprit is caught – but it is ineradicable. *Gu*-poisoning indicates a presence of distrust outside the home. Any stranger may resort to it, and you should be careful. Hence, *gu*-poisoning is also a sign of suspicion. It may be a Chinese variant of concepts related to envy in other civilisations, such as the Evil Eye or even potlach. Exorbitant wealth in the hands of an individual or his family may be destructive to social cohesion. Aside from the sudden acquisition of wealth, however, there are other reasons, too, that raise the question of whether someone can be suspected of having used the *gu*-worm for their purposes. *Gu*-poisoning appears very often in the texts quoted by Li Shizhen, and there is little reason to assume that he himself was not convinced of its reality.

Li Shizhen attests to certain customs having, whether good or bad, a country-wide distribution. He also refers to examples of behavior demonstrated by groups or individuals. We read of recipe experts who practice evil arts, of children who use an herb to form a sticky mass enabling them to pick up cicadas, and we are informed of an Emperor who found pleasure in having sex with court ladies who would enchant him with a specific ornament on their dresses. Readers are told that the common people appreciate what comes from afar and despise what is near, and that at least one monk once intoxicated an entire family, resulting in a mass killing, only so as to be able to conduct shameful intercourse with the landlord's wife. We also learn that one person's chronic ailment can bankrupt the entire family. Family members may send a patient away who has become a burden, or they may offer huge sums of money as a reward to attract a competent healer. Persons of lower social status may use substances to aggravate a bruise and cause it to appear as a serious injury following a brawl.

In this way, the *Ben cao gang mu* allows insights into many levels of Chinese society. At the same time, Li Shizhen conveys his notion of permanent change. Physicians no longer know the drugs they use, merchants no longer know the items they deal with. Also, the principles, Li Shizhen writes, underlying ancient and contemporary therapies differ as they have undergone myriad changes.

Chinese clematis root
Clematis chinensis Osbeck. Vol. V, 18-39-01.[18]

Formerly, a person in Shangzhou suffered from a paralysis of hands and feet. For tens of years he was unable to walk on the ground. Good physicians had exhausted their skills but could not heal him. His relatives positioned him at the roadside to find help. Then a monk from Xin luo saw him and told them: "With this illness, there is one pharmaceutical drug that can return life to him. But I do not know whether it is available here." Hence, they urged him to go into the mountains and search for it. Eventually he got hold of it, and that was Chinese clematis root. They let the patient ingest it and after several days he was able to walk. Later, Deng Siqi, a man living in the mountains, learnt of this and spread the message.

Meat of black grass snakes
Zaocys dhumnades Cantor. Vol. VIII, 43-14-01

The *Complete Records from Court and Commonality* states: In Shangzhou was a man who suffered from massive wind/leprosy. His family abhorred him and built a thatched hut for him in the mountains. One day, without the patient noticing it, a black grass snake fell into his wine jar. He drank the wine and gradually was cured. Eventually he saw the bones of the snake on the bottom of the jar, and then he realized the cause of his recovery.

Chinese white pine
Pinus armandi Franch. Vol. VII, 34-02

As Ge Hong in his *The Master Embracing Simplicity* states: "Zhao Qu of Shangdang suffered from repudiation-illness for several years. When he was about to die, his family abandoned him and put him in a mountain cave. Zhao Qu felt bitter and wept for a whole month when a hermit/im-

---

18 This excerpt from the full text of the *Ben cao gang mu* translation refers – if available – with the colloquial, English designation and with Latin-scientific approximation to the monograph of the substance from which it is taken. Vol. V, 18-39-01 refers to Volume V of the English edition of University of California Press, chapter 18, substance 39, single part (here root) 01. The same applies to all further excerpts.

mortal saw and pitied him, and gave him a bag with medication. Zhao Qu ingested it for more than 100 days, and eventually all his repudiation-illness sores were cured. His complexion was fine-looking and he was happy. Muscles and skin were like glossy jade. When the hermit/immortal passed by again, Zhao Qu thanked him for his generosity that had saved his life and asked him for the recipe. The hermit/immortal said: 'This is pine resin. There is so much of it in the mountains. When this item is refined and ingested, it is able to extend your years of life and prevents death.' Zhao Qu went back home and ingested pine resin for a long time. His body was relieved of its weight and the strength of his qi was increased a hundred times. He climbed steep heights and took all types of risks. All day long he did not feel tired. At an age of more than a hundred years his teeth had not fallen out, and his hair had not turned white. One night during his sleep he suddenly saw a light in the room, as big as a mirror. After a long time the entire room was illuminated as if it were daytime, and he saw on his face two girls in colorful garments playing around his mouth and nose. Later he entered Mount Bao du and became a hermit/immortal on earth. As soon as people learned of Zhao Qu's ingesting this resin, they all wished to ingest it. Transported by carts or carried by donkeys, they filled their homes with it. When after one month they recognized no benefit, they all ended ingesting it. Such was the weakness of their determination." Zhang Gao in his *Medical Anecdotes* has a method how to ingest "pine elixir."

Mirabilite
Vol. II, 11-09-03

To facilitate the binding of a girl's feet. The "decoction to soften bones." Boil one mace of bitter apricot seeds and four maces of the root bark of white mulberry in five bowls of water in a new jar down to three bowls. Add five maces of mirabilite and one mace of frankincense, close the jar's opening and boil it until all substances are transformed into a liquid. Place the girl's foot on the jar, steam it first and then wash it. Do this once in three days. After more than ten such applications, the bones will have become as soft as a bundle of silk floss. *Arrangements for the Ladies' Chambers*.

Mirabilite
Vol I, 04-22-09

For binding the feet of females, boil it together with apricot kernels, white bark of mulberry tree roots and frankincense and soak the feet in the hot liquid. This will soften them.

Fei fei
Vol. IX, 51-55

Chen Cangqi: *Fei fei* originate from the land of the Yi in the South-West. The *Examples of Refined Usage* states: "*Fei fei* are like humans covered with hair. They run fast and eat humans." The *Classic of Mountains and Seas*: "They have a human face, long lips and a black body. They have hair and their heels are inverted. When they see humans, they laugh. When they laugh, their upper lip covers their eyes."

Guo Pu states: "In Jiao and Guang and in the mountains of the Nankan commandery such creatures may be found, too. Big ones may be more than one fathom tall. They are commonly called "mountain dwellers." During the reign period "filial devotion installed" (454 – 456) of the Song dynasty, the Liao people submitted a pair of one male and one female. The emperor asked a local named Ding Luan about the animal. Luan responded: "Their face resembles that of humans. They are of red-crimson color. Their hair/fur resembles that of macaques, and they have a tail. They are able to speak like humans, but they sound like birds. They know of survival and death, and they are strong enough to carry 1,000 pounds. Their heels are inverted, and they have no knees. When they sleep, they lean on something. When they catch a human, they laugh at first, and then they eat him. This is why hunters proceed as follows. They insert one arm into a bamboo tube to attract a *fei fei*. The *fei fei* will grab the bamboo tube, believing it caught a human. Once the hunters see it laughing, they withdraw their hand from within the bamboo tube and nail the animal's upper lip to its fronthead. Then they wait until it has died and take it away. Their hair is very long and can be used to make wigs. Their blood can be used to dye boots and silk fabrics. When humans drink it, they will see demons." The emperor then ordered an artist to prepare a drawing of the animal.

Li Shizhen: According to *An Overall Survey of the Earth*, "*fei fei* are also found in the mountains of Xishu and Chuzhou. There they are called 'human bears'. The people eat their paws, and peel off their skin. They exist in the You mountains of Shaxian in Min where they are more than one fathom tall. When they encounter humans, they laugh. There they are called 'big mountain people' or 'wild people', and 'mountain elfs'." The *Records of Nankang* by Deng Deming states: "They resemble in their physical appearance the people from Kunlun, with hair growing on their entire body. When they see a human, they usually close their eyes, and they open their mouth as if they were laughing. They are good at turning over stones in deep rivers to look for crabs for food." Comment by Li Shizhen: The creatures described above by Mr. Deng Deming are mountain monsters. They are listed here as an appendix for further study and verification.

Rat/mouse
Ratus ratus L. Vol. IX, 51-39

Tao Hongjng: For medicinal purposes one resorts to male rats/mice. These are the "elder man rats/mice." When they die, their gallbladder dissolves immediately; it is not easily obtainable.

Li Shizhen: Rats/mice resemble hares/rabbits, but they are smaller and of greenish-black color. They have four front teeth, but no molars. They have long whiskers and bare eyes. At their front feet, they have four claws; at their hind feet they have five claws. Their tail looks like it is woven; it has no hair; it is as long as their body. The five long-term depots are complete. Their liver has seven lobes; the gallbladder is situated between the short lobes of the liver. Its size is that of a yellow bean, and it is of a purely white color. It is firmly attached there and does not drop. How can it be that the *Recipes for Protecting Life, Treasured by the Family* says that the gallbladder is of red color? Rats/mice are pregnant for one month and then they give birth, at the most to six or seven young ones. In Huizhou, the Liao people take newly born rats/mice with their eyes still closed and who have no hair yet. They raise them with honey and present them to relatives and esteemed guests. When they are squeezed alive and eaten, they emit cries like chirping. This is called "chirping honey."

The gall bladder/bile of the python
Python molurus L. Vol. VIII, 43-11-01

Duan Chengshi: Their gall bladder is close to the python's head during the first ten days of a month. It is close to the heart during the central ten days of a month. It is close to the python's tail during the final ten days of a month.

Su Song: The *Records from Lingbiao* states: "In Leizhou, households raising snakes each year on the fifth day of the fifth month lift a snake and take it to the authorities. There the gall bladder is removed, dried in the sun and offered as a local tribute. To this end, the snake is fastened with soft straw in a basket where it lies in a curled up position. Then it is taken out and placed on the ground. Ten persons with forks turn it around to expose its abdomen. They fix it and make a short incision to remove its liver and gall bladder. The gall bladder is shaped like a duck egg. When this is completed, the liver is inserted back into the abdomen, the incision is sewed up with stitches, and the python is carried back to be set free. Some say that pythons whose gall bladder was removed, when they are caught later on, from afar they will display the wound on their abdomen to demonstrate that they have no gall bladder. It is also reported, that once the gall bladder is removed they can live on for another three years. It is unclear whether this is so, or not."

Li Shizhen: The people in the South are addicted to eating snakes. Do they really open their caves to catch them and then let them live on to expose their abdomen?

Hardneck garlic
Allium sativum L. Vol. VI, 26-09

Qi and Flavor. Acrid, warm, poisonous. Eaten over a long time it injures one's eyes.

Tao Hongjing: By its nature it is very strong-odored. It cannot be eaten. Common people make it into minced pickles to eat it with minced meat. This is detrimental to their nature and jeopardizes their life. There is nothing that has as severe an effect as this item. It can only be eaten raw; it must not be boiled.

Su Gong: This item is boiled to serve as a wonderful condiment in thick sauces and broths. Still, Tao Hongjing states that it should not be boiled in water. Obviously, he did not test it.

Chen Cangqi: At first when it is eaten, it is not good for the eyes. Eaten in larger amounts, it brightens the eyes. Eaten over a long time it clears the blood and turns body hair and the hair on the head white.

Li Shizhen: Eaten over a long time, it harms the liver and injures the eyes. This is why Ji Kang in his *Book on Nurturing Life* states: "Strong-odored, acrid items harm the eyes." That is extremely so. Today, people in the

North are addicted to garlic and they spend the night on heated brick beds. Very often, this leads to blindness.

Dried ginger
Zingiber officinalis L. Vol. VI, 26-18

Cough with rising qi. Prepare dried ginger from Hezhou, baked in a pan, *gleditsia* pods, baked in a pan, with the skin and the seeds and also those infested by moths removed, and shaved cinnamon bark, specimens purple in color with the skin removed. Pound equal amounts of all these substances, pass them through a sieve and mix them. Blend the mixture with heat-refined white honey and pound it 3,000 times. Form pills the size of *firmiana* seeds. Each time ingest with a beverage three pills. Ingest them at the moment of a cough. Ingest them three to five times a day. During this therapy, onions, wheat flour, oil, and items with a fishy smell should not be eaten. The effects are divine.

When I, Liu Yuxi, in Huainan shared an office in the government with Li Ya, Li cured others but never revealed his recipe. Eventually he was accused of being stingy. Li said: "When someone suffers from cough, they often let the patient take cold medication. When the patients see on a recipe that in this recipe I use hot and drying pharmaceutical drugs, they are definitely unwilling to ingest them. For this reason I give out only the medication not the recipe, and it is often effective." I tried it and it was as he had said. Liu Yuxi, *Transmitted Core Recipes*.

Tapestry moth
Tinea tapecella or allied spec. Vol. VIII, 42-23

Li Shizhen: According to Chen Cangqi, in ancient times brocade ashes were used to heal *gu*-poisoning caused by bugs eating brocade. His commentary states: "These bugs curl up like a finger ring and they eat red brocade just like silkworms eat mulberry tree leaves." According to recent research, these bugs are "golden silkworms." The *Cai Tao's Collected Talks* states: "Golden silkworms were found in Shuzhong first. More recently, large numbers have invaded Hu, Guang, Min, and Yue. They are shaped like silkworms, but they are of golden color. Everyday they eat four *cun* of Shu brocade. The people in the South rear them, and they use their excrements to put it into beverages and food to poison other people. These people will die.

When these silkworms get what they want, they daily put down at their owner's disposal the wealth of the others poisoned, and this way they make that person suddenly rich. However, to get rid of them is very difficult. Neither water nor fire or weapons will harm them. There is only one way. One must set up a chest or basket with twice as much gold, silver, and brocade as one had acquired, place the golden silkworm amidst of it, and put this on the roadside. If someone else happens to pick it up, the golden silkworm will follow him. This is called 'to marry a golden silkworm'. If one does not get rid of them this way, they will enter their host person's abdomen and stomach. When this is completed, they will leave that body similar to corpse bugs.

Once there was someone who held an official position in Fuqing. He was accused of possessing a golden silkworm poison. He was searched, but nothing was found. Eventually someone suggested to send two hedgehogs into his house where they would certainly find the bug. The hedgehogs, indeed, captured it in a crevice in the wall underneath his bed. Now, golden silkworms are very poisonous, as if they were demon spirits. How can it be that hedgehogs are able to check them?"

Also, the *Records from the Leisure Time at the Prefect's Office* states: "In Chizhou, the scholar Zou Lang's family lived in poverty. One day, when he opened the door he found a small chest filled with silverware. He took it up and went back into his house. There he felt that there was an item on his thigh, wriggling like a silkworm. It was of golden color and looked rotten. So he wiped it away with his hand. But it remained at the same place. He trampled on it, and he cut it, he threw it into water and into a fire, but it always remained unaffected. Lang went to a friend to ask him what to do, and his friend said: This is a golden silkworm. And he told him what this meant. Lang returned home and said to his wife: 'I cannot do as I should and send it to some poor family. How could they continue to live?' Then he swallowed it. Everybody in his household said that he was bound to die. But he never suffered from anything, and eventually led a long life. Could it be that in view of such extraordinary honesty, even goblins are unable to overcome righteousness?"

Li Shizhen: I say, the destruction caused by a golden silkworm is extreme. Hence I have recorded these two episodes. In the first it is obvious that the *gu* fear hedgehogs. In the other, utmost honesty overcomes evil. *The Records of Yijian* states: "If one was struck by such golden silkworm and feels a sweet flavor when he sucks alum, and will not sense a fishy smell when he chews black beans, then he should ingest a decoction of the bark of pomegranate roots and this will cause him to throw up the golden silk-worm." The *Orthodox Transmission of Medical Studies* recommends to ingest "a decoction of camphorwood scraps to throw them up." This, too, is a method. My own humble opinion is to cure this with the skin of a hedgehog, because it will overcome its natural enemy.

Mountain otter
Lutra lutra chinensis Gray. Vol. IX, 51-34

Li Shizhen: Mountain otters originate from the region of the Liao, the cave people in Yizhou in Guang, and from Nandanzhou. The locals call them "those that raise their tail." Their nature is of a fierce licentiousness. Wherever in the mountains these creatures exist, all other female animals stay away from them. If these otters do not find a mate, they embrace a tree and wither as they lose their seminal fluid there. In spring, the girls of the Yao go in groups into the mountains to collect herbs. When otters smell the qi of these females, they will jump onto and embrace them. They then penetrate the bones of these girls with a hard penis so firmly that they cannot be separated. Hence the people strangle the animal and carry it back home. There they remove the penis and sell it for one ounce of gold. If they find a mountain otter that has died while embracing a tree, it is even more valuable.

The Liao people in the caves value them highly. If a hunter carries one personally away from that region, he will be punished with death. Because even there, they are rather rare. Recipe masters often fake them with moist mice/rats and monkey fetuses. To test whether it is a genuine otter penis, have a woman rub the item until it is very hot. Then place it into her palm and have her breathe out onto it. As a result a genuine one will jump and move. This is because it is excited by the woman's yin qi. This report originates from Fan Shihu's *Treatise of the Supervisor and Guardian of the Cinnamon Sea*, and from Zhou Caochuang's *Rustic Conversations from East of Qi*. The physical appearance of the animal is not recorded. Some text is missing.

Grasshopper
Podisma mikado Boliv. Vol VIII, 41-28-A05.

Li Shizhen: The *Records from Beihu* states: "In Lingbiao is a crane herb. This is a creeping plant with flowers that open in summer. Its physical

appearance is reminiscent of flying cranes, complete with wings, feathers, beak and spurs. It is said to be an aphrodisiac herb. The people collect it and dry it in the sun and use it to eliminate facial moles. In spring, pairs of bugs live on the vine, and eat the leaves. The people store them to add them to a bride's trousseau. They feed them with leaves. When they grow older, they shed their shell and become butterflies of red-yellow color. Girls keep them and wear them on their garments, resembling the skin of delicate birds. This lets them become more enchanting and pleasant. They are called enchanting butterflies." The *Records of Entering the Netherworld* states: "During the reign of Emperor Wu of the Han dynasty, the country Lebi submitted to the throne delicate birds as small as flies, and shaped like parrots. Their daily activities were as regular as if one were watching the movement of the shadow on a sun dial. Later they all died. When the palace ladies wore their skin on their garments, the Emperor found pleasure in having sex with each of them."

Indigo plant
Polygonum tinctorium Lour. Vol. IV, 16-43

When Zhang Jian served as a judge under Zhang Yanshang in Jiannan, he was suddenly bitten by a multi-colored spider on his head. During the night two paths of red color developed from the location of the bite. They were as fine as chopsticks and formed a circle on his head. Then they extended from the frontside of his chest to his central region. After the second night his head and face were affected by painful swelling the size of a bowl of several pints, and his belly slowly swelled. He came close to a status where he could not be rescued. Mr. Zhang Yanshang took out 500,000 cash and Zhang Jian's family added another several hundred thousand to attract someone who could heal him. Then without prior notice a man responded to the call, stating that he could cure Zhang Jian. Mr. Zhang did not believe him and wanted to examine his recipe. That man stated: "I do not hesitate to unveil this recipe. My only intention is to rescue this person's life." Then he took a bowl of large leaf indigo plant juice and tossed a spider into it. As soon as it came into contact with the juice it died. Then he took additional indigo plant juice, added musk and realgar and once again gave a spider into it. It was immediately transformed to water. As a result, Mr. Zhang Yanzhang considered this recipe to be something special and had the liquid dripped on the location of the bite. Within two days the swelling flattened. A small sore formed, and the patient was healed.

Soil mushroom, unidentified
Vol. VI, 28-28

Li Shizhen: According to the *Mushroom Treatise*, "soil mushrooms grow in the soil and are confused with the 'goose paste mushrooms' in the mountains. A common saying is that they are generated by the qi of poisonous snakes/worms. When they are eaten, they kill that person. They are delicious, and yet they are malign. People eat meat, but they do not eat horse liver. That does not mean that the flavor of horse meat is unknown. Those poisoned must laugh all the time. This is resolved by swallowing a mixture of bitter tea and alum with newly drawn water. This is always immediately effective."

Also, according to Yang Shiying's *Straightforward Guide to Recipes*, "people in Guangnan kill poisonous snakes. They cover them with herbs and pour water on them. After several days mushrooms grow. They collect and dry them. They grind them into a powder, add it to wine and use it to poison someone. If that person later drinks wine anywhere else, the poison will be activated and this person will die instantly."

Also, Mr. Chen Cangqi in his *Supplementary Amplifications on the Materia Medica* states: "In Nanyi they fatally poison people with *gelsemium* herb and hang the corpse of the victim in a tree. Where its juice drips on the ground a mushroom grows. They store it and call it 'mushroom medication.' It is an extremely violent poison for humans."

All this must be known. Therefore these things are recorded here.

Garments worn during the monthly period
Vol. IX, 52-16

The *Monograph on a Wide Range of Things* states: "In the country of Funan, they practice a strange art. Menstruation liquid is smeared on the blade of a knife and it will kill a victim without having hacked him. This happens because the filthy fluid destroys a person's spirit qi. Hence it must not be touched during the preparation of medicinal drugs." This is a most reliable statement. Nowadays, there are recipe experts who practice evil arts to mislead ignorant people. Their method is to obtain the first menstrual liquid of a young girl and have their clients ingest it. They call it red lead preceding heaven. They give it deceitful names, and add it to many recipes. When they refer to the Golden Bloom from the *Token of the Agreement*, or to the "first monthly period" from the *Writings on Awakening to the Truth*, then this is always this item. Ignorant people believe them. They gulp down filthy dregs and assume them to be secret recipes. Often enough they develop cinnabar-red rashes, and this is truly horrible.

Heartbreak grass
Gelsemium elegans (Gardn.et Champ.) Benth. Vol. IV, 17-47

Li Shizhen: Ji Han in his *Forms of Herbs and Trees from the Southern Regions* states: "*Gelsemium elegans* grows as a creeper. The leaves are similar to those of sweet basil. They are shiny and thick. Another name is herb of the Hu and Man people. The people there mix it with fresh vegetables to poison others. They die within half a day."

Duan Chengshi in his *A Miscellany from Youyang* states: "*Gelsemium* grows as clusters in the region of Yongzhou and Rongzhou. The flowers are flat like those of mountain *gardenia*, just a little bigger. The flowers do not form clusters; they are yellow-white. The leaves are somewhat black."

Also, according to the *Recipes from Lingnan to Protect Life*, "the leaves of *gelsemium* are similar to tea leaves. The flowers are yellow and small. When only one leaf enters the mouth, blood will spill out of one hundred orifices. Such a person will not be brought back to life."

I, Li Shizhen, visited people in the South to ask them about this herb. They stated: "*Gelsemium* ... is the one called by people the herb that severs intestines today. It grows as a creeper. The leaves are round and shiny. In spring and summer the tender seedling is extremely poisonous. In autumn and winter it has dried, is old and the poison is a bit slower."

Cucumber herb
Trigonotis peduncularis (Trev.) Benth. ex Baker et Moore. Vol. VI, 27-08

Tao Hongjing: This herb is also found in the gardens of private homes. Children rub it in their hands and mix the juice with spider webs to make a very sticky mass that allows them to pick up cicadas. Su Gong: This is chickweed; it is a subsection taken out of the chickweed entry.

Li Shizhen: Cucumber herbs grow on low-lying marshland. They develop a seedling in the second month. The leaves resemble those of chickweed, but their color is slightly more intense. The stem is tinted slightly purple; it is neither hollow nor does it have a wisp. In the fourth month the short stem opens small, purple flowers with five petals. They form small fruits with fine seeds inside. The seedling can be prepared as a vegetable, but it does not reach the quality of chickweed. For this reason, the *Supplementary Records by Famous Physicians* lists chickweed in the section on vegetables, while the item discussed here is listed in the section on herbs. Su Gong did not know it; he assumed chickweed and cucumber herb to be one and the same item. That is wrong. When fresh cucumber herb is chewed, it forms a smooth sticky saliva that can be used to pick up cicadas. When fresh chickweed is chewed no such sticky saliva forms; this, too, can be used to distinguish one from the other.

Japanese plum tree leaf
Armeniaca mume Sieb. Vol. VII, 29-04-06

For dormant free-flux illness and cholera, boil plum tree leaves in water to generate a thick juice and drink it. Da Ming.

Chen Cangqi: Songyang zi says: "Soak plum tree leaves in clear water and use it to wash garments made of banana or *pueraria* leaves to prevent them from becoming brittle in the summer."

Li Shizhen: In summer garments develop dots of mildew. Boil plum tree leaves in water and use it to wash them. This removes the mildew. Very wondrous.

Daphne flower
Daphne Genkwa Sieb. et Zucc. Vol. IV, 17-36

Li Shizhen: Gu Yewang in his *Jade Chapters* states: "Daphne wood comes from Yuzhang. Fruits and eggs do not decay when processed with the juice obtained by boiling it in water."

Hong Mai in his *Informal Notes of Hong Rongzhai* states: "Today it can be found everywhere in Raozhou. Its leaves and trunk are not pure wood. When someone of lower status has fought in a brawl, he rubs his skin with the leaves. Then his skin swells and turns red and he falsely accuses his opponent of having injured him. If you apply it to an egg with salt, its exterior appears brown in color."

Japanese ginger
Zingiber mioga (Thunb.) Rosc. Vol. IV, 15-43

Tao Hongjing: Let a person struck by *gu*-poison ingest Japanese ginger herb juice. Then he is to lie on Japanese ginger leaves and he will call the name of the person in control of the *gu*. Eaten in large quantities, it decreases the strength of medication taken simultaneously, and it is not beneficial for leg movement. People plant it; they also claim that it keeps snakes away.

Su Song: According to Gan Bao in his *Records of Searching for the Supernatural*, "Jiang Shixian, husband of his elder sister, fell ill with blood discharge. It was said that he was struck by *gu*. His family secretly placed Japanese ginger under his mat. Suddenly he laughed and shouted with a loud voice: 'The one who has plagued me with *gu*-poison is Zhang Xiaoxiao.' They went to get Zhang Xiaoxiao, but Zhang Xiaoxiao had already disappeared; he had run away. Since then Japanese ginger juice and leaves are often used as medication to resolve *gu* poison, and this has been successful again and again."

According to the *Rites of Zhou*, "Mr. Shu used the *jia*嘉 herb to remove *gu*-poison," and Zong Lin said: "*Jia* herb is Japanese ginger." This is correct. Chen Cangqi states: "Japanese ginger and madder root are the very best items to control *gu*-poison."

Li Shizhen: The Japanese ginger listed in the *Supplementary Records by Famous Physicians* in the section "vegetables" is the root, while the Japanese ginger listed in the section "herbs" refers to the leaves. Their potentials of therapeutic control are quite similar. Here now they are discussed in one entry.

Henbane
Hyoscyamus niger F.W.Schmidt. Vol. IV, 17-11

Tao Hongjing: Henbane is used in recipes to heal peak-illness and madness. However, it must not be administered excessively. Ingested over a long time, henbane is unproblematic. It lets one communicate with spirits and walk strongly. It is of sufficiently great benefit but its use is rarely seen in the classics of hermits/immortals.

Zhen Quan: Boil them in lime for one full day. Pick up a handful, remove the shoots and dry them in the sun. With *aconitum* accessory tubers, dried ginger, long-stored tangerine peels, shaved cinnamon bark, and *magnolia* bark prepare pills that are to be ingested. They serve to remove all types of cold qi and qi disorder free-flux illness accumulated over years. They are very warm and warming. They must not be ingested raw/unprepared. They harm one and let him see demons. Patients seem to stitch some tissue with a needle, and are confused.

Li Shizhen: I have not seen any of the therapeutic effects henbane is said to have. But the seeds are very poisonous. When they are boiled for one or two days they grow shoots. This shows what type of items they are. Henbane, Mysore thorn, *peucedanum* root, and Indian pokewee root are all capable of letting one turn mad and see demons. The ancients had not uncovered the meaning underlying these effects. The fact is, all members of this group are poisonous, and they can send phlegm to fill the openings of the heart. This way they hide one's spirit brilliance and this is the reason behind one's confusion in what one sees and hears.

During the Tang, An Lushan led a campaign against the Xi and the Qidan. He let them drink henbane wine to intoxification and entrapped them.

Also, in the 43rd year of the reign period "splendid peace" (1564), an itinerant monk Wu Ruxiang in Shaanxi practicing black art reached the home of Zhang Zhu in Changlixian. There he saw the beauty of Zhang Zhu's wife. The monk arranged a meal and asked the entire family to sit together. He added a red powder to the food and let them eat it. After a short while, everybody was clouded with confusion, and the monk carried out his shameful activity on the woman. Also, he applied a terrifying method by blowing the powder into Zhang Zhu's ears whereupon Zhang Zhu turned mad. He recognized all his family members to be goblins and demons and went to kill them all, 16 persons. But there were no traces of blood. A judicial official arrested and imprisoned him. Ten days later, Zhang Zhu spat out more than two bowls of phlegm. When he learned why he was in prison, he realized that he had killed his father and mother, his elder brother and his sister-in-law, his wife and his children, his sister and his niece. Zhang Zhu and Wu Ruxiang were both sentenced to death. Emperor Shi zong Su issued a decree to be publicized in the entire empire. A view on this bewitching medication shows that henbane is part of it. When the phlegm has its confusing effect, other people appear as demons. Is it at all possible not to be familiar with the methods to resolve these effects?!

Vitis flexuosa Thunb. Vol.V, 18-60

Kou Zongshi: During the Tang era, at the end of the reign period "To Open what is Foundational" (713 – 741), Jiang Fu, an hermit, several hundred years of age, was invited to the Academy of Scholarly Worthies. He said "to ingest *vitis flexuosa* lets white hair turn black again, and enables a long life. The vine grows at Lake Tai hu and on Mount Zhongnan." The Emperor sent someone there to gather large quantities and gave them to his older officials. He also ordered that everyone should search for it for his personal use. He promoted Jiang Fu to "Glorious Grand Master Yin Qing," and gave him the alternative name "Mr. Decoction Mixer." Jiang Fu also said that "on Mount Zhongnanshan there was a drought lotus that, when eaten, extends the years of life. It is shaped similar to *pueraria.*" The Emperor had it gathered, ordered to prepare cakes and distributed them to his senior officials. Valiant Cavalry General of the Right Gan Shoucheng stated: "*Vitis flexuosa* and drought lotus, i.e., paris root have not been used by recipe experts for a long time already. Hence, Jiang Fu changed their name and declared them to be divine." Following the suggestion by the Emperor, the people soaked the vine in wine and drank it, and many died a sudden death. Then this suggestion was stopped. Jiang Fu lost the Court's favor and requested to search for pharmaceutical drugs on Mount Laoshan. Then he fled. This is recorded here to make everybody suspicious of such claims.

Honeysuckle
Lonicera japonica Thunb. Vol. V, 18-61

Tao Hongjing: Honeysuckle boiled, brewed into wine and the liquid drunk supplements depletion and heals wind intrusion. As this item extends the years of life and boosts longevity qi, it can be collected and ingested permanently. Still, it is rarely used in the classics of hermits/immortals. All herbs that are easily obtainable are often neglected by people. They care more about those that are hard to come by; they appreciate what comes from afar and despise what is near. That is the attitude of common people.

Li Shizhen: The therapeutic potential and usage of the stem, the leaves, and the flowers of honeysuckle are identical. The ancients regarded it as an important pharmaceutical drug for its ability to cure wind intrusion and eliminate abdominal distension, to resolve free-flux illness, and repel corpse qi. But in later times it was no longer known how to use it for these ailments. People in later times regarded it as an important pharmaceutical drug for its ability to dissolve swelling, disperse poison, and cure sores. But the ancients had never mentioned such therapeutic indications. From this it is clear that the principles underlying ancient and contemporary therapies differ as they have undergone myriad changes. They cannot be subsumed under one idea!

According to Chen Ziming in his *Essentials of the Discipline Concerned with External Diseases and Treatments*, "honeysuckle wine serves to cure obstruction-illness and impediment-illness with an effusion on the back. When they have just begun to emerge, this item must be ingested. Its effects are extraordinary, even superior to those of *polygonum multiflorum*. In the recipe books compiled by Han lin academician Hong Mai and Han lin academician Shen Gua, this is recorded in great detail.

The recipes that have shown to be extraordinarily effective in healing obstruction-illness and impediment illness with an effusion on the back, recorded by ulcer physicians such as a monk from Dan yang, Jianqing, a monk from Jiang xi, Wang Qi, and Commandant Wang Zijun from Jinling, as well as Cultivated Talent Liu Chunchen of Haizhou, they all have used this item. Hence, when Minister Duke Zhang states: 'Who knows that in the midst of the most despised items there are those that have the most unusual effects,' that is applicable here."

Garden shallot bulbs
Allium macrostemon Bunge. Vol. VI, 26-06-01

Xue Yongruo in his *Records of Qixie* states: "In An lu, the elder brother of Guo Tan developed a great appetite in the aftermath of an epidemic disease. Every day he ate up to one bushel of cooked rice. Within five years his family was impoverished and he went begging. One day he was very hungry. He reached a garden and ate all the shallots from one bed and all the garlic from another bed. He immediately felt an extreme heart-pressure and lay down on the ground where he spat out an item that looked like a basket and gradually decreased in size. Someone dropped cooked rice on it whereupon it was dissolved into water. That person's disease of hunger subsided and he was cured." This, then, is proof of the ability of shallots to disperse nodes and of garlic to dissolve concretion-illness.

(This is an abbreviated version of a more elaborate anecdote. The original text is recorded in *Medical Anecdotes* ch. 7, "strange illnesses," "the basket that dissolved cooked rice." It reads:

In An lu, commandery Jiang xia, a man with his family name Guo and personal name Tan lived with his elder and younger brother, three persons. The eldest having recovered from an epidemic disease developed a massive appetite. Every day he ate one bushel of rice. The family could deliver so much for five years. Then their resources were exhausted and they were impoverished. He went begging to the front door of a house and after he had received some food, he again went begging to the back door. The person from that household said to him: "You have already come to eat at the front door, and now you are coming back to us from the back door!" That man responded: "Obviously I did not know that your house has two doors. My abdomen is so very hungry; it is unbearable." At the back door were three beds with garden shallots and one bed with garlic. Then he ate everything from two fields and immediately experienced an extreme heart pressure. He lay down on the ground and after a short while began to vomit severely. He vomited something that looked like a basket. As it had come out and fell to the ground it decreased in size. The landlord had brought out some food, but the beggar did not eat it. Instead, he took the food and placed it on top of the object he had vomited. There it was dissolved into water. Soon after this, his disease was gone.)

Where pharmaceutical drugs come from, whether they are real or fakes,
and whether they are stored for a long time or are used fresh,
for all these facets standards exist. Vol. I, 01-05-09

Physicians no longer are familiar with pharmaceutical drugs; they only listen to merchants. The merchants do not examine the pharmaceutical drugs themselves; they entirely rely on information given by those who collect them. It is not possible to measure whether conventional methods of processing pharmaceuticals lead to genuine or counterfeit products, to good or bad pharmaceuticals. Hence, stalactites are boiled in vinegar to make them whiter. Chinese wild ginger is soaked in water to make it straighter. Yellow vetch is steamed with honey to make it sweeter. Chinese *angelica* is sprayed with wine to enrich it with moisture. They paint the feet of centipedes with cinnabar to let them appear red. They attach mantis larvae to the twigs of mulberry trees. They pass off common *cnidium* as young leaves of *ligusticum chuanxiong*. They confuse apricot leaf ladybell with ginseng root. These activities serve to adulterate facts.

Giant Panda
Ailuropoda melanoleuca. Vol. IX, 51-04.[19]

Pandas have the nose of an elephant, and the eyes of a rhinoceros, the tail of an ox and the feet of a tiger. They often eat from the cooking vessels

---

19   Pierre Abel-Rémusat (1788–1832) was the first to identify an animal named *mo* 貘 in ancient China as "tapir." In my translation of ch. 51 of the Ben cao gang mu I followed this – still widely transmitted - error unaware of Donald Harper's study THE CULTURAL HISTORY OF THE GIANT PANDA (*AILUROPODA MELANOLEUCA*) IN EARLY CHINA. *Early China* 35–36, 2012–13, 185 – 224.

and cauldrons of the local population. They cause considerable suffering to those living in the mountains. When they catch them, they use them for medicinal purposes. Their teeth and bones are extremely hard; they break the iron of knives, hatchets, and hammers. In a fire they cannot be burned. The people fake them as teeth and bones of Buddha, and deceive those who are ignorant.

Li Shizhen: It has been transmitted for generations that with an antelope's horn one can break a diamond. This is a similar assumption of how things are afraid of each other. According to the *Explaining Single and Analysing Compound Characters*, pandas resemble bears. They are of yellow and white color, and they come from Shu.

The *Gazetteer of the South Central Area* states: "Pandas are as big as donkeys, and their appearance is that of bears. They are of gray and white color, and they are very strong. When they lick iron, they dissolve 1,000 pounds. Their hide is warm."

The *Increased Examples of Refined Usage* states: "Pandas look like bears. They have the head of a lion, and the hair of a Asian wild dog. They have a sharp mane and small legs. When their feces is applied to a weapon, it will be able to cut jade, and their urine is able to dissolve iron to water."

Ceylon ebony wood
Diospyros ebenum Koen. Vol. VII, 35-39

Li Shizhen: Ceylon ebony wood comes from Hainan, Yunnan, and Nanfan. The leaves resemble those of windmill palms. The wood is lacquer black. Its body is heavy, hard, and dense. Chopsticks and utensils are made from it. The trees found along the roads are of tender wood. People in the South dye *ji* – wood (unidentified) to present it as fake ebony wood.

The *Forms of Herbs and Trees from the Southern Regions* states: "Ceylon ebony wood trees are seven to eight feet tall. They are truly black, similar to water buffalo horns. They are made into horse whips. They are present in Rinan."

The *Notes on Things Old and New* states: "Ceylon ebony wood comes from Persia. The ebony wood brought here on ships is rotten. It also comes from Wen, Kuo and Wuzhou." It is always the item discussed here.

Fibrous gypsum
Alabaster. Vol. II, 09-10

Su Gong: This mineral is situated between two layers of other minerals, like mineral vessels, and to prepare it for therapeutic use it is struck out of its environment. Or it grows in the soil in repeated layers. It has a genuinely red skin and a white meat with a line design of needle-like structures. It does not resemble gypsum at all. Some of the market traders remove its skin and substitute fibrous gypsum for gypsum, and also for arsenolite. In both cases, these are fakes.

Natural Indigo
Prepared from Chinese Indigo plants. Vol. IV, 16-45

Ma Zhi: Natural indigo comes from Persia. Today, in Taiyuan and also in places such as Luling and Nankang the purple greenish-jade-bluish foam on indigo dye vats is used instead. Its therapeutic potential is identical to that of natural indigo.

Li Shizhen: Persian greenish indigo is a foreign indigo plant. As it cannot be obtained easily, indigo from China can be used, too. If it is out of reach, the juice in which a greenish indigo fabric was soaked may be used instead. Merchants repeatedly pretend dry indigo sediments to be natural indigo. However, these sediments contain lime. Hence one should take a close look at indigo before adding it to food or medication.

Aloes wood containing resin
Aquilaria agallocha (Lour.) Roxb. Vol. VII, 34-10

Ding Wei in his *Tradition of Heavenly Aromatic Substances* states: "This aloes wood includes very many strange substances. Four items named aloes aromatic with four different names and twelve different shapes all originate from one tree. The trunk of the tree is similar to that of poplars. The leaves are similar to those of evergreen trees, but they are smaller. Dou, Hua, Gao, and Leizhou in Haibei are all places where aloes wood comes from. But its quality is inferior to that of aloes from Hainan. The qi they are endowed with are not the same. Also, there are many who sell them and seek to get them quickly so that there is not enough time for their fragrance to mature. The merchants run after profit and are deeply involved in murder and robbery. This is different from the common people in the region administered by Qiong. When it is not yet the right time they do not cut the trees too quickly, and the wood applied there does not cause the suffering of early death."

Sea silkworm. Vol. VIII, 39-20

Li Xun: According to the *Records of Nanzhou*, "sea silkworms live among the mountain rocks of the Nanhai. Their appearance resembles that of silkworms, and their size is that of a thumb. Their excrements are extremely white, like powdered jade. They have no nodes, and it is difficult to obtain genuine ones. The people there prepare fake specimens from *pueraria* flour and lime, and they form them with the teeth of a comb so that they look like genuine specimens. To ingest them is of no use; on the contrary they may harm one. One should be careful."

Bile of the python
Python molurus L.43-11-01

Tao Hongjing: Genuine gall bladders are narrow and long, and entirely black, with a very thin membrane. When dried bile is licked, it tastes sweet and bitter. Rubbed and given into water, it sinks down and does not disperse.

Su Gong: A method to test whether they are genuine. Remove a small piece of millet grain size of dried bile and give it into clear water. If it floats on the surface and quickly circles around, it is genuine. If it goes straight down, it is the blood of a gall bladder. One must not give too big a piece into water, because even a genuine specimen will sink down and disperse. Tao Hongjing was not yet aware of this method.

Meng Shen: The people often fake them with dried bile taken from pig gall bladders and tiger gall bladders. They, too, move in water, but their circling movement is slow.

Musk deer
Moschus moschiferus L. Vol. IX, 51-20

Musk originating from Yizhou is flat and it is wrapped in skin and membranes. It is often faked. It is always such that one part of genuine musk is divided into three or four parts. A bloody membrane is cut and the musk is mixed with some other things. This is then wrapped in the skin from the knees of the four legs and sold. The merchants then further adulterate it. The people there say that one must break open one piece and inspect it.

Those with hair inside are best. Today the only way to be sure that musk is genuine is to obtain a living musk deer and to watch the removal of musk. This will certainly be genuine.

Su Song: Musk deer are present everywhere in Shaanxi, Yizhou, Lizhou, and all the mountains in the Hedong region. And there are particularly many in the Man regions of Qinzhou and Wenzhou. Sometimes they also appear in Qizhou and Guangzhou. Their musk is very small. One piece is just as big as a bullet. But it is mostly genuine because the people there are not very much into producing fakes. Their aroma/musk is available on three levels. The first is fresh aroma/musk. It is called "bequeathed aroma/musk." It is picked out by the musk deer themselves. But it is very difficult to obtain. Its price is that of shining pearls.

Where the aroma collects on the ground, no herbs or trees will grow nearby or far away, or at least they will burn and assume a yellow color. When someone who carries musk passes through a garden or forest, no melon or fruit will ripen. That is the evidence that he has obtained musk of best quality. The next level is that of "navel aroma/musk." It is obtained from an animal that has been killed. The third level is that of "musk nodes from the heart." When a musk deer realizes that a large animal pursues it to catch it, it is extremely frightened, loses control over its heart, runs away madly, falls down and dies. When someone finds it, the blood from the broken heart has flown out onto the spleen where it has coagulated to form lumps of blood. They are not suited for medical use.

3. Visions of associations:
From magic correlations observed in equal appearances and functions to systematized correspondences of the yin and yang and Five Phases doctrines

At some point in the distant past, some individuals no longer accepted as such the reality into which they were born and which they would ultimately have to leave through death. They had noted correspondences connecting different phenomena. Eventually they came to believe in a potential inherent in these correspondences that would allow humans to influence reality in their own interest. A bowstring serves to shoot an arrow from a bow. Why should this potential be limited to its application with a bow? A bowstring tied around the abdomen of a woman giving birth may have the same "shooting" effect. Lice are removed from the hair with a comb. Why should a comb, ingested as ash, not be able to eliminate lice causing discomfort in the stomach?

To be sure, nature is permeated with connections, some obvious, others hard to discover, still others remaining forever hidden. They are based on principles guiding all types of generation, growth, change, transformation, decay, and disappearance. It was recognized as the task of "seers" to pay attention to these connections and examine their underlying principles. On the basis of their knowledge these seers were supposed to interpret and manage human existence. Explanatory models emerged that traced natural and life events to numinous forces, whether deceased persons, human-size or animal-type spirits, or omnipotent and omniscient gods. In addition, a sense of purely natural correspondences, unaffected by numinous forces, found enough acceptance to be transmitted through the ages and to eventually result in a secular science.

An awareness of innumerable pairwise correspondences was extended by two all-encompassing systems of correspondences. One is known as the yin and yang doctrine; the other is known as the Five Phases doctrine. Both resonate with the time of their inception. Conceptualized during the Warring States period, they reflect an understanding of natural processes and social events as signs of the normality of violence. Harmony between opposing aspects is not achieved by having them co-exist peacefully. Rather, harmony is achieved in nature when winter, i.e., a manifestation of yin qi, eliminates summer, i.e., a manifestation of yang qi, and when after a while yang qi regains enough strength to come back and subdue yin qi in turn.

Defeat and revenge are two alternating realities of social life and natural processes. Winter/night and summer/day cannot co-exist in harmony. If there were only winter/night, this would be a disaster; if there were only summer/daylight, this, too, would be a disaster. Everything would come to a standstill.

The dualistic normality of violence in the yin and yang doctrine and the pentic interpretation of mutual overcoming and generation conceptualized in the Five Phases doctrine became the dominant models in the *Yellow Thearch's Inner Classic*'s interpretation of health and disease. Human culture is aware of an eternal normality of violence in nature. Human culture is continuously being further developed to help man to meet the challenge of violence, to survive it and to generate harmony in social life. Li Shizhen uses an example as simple as wheat to clearly show the difficulties and limitations of distinctly classifying the individual substances used medicinally within the theoretical framework of the yin yang and Five Phases doctrines.

The *Ben cao gang mu* is a fascinating panopticum of all levels and applications of such explanatory models developed and accepted in China over time. In the very first chapter of his encyclopedia, Li Shizhen explains the principles at work in what we identify as the "magic of correspondences." For Li Shizhen such explanatory models represented a natural science requiring an explanation but not a justification, or even an excuse: "The nature of snakes is to slither upwards, and thus they serve to guide pharmaceutical drugs to a specific, diseased part of the body. The nature of a cicada is to throw off its outer skin, and this serves to remove clouding of the eye. Gadflies drink blood and are used to cure blood diseases. Mice/rats are good at burrowing and are used to cure the leaking of body fluids. These are examples of things being utilized because of their intrinsic nature. The tooth-like trigger of a crossbow causes the quick release of a bolt. Thus, it triggers an outpouring of fluid and does not does not lead to a concentration of things. The granules under a pestle can clear the throat of a patient choking on something because a pestle is active in a downward movement. These are examples of what are referred to as things that can be applied in ways corresponding to their original usage."

The "doctrine of signatures" known in ancient and medieval Europe had its counterpart in China. The principle of correspondences appeared obvious, for example, in the identical shapes of certain beans and the kidneys.

Obviously, these beans should be brought into contact with the kidneys so as to cure a disease affecting the latter. Both, the beans and the kidneys, are linked by identical qi. Items categorized as belonging to one of the Five Phases have the same qi, and this is why hemp, a cereal associated with the phase wood, serves to cure intrusive wind. Wind, too, is associated with the phase wood, and, as we read in the *Ben cao gang mu*, "identical qi look for each other."

"Group correspondence" and "stimulus and response" among related objects in nature are encountered sporadically in the *Ben cao gang mu*. This, however, does not exclude numerous references to the influences of gods, spirits and demons. If Li Shizhen had a value system that accords any of the natural or numinous forces a higher degree of suitability and truth, he certainly does not reveal it to his readers.

Iron lock
Vol. II, 08-28-12

Nasal congestion with an inability to smell aroma and stench. Grind an iron lock on a rock to obtain a powder. Mix it with lard, wrap it in silk floss, and insert this into the nostrils. After one day, tumorous flesh will come out, and this is the cure. *Recipes for Universal Benefit*.

Combs
Vol. Vol. VIII, 38-48

Gullet occlusion with blockage. Burn a wooden comb of a widow to ashes and let the patient send down two maces mixed with a decoction of a key. *Compilation for Engendering Life*.

Iron saw
Vol. II, 08-28-08

If someone has inadvertently swallowed bamboo or wood, that have entered his throat. Heat an old saw until it is hot, steep it in wine and let the patient drink the hot liquid. Chen Cangqi.

String of a spinning wheel
Vol. VIII, 38-44

For obstruction-illness resulting from horse riding burn it to ashes and apply it to the affected region. Li Shizhen. Whenever a person has run away, wind some of his/her hair around a spinning wheel contrary to its direction on rotation. This will make that person confused and he does not know where to go. Chen Cangqi.

Hemp shoe
Vol. VIII, 38-20

Anal prolapse of the large intestine. Roast the sole of a hemp shoe and repeatedly press it on the prolapsed intestine to let it enter the body again. Also burn the sole of an old hemp shoe together with one head of a fresh-water turtle, grind the residue to powder, and apply it to the prolapsed intestine. Exert pressure on the prolapsed intestine until it enters the body, and it will not come out again. *Recipes Worth a Thousand in Gold.*

Chinese chastetree
Vitex negundo L. var. *cannabifolia* (Sieb.et Zucc.) Hand.-Mazz
Vol. VII, 36-28

Li Shizhen: In Ningpu is a male Chinese chastetree that is used to point at a patient and this results in a cure. If no section of wood is at hand that fits the size of the patient, wait for a time when there is a lunar halo, cut a piece corresponding to the length of the patient's body, and place it under his bed. Even if the disease is dangerous, it will not cause harm."

Snake slough
Periostracum serpentis. Vol. VIII, 43-10

Painful fetus with an impending birth prior to the due date. Fill one complete slough into a tough silk pouch and wind this around the pregnant woman's waist. *Recipes Worth a Thousand in Gold.*

Crabs. *Eriocheir sinensis* H. Milne-Edwards
Vol. VIII, 45-16

"Armed warrior moving sideways," *Crab Treatise.*

Zhang Ding: When a pregnant woman eats them, the child will be born in a transverse position.

Aconite paste "to cast a net."
Aconitum carmichaeli Debx. Vol. IV, 17-21-02

Wang Ji: An aconite tuber is shaped like a crow's beak. Its qi are very sharp. That makes it suitable for use as a medication to penetrate conduits and network vessels, to free the movement of/through joints, and to find paths and access tracks leading pharmaceutical drugs directly to the location of a disease. Boiled to a paste it is called "a net cast" and can kill fowl and animals. If it were not for the fast actions of its sharp qi, how could it have such effects?

Mung bean
Vigna radiata (L.) R. Wilczak. Vol. V, 24-06

To prevent smallpox from getting into the eyes. Take seven mung beans and let the affected child itself toss them into the well. The child is to look at them seven times and then is brought back home.

Black soybeans
Glycine max (L.) Merr. Vol. V, 24-01-01

Tao Hua boiled black beans with salt and regularly ate them for quite some time. He states: "They can supplement kidney qi." The fact is, black soybeans are a grain for the kidneys. Their shape resembles that of kidneys, and with their black color and guided by salt they penetrate the kidneys. Hence their effects on the kidneys are wondrous.

 Li Shizhen: According to the *Book of Nourishing the Elderly*, "Li Shouyu swallowed two times seven black beans every morning, calling them 'grain of the five longterm depots.' Even in old age he was not weakened." Now, the beans appear in five colors, and each of them serves to cure one of the five long-term depots. But black beans are associated with the phase water and their nature is cold. They are a grain for the kidneys, and when they enter the kidneys, their therapeutic effects are many. Hence they can cure water accumulation, dissolve swelling, and send down qi. They check heat related to wind intrusion, quicken the blood flow, and resolve poison. This is a case of "identical qi look for each other."

Cowpea
Vigna unguiculata (L.) Walp. Vol. V, 24-11

Li Shizhen: The flower opened and the pods formed by cowpea always hang down in pairs of two. They reflect the idea of "doubled danger." The bean seeds are slightly bent, similar to human kidneys. When beans are called "kidney cereal," that is based on this agreement. Formerly, Lu Lianfu taught people how to supplement their kidney qi. Every day they should eat, on an empty stomach, cowpea boiled in water with a little salt added. That was based on this principle.

Northern pipevine
Aristolochia contorta, Bunge. Vol. IV, 18-10

Li Shizhen: Northern pipevine has a light and hollow body. When the fruits are ripe they remain suspended and open on four sides, resembling the image of a lung. Hence they are capable of entering the lung. Its qi are cold; the flavor is bitter and slightly acrid. The cold qi can cool the lung heat; the bitter-acrid flavor can cause lung qi to descend.

Tangerine kernels
Citrus reticulata Blanco. Vol. VI, 30-17

Li Shizhen: Tangerine kernels enter the foot ceasing yin conduits, and their therapeutic potential is identical to that of greenish tangerine skin. Hence, that tangerine kernels serve to cure diseases in the lower body parts, such as lower back pain, prominence-illness with elevation-illness, is not just based on a reflection on the nature of these diseases in the shape of the kernels.

Lychee
Litchi chinensis Sonn. Vol. VI, 31-01

Li Shizhen: Lychee kernels enter the ceasing yin conduits and stimulate the dispersion of stagnant qi. The fruits form twins and the kernels resemble the testicles. This is why they are resorted to cure breakdown-illness with elevation-illness and swollen testicles. The underlying idea is to rely on a group of items with similar appearance.

Luffa gourd
Luffa cylindrica (L.) Roem. Vol. VI, 28-10-01

Abdominal swelling. Remove the skin from an old luffa gourd and cut it into small pieces. Stir-fry them together with 14 *croton* bean grains. Once the *croton* beans have turned yellow, remove them. Then take the gourd and stir-fry it again, this time with long-stored husked rice from a granary, until done. Remove the gourd and grind the rice into a powder. With wheat flour make a paste and form pills the size of *firmiana* seeds. Each time ingest 100 pills, to be sent down with clear, boiled water. The fact is, the husked rice absorbs stomach qi. The *croton* beans remove water. The luffa gourd reflects the image of a human vessel network. It adopts the qi of the other items and leads them to the affected region. This is a recipe of the famous Yuan era physician Song Huizhi. Xianyu Shu, *Exploring the Profound.*

Eggplant
Solanum melongena L. Vol. VI, 28-01-01

Eggs/scrotum affected by prominence-illness, with a hemilateral sagging of testicles. Hang a double fruit base eggplant above the door of the house. When leaving and entering, always look at it. As the eggplant fades, the suffering fades, too. When the eggplant has dried, the prominence swelling has dried, too. Another method. Hang a double fruit base eggplant above the door. Everyday hold the child and let it look at it. Two or three times puncture the eggplant with a needle. After ten or more days, the swelling is dissolved. A recipe recorded in Liu Songshi's *Tried and Proven Recipes from the Hall of Preserving Long Life.*

Hedge bindweed
Calystegia sepium (L.) R. Br. Vol. V, 18-14

Li Shizhen. All plants that are vines and creepers resemble human sinews. Hence they often serve to cure sinew diseases. The roots of *xuan hua* are as fine as sinews, and they are edible. Hence the *Supplementary Records by Famous Physicians* says that "ingested for a long time they prevent hunger." When I, Li Shizhen returned from the Capital, I witnessed charioteers with every one of their vehicles loaded with them. When asked they stated that "after returning home in the evening they prepare a decoction that can supplement qi in the case of conditions of injury and other harm."

This serves as evidence for the claim that it boosts the qi and reconnects sinews.

Eggplant fruit base/calyx
Solanum melongena L. Vol. VI, 28-01-02

Li Shizhen: To cure white and purple patches wind, dip an eggplant fruit base into sulphur and the powder of *aconitum* accessory tuber and rub this on the affected region. That is taking advantage of its ability to disperse blood. For white patches use the fruit base of white eggplants; for purple patches use the fruit base of purple eggplants. These, too, are examples of therapies in accordance with group correspondence.

Flower, leaf of Japanese salvia
Salvia japonica Th. Vol. IV, 16-35-01

Mouse fistula with alternating sensations of cold and heat. Unending discharge of pus and blood with frailness. White flowers control white discharge; red flowers control red discharge. *Supplementary Records by Famous Physicians*. They control malaria ailments and water *gu*-poison. Li Shizhen.

Frost of the hundreds of herbs. Soot scratched from within a chimney of a furnace where all types of herbs had been burned
Vol. II, 07-53

Accumulation free-flux illness of children. The "pills that bring a cart to a halt." Grind two maces of "frost of the hundreds of herbs" and one mace of *croton* seeds, slowly cooked with the oil removed, to an even mixture, and form with a fine flour-water paste pills the size of mung beans. Each time let the patient ingest three to five pills. For red free-flux illness to be sent down with *glycyrrhiza* root decoction. For white free-flux illness to be sent down with a rice beverage. For red and white free-flux illness to be sent down with a ginger decoction. *Heart Mirror of Healing the Young*.

Tinder fire
Vol. II, 06-02

Li Shizhen: A Mr. Sacrificial Fire Manager handled the fires in the country in accordance with their changing nature in the course of the four seasons to protect the people from seasonal illness. In the final month of spring, he came forward with fire; in the final month of autumn, he took the fire in again. All the people followed him. The fact is, the extent to which the preparation of food is based on fire is related to the people's illnesses and diseases and longevity, to their dying young and surviving until a late death. As long as, in the course of the four seasons, tinder wood is drilled to obtain a fresh fire which then is used to prepare beverages and food, and as long as excesses and shortages are avoided by acting in accordance with the changing nature of qi in the course of the four seasons, the people are protected against those illnesses that are associated with the qi of the seasons.

Elms and willows turn greenish prior to the hundred other trees. Hence they are resorted to as firewood in spring, and the fire lit with them is of a greenish color. The heart of apricot and date trees is red. Hence they are resorted to as firewood in summer, and the fire lit with them is of a red color. *Xylosma* and oak wood are white inside. Hence they are resorted to as firewood in autum, and the fire lit with them is of a white color. *Sophora japonica* wood and sandalwood have a black heart. Hence they are resorted to as firewood in winter, and the fire lit with them is of a black color. Mulberry trees and *maclura* trees have yellow wood. Hence they are resorted to as firewood in the last month of summer, and the fire lit with them is of a yellow color.

Chinese *angelica* root
Angelica sinensis (Oliv.) Diels. Vol. III, 14-01-01

Lei Xiao: Whenever the root of Chinese *angelica* is to be used for therapeutic purposes remove the reed/rhizomes and the head and soak it in wine for one night before supplying it as a pharmaceutical drug. The abilities of its head and end in stopping bleeding and breaking through accumulations of stagnating blood differ. If one intends to break through an accumulation of blood, he should apply a hard and solid section from the head. If one intends to end pain and to stop bleeding, he should use the tail. If both head and tail are used together, they remain without effect even if consumed as food. Then it is better not to use them at all. Their wondrous effects are achieved only if head and tail are used separately.

Zhang Yuansu: The head of Chinese *angelica* roots stops bleeding. The tail breaks through accumulations of stagnating blood. The body harmonizes blood. When it is used in its entirety, it both breaks through accumulations of blood and stops bleeding. First wash off with water the soil. To cure diseases in the upper section of the human body soak it in wine. To cure diseases in the outer section it is to be washed with wine. It may be dried over a fire or in the sun, and is then added to medication.

Li Gao: The head ends bleeding and moves upward. The body nourishes the blood and protects the center. The tip breaks through accumulations of blood and flows down. The complete root quickens the blood and does not move.

Li Shizhen: The statements of Lei Xiao and Zhang Yuansu on the potential and effect of the root's head and tail differ. For the roots of all items the following applies. The upper half moves upward in the qi vessels; it is modelled after heaven. The lower half moves downward in the qi vessels; it is modelled after the earth. The human body is modelled after heaven and earth. Hence, to cure diseases in the upper section requires to use the head of a root. To cure diseases in the central section requires to use the body of a root. To cure diseases in the lower section requires to use the tail of a root. If a cure is directed at the entire body, the entire root is to be used. This is a firm principle.

Seeds of siler
Saposhnikovia divaricata (Turcz.). Vol. III, 13-07-03

Zhang Yuansu: Siler is generally applicable to cure wind intrusion. If the upper half of the body is affected, use the body of the root. If the lower half of the body is affected, use the small ends of the root. It is an immortal's drug to cure wind intrusion and eliminate moisture. This is so because wind is able to overcome moisture.

Toad
Bufo bufo gargarizans Cantor. Vol. VIII, 42-01

Supplementary Records by Famous Physicians: Toads live in rivers and lakes, in ponds and marshlands. On the fifth day of the fifth month gather those moving eastward, dry them in the shade, and use them for medicinal therapies.

Tao Hongjing: These are those that have a large abdomen and many bumps on their skin. The juice emitted by their skin is very poisonous. When a dog bites a toad, its mouth will be completely swollen. On the fifth day of the fifth month gather five specimens moving eastward, turn them over, bind them and seal them in a tightly closed room. The next morning, see which of them have freed themselves and they can be used for the arts of the Daoists. They can cause people who have been bound to free themselves.

Xiao Bing: Those that have the character "eight" written with cinnabar below their abdomen, and that draw writings on the ground with their feet, they are genuine toads.

Teeth of the python
Python molurus L. Vol. VIII, 43-11-04

Worn on one's garments python teeth drive away inauspicious qi and demons. This is of benefit on long journeys. Li Shizhen. *Records of Extraordinary Things.*

Water beetles
Dytyscidae family, esp. *Cybister chinensis.* Vol. VIII, 40-01

The *Records of Searching for the Supernatural* states: "In the South there are worms/bugs named *dun yu*. From their appearance and size they resemble cicadas. Their flavor is acrid and they are delicious; they can be eaten. Their eggs are attached to the surface of herbal leaves like the eggs of silkworms. If one removes their eggs, the mothers will fly by. Even if the eggs had been taken to some hidden place, they still know their location. If one kills the mother and smears it onto a coin, and if one takes the eggs and smears them on a string of cash, after the coins are spent, they will return by themselves."

The Master of Huainan, chapter "All the Ten-Thousand Arts," states: "Water beetles let one's money come back." In his commentary, Gao You states: "If one puts equal numbers of eggs and mothers of water beetles into two separate jars and buries them underneath a wall on the East, and if one opens them after three days, the mothers and eggs will have found each other. If one smears the blood of the mothers on 81 coins and if one smears the blood of the eggs on another set of 81 coins, if one keeps the eggs, and uses for payment the mothers, and if one keeps the mothers, and uses for payment the eggs, all those spent will return automatically."

Li Xun: According to the *Records of Extraordinary Things*, "they are present in all the mountains of Nanhai. Males and females live together permanently at one location; they do not leave each other. They are of greenish-gold color. The people gather them and use a specific method to grind them to powder which they use to smear on coins that they spend in trading with other people. The coins spent during the day will have returned by night. In addition water beetles can block the ejaculation of essence/ sperm and restrict urination." They are hard to obtain.

Li Shizhen: According to the *Records of Extraordinary Things*, "the water beetles have an appearance reminiscent of cicadas, but are longer. Their eggs resemble shrimp roe; they are attached to greenish leaves. If one gathers their eggs, the mothers will fly by. Consumed fried, they taste very acrid and are delicious."

The *Spirit Book of Gou lou Mountain* states: "Water beetles resemble small cicadas, and also gadflies. They are of greenish color and glossy. They live in lakes and marshlands, and they often gather on the leaves of cattails. In spring, they generate eggs on the cattails, always in lines of eight each, or in lines of nine each, resembling large silkworm eggs, but round. If one takes the blood of the mothers or the blood of the roasted eggs and smears it on coins used on the market, they will return by themselves. One spends them and will never be out of money. This is truly an art of the hermits/ immortals."

All statements on this more or less agree.

Safflower
Carthamus tinctorius L. Vol. IV, 15-27

Li Shizhen: The blood is generated in the heart enclosing network. It is stored in the liver and it is associated with the throughway and controller vessels. Safflower (lit.: "red flower") juice belongs to the same group as blood. Hence it is able to pass through the blood vessels of males and to open the flow of menstruation of females. Large amounts stimulate the movement of blood. Small amounts nourish blood.

According to the *Literary Notes Written During Recuperation*, "the wife of Mr. Xu in Xi chang had died of the disease blood induced brain movement following delivery. Still, there was some heat left in her chest and diaphragm. The famous physician Mr. Lu said: 'This is blood-related heart-pressure. With tens of pounds of safflower she can be brought back to life.' Hence, a large quantity was purchased and boiled in a huge cauldron. The resulting decoction was filled into three buckets that were then placed underneath the window. The woman was lifted and placed on the buckets to be steamed by the vapors of the hot decoction. When the decoction cooled, hot liquid was added again. After a short while her fingers began to move. After half a day she awoke." Now, this was an application of the same method used during the Tang era by Xu Yinzong to treat the wind disease of the empress dowager Liu tai hou by steaming her with an *astragalus* root decoction.

White root bark of tallow trees
Sapium sebiferum (L.) Roxb. Vol. VII, 35-46-01

Li Shizhen: The roots of tallow trees sink by their nature and make other items descend in the body. They are a yin in yin item. They free the flow of water and open the passage through the intestines.

Lycium seeds/fruit
Lycium chinense Mill. Vol. VII, 36-24-03

The 13 kinds of pin-illness swelling. On the first *jian* 建 day of the three months in spring collect the leaves. They are named celestial essence. On the first "Set up" day of the three months in summer collect the twigs. They are called "wolfberry." On the first "set up" day of the three months of autumn collect the seeds/fruits. They are called "defender against aging." On the first "set up" day of three months of winter collect the root. It is called "ground bone." Dry all of them in the sun and grind them into a powder. If it is impossible to collect them in accordance with this method, to obtain only one kind is possible, too. Wrap the medical powder in a piece of red silk fabric. Grind cow bezoar, a piece the size of a *firmiana* seed, three times seven reverse hook jujubes, and seven red mung beans into a powder. First, place a lump of dischevelled human hair, the size of an egg, on a piece of silk fabric. Then apply the powder of the cow bezoar and the other items (i.e., the jujubes and the mung beans) to the hair and form a roll. Fasten it with hair and simmer it on a flat iron until it boils. When the boiling has ended, scrape it off the flat iron and grind it into a powder. Take the amount held by a square inch spoon and mix it with two spoons of the aforementioned *lycium* powder. Ingest two and a half maces with wine on an empty stomach. To be ingested twice a day. *Recipes Worth a Thousand in Gold.*

Ginseng root
Panax ginseng C. A. Meyer. Vol. VII, 12-03

Li Yanwen: When ginseng root is used unprocessed, its qi are cool. Used prepared with heat its qi are warm. Sweet flavor supplements yang qi; a slightly bitter flavor supplements yin qi. The qi control the generation of items; they are based in heaven. Flavors control the completion of items; they are based in the earth. Generation and completion by qi and flavors, this is the creation and transformation by yin and yang. Cool qi are the clear and stern qi of mid-autumn. They are the yin qi of heaven. Their nature is to descend. Warm qi are the generating and effusing qi of spring. They are the yang qi of heaven. Their nature is to rise. Sweet flavor is the flavor of moist soil that transforms and generates. It is the yang qi of the earth. Its nature is to float on the surface. Slightly bitter flavor is the flavor resulting from an interaction of fire and soil. It is the yin qi of the earth. Its nature is to sink into the depth.

The qi and the flavor of ginseng root are weak. That which is of weak qi descends as long as it is unprocessed and rises when it is prepared with heat. That which is of weak flavor rises as long as it is unprocessed and descends when it is prepared with heat. For example, in the case of diseases with soil (i.e., spleen qi) depletion and fire (i.e,. heart qi) abundance, it is advisable to use unprocessed ginseng root with its weakly pronounced cool qi to drain the fire and supplement the soil. This is to exclusively make use of its qi. In the case of a disease of spleen depletion and lung timidity, it is advisable to use ginseng root prepared with heat. Its sweet flavor and warm qi will supplement the soil (i.e., spleen qi) and generate metal (i.e., lung qi). This is to exclusively make use of its flavor.

White persimmon
Diospyros kaki Thunb. Vol. V, 30-13-02

Zhu Zhenheng: Dried persimmons are associated with the phase metal and contain the qi of the phase soil. They are associated with yin and that includes the idea of collecting. Therefore, they can be also of assistance to medication designed to end bleeding and cure coughing.

Li Shizhen: Persimmons are a fruit for the blood section of spleen and lung. Their flavor is sweet and their qi are balanced. Their nature is astringent and they are capable of collecting. For this reason they have a potential of strengthening the spleen and astringing the intestines, of curing cough and of stopping bleeding. The fact is, the large intestine is an adjunct of the lung (associated with the phase metal) and the child of the stomach (associated with the phase soil).

Ginseng root
Panax ginseng C. A. Meyer. Vol. III, 12-03

Li Shizhen: Ginseng (Chinese: *ren shen*) is present in different "ranks." Hence, it is called "human rank." This herb turns its back on the yang and reaches out toward the yin. Hence it is called "demon's canopy." As there are five different herbs called *shen*, ginseng root with its yellow color associated with the phase soil, and supplementing spleen and stomach and generating yin blood, is called "yellow *shen*," and "blood *shen*." It is endowed with the miraculous essence power of the earth, hence it is also called "essence of the soil" and "essence of the earth."

Wheat
Triticum aestivum L. Vol. IV, 22-04

Li Shizhen: Zhu Gong in his *The Book from Nan yang for Saving People's Lives* recommends to "cure yang poison, warmth poison, extreme heat resulting in madness, macule development, and massive thirst twice as serious as usual with the 'black slaves pills,' with one pill ingested dissolved in water. Once a sweating occurs, or a mild free flow, a cure is achieved. The recipe advises to grind equal amounts of *mai nu*, dust from a beam, coal/soot from the bottom of a cauldron, ink/soot from the chimney of a furnace, together with *scutellaria* root, *ephedra* herb, mirabilite, and sulphur into powder and form with honey pills the size of a bullet."

The fact is, in that it makes use of items transformed by fire, this treatment is based on the meaning of a therapy in conformity with the nature of the disease. Wheat is the grain of the heart; it is associated with the phase fire. *Mai nu* is the black mould found on wheat fruits that are steamed with moisture and heat when they are just about to mature. Their underlying principle is identical with that of coal/soot on the bottom of a cauldron and the ink/soot found in a chimney.

Li Shizhen: According to the *Basic Questions*, "wheat is associated with the phase fire; it is the grain of the heart."

Zheng Xuan states: "Wheat is protected by a shell; it is associated with the phase wood."

Xu Shen states: "Wheat is associated with the phase metal. When the phase metal rules, wheat grows. When the phase fire rules, it dies." These three statements differ.

The *Supplementary Records by Famous Physicians* states: "Wheat nourishes the liver qi." That is in agreement with the statement of Zheng Xuan.

Sun Simiao states: "Wheat nourishes the heart qi." That is in agreement with the statement in the *Basic Questions*.

Let us take a look at the therapeutic potential of wheat. It eliminates vexation, ends thirst, holds back sweat, frees urination, and ends bleeding. These are all heart diseases. Hence, the *Basic Questions* should be considered authoritative. The fact is, Xu Shen takes the time, Zheng Xuan takes the physical appearance and the *Basic Questions* takes the therapeutic potential and nature of wheat as a starting point to identify the nature of wheat. Therefore, their theoretical conclusions differ.

Vol.1: 01-09-11

Hence, heaven and earth bestow physical appearance, and this never leaves the framework of yin and yang. Physical appearance and color are always reflections of the patterns underlying the universe. Hair and feathers form a group that grows in the yang but is associated with the yin. Scales and shells form a group that grows in the yin but is associated with the yang. Malachite reflects the pattern of wood; its color is greenish and it controls the liver. Cinnabar reflects the pattern of fire; its color is red and it controls the heart. Muscovite reflects the pattern of metal; its color is white and it controls the lung. Magnetite reflects the pattern of water; its color is black and it controls the kidneys. Yellow halloysite reflects the pattern of soil; its color is yellow and it controls the spleen.

Hence, if this is extended by analogy to all other items, there is nothing that is not within the principles underlying nature. Those who wish to serve as physicians, above they should know the markings in heaven and below they should know the principles pervading the earth. In the middle they should know the affairs of humans. If one is familiar with all three, an understanding of the diseases of humans is possible. Otherwise, this is as if one were to travel blind in the night, and to climb on a hill or wade through a water without feet. One would fall and get hurt as soon as he moves. And if such people wish to cure illness, they would never achieve an effect.

Fine husks of grain at the tip of the pestle in a mortar
Vol. V, 25-29

Tao Hongjing: To use these fine husks of grain at the tip of the pestle in a mortar as a pharmaceutical drug to cure gullet occlusion, is based on the concept of pounding in a mortar. The principle underlying events in the world is often one of mutual reflection, similar to that shown here.

Indian lotus leaf
Nelumbo nucifera Gaertn. Vol. VI, 33-10-09

As Li Dongyuan in his *Tested Efficacious Recipes* states: "In the case of thundering head wind conditions with painful lumps and swelling on the head and in the face, an aversion to cold and an effusion of heat, similar in their appearance to harm caused by cold, the disease is situated in the three yang conduits and it is not appropriate to apply excessive doses of preparations of cold medication. This would be punishment without crime. Once a patient suffered from this and all types of medication showed no effect. I prescribed the "decoction to clear up a thunderbolt" and he was cured. That is, one lotus leaf, five maces of *cimicifuga* rhizome, and five maces of *atractylodes lancea* rhizome are boiled in water, and the liquid is ingested warm. The fact is, the trigram "thunderbolt" of the *Classic of Changes* equals "thunder," and the shape of lotus leaves reflects the shape of the trigram "thunderbolt." Also, their color is greenish. That is, the idea that objects form a group that reflects similar shapes comes into play here.

Chestnut wedge
Castanea molissima L. Vol. VI, 29-07-02

Li Shizhen: Among the five fruits, Chinese chestnuts are the ones associated with the phase water. In years of heavy rain/flooding, chestnuts do not ripen. This is so because of the correspondences within one group. Once someone was affected by internal cold. Suddenly he experienced an outflow as if a liquid was poured out. They let him eat 20 to 30 simmered chestnuts and he was cured immediately. The kidneys control massive relief (i.e., defecation). As Chinese chestnuts are able to pass through the kidneys they successfully deal with such an ailment.

Cooked rice/millet
Vol. V, 25-05

Li Shizhen: When a cooked rice meal is prepared with non-glutinous rice using a lotus leaf decoction, it widens the center. Using a black mustard leaves decoction, it opens phlegm. Using a *perilla* herb decoction it stimulates the movement of qi and resolves muscle tension. Using a mint decoction, it eliminates heat. Using a bland bamboo leaf decoction it keeps away summer heat. All these effects can be deducted from group associations.

Phellodendron wood/tree
Phellodendron amurense Ruppr. Vol. VII, 35-01

Wang Haogu: *Scutellaria* root and *gardenia* fruits enter the lung. *Coptis* rhizome enters the heart. *Phellodendron* qi enter the kidneys. When they return to locations of dryness and moisture, this is always in correspondence with their group association. Hence, the "decoction with four items to resolve poison" recommended in the *The Book for Saving People's Lives* combines pharmaceutical drugs that are capable of curing ailments affecting the upper and the lower, the inner and the outer body parts.

Algae
Spirogyra nitida (Dillw.) Link. Vol. V, 21-01

Su Song: Dried algae are prepared as a vegetable. Consumed with a spicy broth it is especially delicious. The group of mosses comprises "mosses in wells," "clothes of walls," "ancient evil," and "roof walker." Their therapeutic functions are basically the same. … They are grouped differently, by they all alike grow endowed with the qi of roof tiles and stones. Hence, that is their group association from which their therapeutic potential is derived.

Peaches remaining on the tree throughout winter
Amygdalus persica L. Vol. VI, 29-06-05

When eating peaches results in disease. Burn peaches remaining on the tree throughout winter to obtain two maces of ashes. Ingest them with water to stimulate vomiting and achieve a cure.

Lu Guanglu says: "Once someone ate peaches and fell ill when they failed to be dissolved/digested. In the forests I obtained withered peaches, burned them and let the patient ingest the residue. Immediately afterwards he vomited the undigested peaches and was cured. This is an example of how members of the same group attack each other." Zhang Wenzhong, *Recipes for Emergencies.*

Breficaude pit vipers
Agkistrodon halys Pallas. Vol. VIII, 43-19-02

Li Shizhen: Repudiation-illnesses are caused by an exposure to the stern and killing qi of heaven and earth. These are malign illnesses. Pit vipers are born endowed with the poisonous and fierce qi of heaven and earth, of yin and yang. They are malign items. When poisonous items are used to attack poison diseases, then this is always based on their group correspondences.

Dried fermented red rice
Monascus purpureus Went. Vol. V, 25-17

Li Shizhen: When water and grain enter one's stomach, they are exposed to the moist and hot steam of the central part of the Triple Burner, moving on and spilling out as essence qi. Within a day they are transformed and assume a red color. They spread through the long-term depots, the short-term repositories, the conduits and their network vessels. They are the camp qi, i.e., the blood. This is one of the subtle miracles of the creation of nature. When fermented red rice is made, a cooked meal of white rice is exposed to intense moist, hot steam. It changes and assumes a red color. That is its real color; even after a long time it will not fade. That is an example of man's spying on the skills of creation. That is, the potential of fermented red rice to cure diseases affecting spleen and stomach and camp qi, i.e., blood, is based on the principle of identical qi looking for each other.

Flower of hemp
Cannabis sativa L. Vol. V, 22-03-01

The *Arcane Essential Recipes from the Outer Censorate* says that persons with a pin-illness swelling should avoid contact with hemp flowers, and that if they come into contact with hemp flowers they die. It recommends to grind sesame, iron crumbs, and candle cinder into powder, mix it with vinegar, and apply it to the affected region. I have no idea why hemp flowers and pin-illness sores should be mutually antagonistic. This is similar to what happens to people who come into contact with lacquer and develop sores. The underlying principles are incomprehensible.

Quince
Chaenomeles speciosa (Sweet) Nakai. Vol. VI, 30-05

Tao Hongjing: Quince fruits are extremely capable of healing contorted sinews. In the case of contorted sinews, all that is required is to call out the name quince or to write down the characters for quince, and this always results in a cure. The underlying principle is beyond our understanding. Common people lean themselves on a quince wood walking stick, claiming that this is good for the functions of sinews and vessels.

Phellodendron wood/tree
Phellodendron amurense Ruppr. Vol. VII, 35-01

Epidemic red eyes. Remove the coarse bark of *phellodendron* and grind it into a powder. Wrap it in moist paper. Cover it with yellow mud. Simmer this until it has dried. Each time take as much as the size of a bullet, wrap it with a gauze handkerchief, soak this in one cup of water and steam it above cooked rice until done. Use the hot steam to fumigate the eyes and use the liquid to wash them. Extremely effective. This recipe combines the phases metal (i.e., the steaming pot), wood (i.e., the bark), water, fire, and soil (i.e., the yellow mud). Hence, it is called the "Five Phases decoction." One pill can be used three times or twice. *Nagarjuna's Discourse.*

Greenish ganoderma
Vol. VI, 28-18-01

Li Shizhen: The five colors of *ganoderma* are matched with the flavors of the Five Phases. The fact is, such correspondences exist only in theory. It is not so that the flavor simply follows the five colors. This is similar to the meaning underlying the fact that sheep, a livestock animal, are associated with fire, and apricots, one of the five fruits, are matched with fire, while both are of bitter flavor.

Xu Zhicai: Greenish, yellow, white, black, and purple variations of *ganoderma* all alike have Chinese yam as their guiding substance, and ingested combined with hair, they yield good results. Combined with hemp seeds, wax gourd seeds, and unscraped bark of male cinnamom trees, they benefit humans. Ingested together, they abhor *dichroa* root, and they fear flat malachite and *artemisia scoparia* herb.

Raw cane sugar
Saccharum sinensis Roxb. Vol. VI, 33-07

Explication. Kou Zongshi: Sugar cane juice is clear. Hence, it is boiled and heat refined until it assumes a purple-black color. Today, in the treatment of sudden/violent heat, physicians often resort to it as the prime guiding substance. In addition, patients are advised to eat camel and horse meat to resolve the heat. When children eat raw cane sugar in large amounts it destroys their teeth and generates worms/bugs. The phase soil checks the phase water. Worms/bugs are associated with the phase soil. When they are exposed to sweet flavor they grow.

Zhu Zhenheng: Sugar stimulates stomach fire. That is, moist soil generates heat. It is for that reason that sugar in large amounts destroys the teeth and generates worms/bugs. This has the same underlying meaning as when consuming Chinese dates causes tooth decay. It has nothing to do with the phase soil checking the phase water.

Chinese coffee tree
Gymnocladus chinensis Baill. Vol. VII, 35-22

The *Records of the Mutual Influences of Various Categories of Things* says: "Chinese coffee tree water kills gold fish and keeps ants away. When they see bran they do not come close." This is so because of the nature of things.

Walnut
Juglans regia L. Vol. VI, 30-28.

Li Shizhen: That walnuts check the poison of copper is one of those enigmatic principles in the nature of things.

Musk melon pulp
Cucumis melo L. Vol. VI, 33-01-01.

Zhang Hua in his *Monograph on a Wide Range of Things* says: "A person who is immersed in water up to the knees can eat several tens of melons. Immersed in water up to the neck, even more, and the water releases the melon qi." That melons immersed in water are dissolved, is another example of the nature of things.

Indian lotus rootstock
Nelumbo nucifera Gaertn. Vol. VI, 33-10

The *Records of the Mutual Influences of Various Categories of Things* states: "Insert a lotus stalk into a hole and all the rats/mice leave. A lotus stalk decoction washes the dirt from pewter and lets it appear like new." Such is the nature of things.

Chinese Olive
Canarium album (Lour.) Raeusch. Vol. VI, 31-04

Li Shizhen: Chinese olive trees are tall. When the fruits have ripened insert a wooden pin into them, or put a little salt into the bark. The fruits fall off within one night. This, too, is one of the wondrous principles inherent in things.

Vol. 01-05-14

Tao Hongjing: In delineations of diseases controlled by pharmaceutical drugs, only the name of one disease is mentioned. However, wind stroke exists in tens of variations. The list of pathological conditions associated with harm caused by cold fills more than 20 paragraphs. It is essential to reach the center of such diverse conditions and to identify the group they form. For a general approach, the beginning and the end of a disease is to be understood, and its basic nature is the foundation of a treatment. Then the various illness signs are to be surveyed to assemble the pharmaceutical drugs required. The many different appearances an illness may assume cannot be expressed summarily. It is for this reason that medical recipes are listed in thousands of chapters, and even they do not entirely comprise the principles underlying all these variations.

Vigna umbellata (Th unb.) Ohwi et Ohashi
Red mung bean leaf. Vol. V, 24-04-01

Li Shizhen: Mung beans stimulate urination, while the leaves stop urination. The underlying idea is the same as with *ephedra*. The herb stimulates sweating; the root stops sweating. The principles underlying the activities of items are that strange.

Composite prepared by boiling tamarisk resin, pine resin, *glycyrrhiza* root, and Chinese foxglove rhizome together with hot blood. Vol. VII, 34-25.

Zhang Hua in his *Monograph on a Wide Range of Things* states: "At the time of Emperor Wu di, Yue shi guo in the western regions sent an envoy across the Ruo shui river to present three pieces to the throne. They were as big as swallow eggs, and as black as mulberry fruits. When the great epidemic hit Chang an, the western envoy asked to burn one piece to repel the epidemic. Those in the palace who had fallen ill smelled the fumes and rose again. The fragrance was smelled a hundred miles and did not cease for several days. When those who had died less than three days ago were fumigated, they were all brought back to life. It is a divine pharmaceutical drug that brings you back to life." Such an account borders on the absurd. Yet there are such things that happen outside of our reason. They should not simply be labeled as faulty.

4. Cosmic structures: Numbers, time, and cardinal directions

What signs in nature may have first given early humans hints of an ongoing and perhaps everlasting regularity? Maybe the sequence of day and night? After all, humans' lives often extend over a period of three generations: children, parents, grandparents. It would be unthinkable for the elders to report that one day has once passed into the next day without an intervening night. The sequence of the annual seasons, with an exactly foreseeable beginning and end year after year, is a fact observed in an agricultural setting at the far east end of a vast Eurasian mainland continent. Spring is followed by summer, by autumn and by winter, and returning spring.

The continuing regularity with which a new season occurred give or take a few days may have suggested conclusions about an underlying order different from that in the regions adjacent to the eastern Mediterranean. Here the whims and follies of the gods were seen in a less than perfectly reliable sequence of events. In the far east, however, there was reason enough for a computational approach to better and better grasp the intricacies of regularity in the universal order. Social order and stability came to be seen as closely related to, if not dependent on, the recognized order underlying the sequence of day and night, and of the seasons.

The attempt to integrate into a larger order is motivated by a sense of resonance. Perhaps it is not only the larger order that predetermines the order of social and individual life. Perhaps it is also the order humans achieve in their own social relationships and individual lives that has a bearing on events in nature, that is, on a universal order *per se*. A numerical recording of regularities observed in nature offers a framework for human behavior. Human existence is seen as deeply embedded in a matrix of resonating with the many facets of a reality humans are born into. This may be the oldest pattern of correspondences and associations humans have ever thought of. In particular, during the era of the Empire, the Emperor, as ruler and representative of his subjects, was held responsible for performing the necessary rituals so as to restore humanity's required place in the grand order.

As early as prehistoric times, the numbering of hours, days, months, etc. did far more than fulfill basic arithmetic necessities as they occur in social, economic and administrative spheres. Numbers were given a value as emblems, and in an increasingly complex system these emblems reflected the human connection with time and space. In this context we barely scratch the surface of a very delicate number system of emblems that had evolved in antiquity and which was fully observed and used throughout the Ming period without ever weakening.[20] Whether all the emblematic applications of numbers in the collection, preparation, dosage, and application of pharmaceutical substances and in the performance of therapeutic rituals can still be traced to their original significance is another question.

It is not known when in China, for whatever reasons, certain months, days, and double hours were considered particularly favorable or unfavorable for certain human activities. A complex, hemerological system developed as a science in its own right, with no ties to the yin yang doctrine of systematic correspondences, nor to the temporality of the calendar. The "doctrine of [choosing] the right day" was based on independent cycles of time units that have their own qualities and whose constellations produce their own prognostic rhythm, independent of the astronomical rhythm.

At some point, this doctrine was so consolidated that it became possible to find the right date for preparing medicines and taking remedies. There are numerous references in the *Ben cao gang mu* to advice to this effect.

Let us consider the dates to be followed in the preparation of wine: "It supplements depletion by boosting qi, and removes all types of blockage related to wind intrusion and moisture qi. Ingested over a long time it boosts long life, helps to endure aging, and improves your complexion. The production method: On the third day of the third month collect three ounces and three maces of peach flowers. On the fifth day of the fifth month collect five ounces and five maces of Chinese irish flowers. On the sixth day of the sixth month collect six ounces and six maces of sesame flowers. On the ninth day of the ninth month collect nine ounces and nine maces of yellow, sweet *chrysanthemum* flowers and dry them in the yin (i.e., shade). On the eighth day of the twelfth month obtain three pecks of water collected in the twelfth month. Wait until spring equinox, gather 49 good peach stones, with their outer surface and tips removed, and ten pounds of white wheat flour. Add the stones and the flour to the flowers mentioned above to make a mould ferment, wrapped in paper for 49 days. When the time has come, add one pill from the ferment and one lump of flour to one bottle of clear water and keep it sealed for a long time until the wine is ready. If it is bland, add another pill from the ferment."

---

20 Additional reading: Aihe Wang, *Cosmology and* Political Culture in Early China. Cambridge University Press. Cambridge, 2000.

Similarly, specific hours are to be observed when ingesting medication; different cardinal directions are to be considered, for instance, when acquiring some things in their natural habitat. An explanation for such requirements and many similar ones is not given. Who knows whether by the time of Li Shizhen they had deteriorated to a level of empty conventions, observed simply because they were conventions followed since times immemorial.

Numbers, in the *Ben cao gang mu* especially the number seven, hours, seasons, and cardinal directions formed a fixed spatial-temporal framework, either as an alternative to or integrated into the yin and yang as well as the Five Phases doctrines of systematic correspondences. They allowed clear-cut advice on when and where to perform specific therapeutic activities. Numbers in Chinese medicine as in Chinese culture in general stood for much more than the abstract designation of a quantity. Numbers served to assign a value to groups both of things and also of humans. Numbers reflected in rituals signaled power; in medicine such powers were required to counter the power of evil as manifest in disease and early death.

Cinnabar
Vol. II, 09-01

To ingest cinnabar for food. A recipe of the Three Perfected Primordial Sovereigns: Grind one pound of cinnabar to a powder and repeatedly give it through a sieve. Let it soak in unmixed wine until it has turned into a mud-like mass, and fill this on a copper plate to be placed on an elevated shelf. Do not allow the women to see it. Once it has dried let it soak in wine again until it has turned into a mud, and store this at a shady place where it rains and where winds are swift. After three pecks of wine are used up this way, dry it in the sun. After 300 days it will have assumed a purple color. Abstain from meat, wine etc. and bathe hair and body for seven days, and in a quiet room prepare the cinnabar with cooked rice to pills the size of hemp seeds. Then regularly in the early morning hours face the sun and swallow three pills. Within one month three bugs/worms will leave the body. After half a year, all types of diseases will have been cured. Within one year, beard and hair on the head will be black. After three years the status of a spirit man will have been reached. *The Classic of Mysterious Changes up on High.*

Ink plant herb
Eclipta prostrata(L.) L. Vol. IV, 16-38-01

All eye afflictions. Eye shade blocking vision. It cools the brain and serves to cure headache. It can stimulate hair growth. Prepare the following recipe in the early morning hours of the fifth day of the fifth month. Soak a handful of ink plant herb and a handful of *eupatorium* leaves in one pound of oil. Keep it tightly sealed for 49 days. Each time when going to bed, drip some of it with an iron spoon on the top of the head and rub it into the skin. 49 times. The longer the better. *General Records of Sagely Benefaction.*

Divine water
Vol. II, 5-11

Li Shizhen: The *Records of the Golden Gate* states: "When rain falls at noon on the fifth day of the fifth month, quickly fell a bamboo pole. There must be 'divine water' in it. Let it trickle out to serve as medication."

Newly drawn water
Vol. II, 05-15-02

To ward off warmth epidemics. During the night following the 12th month, drop seven times seven small beans and Sichuan pepper grains into a well, but do not let anyone be aware of this. This can keep away warmth epidemics. Another method. On New Year's day drop three times seven hemp seeds into the well.

Old black roof tile
Vol. II, 07-48

Harm caused by the stings of bees/wasps and scorpions. Rub the surface with a tile, spit on it two times seven times, and replace the tile to where it had been. *Recipes Worth a Thousand in Gold.*

Black soybeans
Glycine max (L.) Merr. Vol. V,24-01-01

Huang Shangu's method of famine relief. Boil one pint each of black beans and *dryopteris* roots in water until they are done, remove the *dryopteris* roots and dry the beans in the sun. Every day take on an empty stomach five times seven beans and each of the hundred types of wood, twigs, and leaves has a flavor when consumed and can satisfy hunger.

Great burnet
Sanguisorba officinalis L. Vol. III, 12-24

Blood discharge caused by bound yin qi, with an unending abdominal pain. For each dose give five maces of a mixture of four ounces of great burnet and three ounces of roasted *glycyrrhiza* root into three small cups of water, add four times seven pieces of *amomum villosum* seeds, and boil this down to one and a half small cups, to be ingested divided into two portions. *Recipes of Illumination.*

Chinese quinine
Dichroa febrifuga Lour. Vol. IV, 17-14

Miasmatic malaria with alternating sensations of cold and heat. Liu Changchun in his *Tried and Proven Recipes* recommends the following recipe. Soak a one inch long piece of Chinese quinine *shan* and one red cardamom fruit in one bowl of hot wine for one night and let the patient ingest the liquid in the early morning hours facing East. Then let him lie down covered warm and he will be healed when he wakes up from the effects of the wine.

Musk melon
Cucumis melo L. Vol. VI, 33-01

Black moles on the face. On the seventh day of the seventh month at noon gather seven melon leaves, walk straight into the northern hall of your house, stand there facing South and with one after another of the seven leaves rub the moles. This will eliminate them. *All the Ten-thousand Arts of Huainan.*

Peach flower
Amygdalus persica L. Vol. VI, 29-06-06

To give the face a shiny splendor. Collect peach flowers on the third day of the third month. Collect chicken blood on the seventh day of the seventh month. Mix them and apply this on the face. Take it off two or three days later, and the complexion will have a shiny splendor. *General Records of Sagely Benefaction.*

Winter aster
Dendranthema indicum (L.) des Moul. Vol. IV, 15-02

The *Easy and Simple Recipes for Protecting Life* recommends to pound one handful each of winter aster flowers, stems, and leaves, and cocklebur herb, give this into a bowl of wine, and squeeze it to obtain a juice that is to be ingested. The dregs are applied to the affected region. Once the patient sweats he is cured. Or, collect cocklebur leaves on the sixth day of the sixth month and winter aster flowers on the ninth day of the ninth month and grind them into powder. Each time ingest with wine three maces. This is possible, too.

Chinese iris
Iris lactea Pall. var. *chinensis* (Fisch.) Koidz. Vol. IV, 15-40

The hundred diseases related to watery free-flux illness. Zhang Wenzhong in his *Recipes for Emergencies* recommends to grind equal amounts of Chinese iris with roasted wheat flour from the sixth day of the sixth month into powder and ingest on an empty stomach with a rice beverage the amount held by a one square inch spoon. If no wheat flour of the sixth day of the sixth month is at hand, normal wheat flour will do, too. The ashes of the bones of oxen can be used, too.

St. Paulswort
Siegesbeckia orientalis L. Vol. IV, 15-44

Su Song: The method of people in Shu to ingest St. Paulswort as a single substance. Collect the leaves on the fifth day of the fifth month, the sixth day of the sixth month, and the ninth day of the ninth month. Discard the root, the stem, the flowers, and the fruit and wash the leaves clean. Then dry them in the sun and give them into a jar. Place them in layers with each layer sprinkled with wine and honey, and steam this. Then dry them again in the sun. Do this nine times. This will result in extremely fragrant qi and a delicious flavor. Heat them, pound them, and pass them through a sieve to obtain a powder to be formed with honey to pills. To ingest them, they say, very much boosts the original qi, cures liver and kidneys affected by wind qi, numbness of the four limbs, cold in the bones, and lack of strength in the lower back and knees. They also stimulate the passage of qi through the large intestine.

"Divine" yeast/ferment
Vol. V, 25-16-2

Mr. Ye in his *Records of Waters and Clouds* states: "On the fifth day of the fifth month, or on the sixth day of the sixth month, or during the three ten-day periods of the hottest season of the year, prepare 100 pounds of white wheat flour, three pints of the natural juice of wormwood herb, three pints each of red mung bean powder and apricot kernel pulp, as well as three pints each of the natural juice of cocklebur herb and the natural juice of *anemarrhena* root. They correspond to the six gods of the stars White Tiger, Blue Dragon, Vermilion Bird, Black Tortoise, Sickle Posture, and Flying Serpent. Take the juices, the wheat flour, the beans, and the apricot kernel pulp and form a cake. Wrap it with hemp leaves or paper mulberry leaves, similar to the method of how yellow bean sauce is prepared, wait until a yellow coating has developed, dry it in the sun, and store it."

Vinegar
Vol. V, 25-23

Li Shizhen: Rice vinegar: Soak one peck of husked granary rice in water during the three ten-day periods of the hottest season of the year, clean it, and steam it until it is cooked. Spread it out to let it cool down, cover it, and wait until a yellow coating has developed. Dry it in the sun and winnow away the chaff. In addition, steam an extra two pecks of husked granary rice to prepare cooked rice, mix the two evenly, and give them into an earthenware pot. Fill it with water, seal it tightly, and leave it at a warm place. The vinegar is ready after three times seven days.

Vinegar made from glutinous rice: On the day of the sacrifices to the god of the land in autumn, rinse one peck of glutinous rice, steam it, and mix it with wheat ferment prepared on the sixth day of the sixth month. Give this, with two pecks of water, into an earthenware pot, seal it, and let it ferment. The vinegar is ready after three times seven days.

Vinegar made from short millet: Wash one peck of long-stored short millet in a pan and soak it in water for seven days. Wash it again, steam it until done, give it into an earthenware pot, and tightly seal it. Stir the contents during the day and during the night. The vinegar is ready after seven days.

Vinegar made from wheat: Soak wheat in water for three days. Steam it until done, cover it, and wait for a yellow coating to develop. Give it into an earthenware pot, submerge it in water, and the vinegar is ready after seven times seven days.

Vinegar made from barley: Soak one peck of barley in water, and steam it until cooked. Cover it, wait for a yellow coating to develop, and dry it in the sun. Pour water over it and evenly mix it with another two pecks of cooked barley. Add water, close the pot tightly, and after three times seven days the vinegar is ready.

Vinegar made from malt sugar: Boil one pound of malt sugar in three pecks of water until the sugar is dissolved. Add two ounces of white ferment powder, seal it in a bottle, and expose it to the sun until the vinegar is ready.

All the other types of vinegar, that is, those prepared from wine brewing residue/sediment and bran, are not added to medication. Hence, they are not described here in detail.

"Wine that lets you hesitate to move forward."
Vol. V, 25-24-10

It supplements depletion by boosting qi, and removes all types of blockage related to wind intrusion and moisture qi. Ingested over a long time it boosts long life, helps to endure aging and improves your complexion. The production method: On the third day of the third month collect three ounces and three maces of peach flowers. On the fifth day of the fifth month collect five ounces and five mace of Chinese irish flowers. On the sixth day of the sixth month collect six ounces and six maces of sesame flowers. On the ninth day of the ninth month collect nine ounces and nine maces of yellow, sweet *chrysanthemum* flowers and dry them in the yin (i.e., shade). On the eighth day of the twelfth month obtain three pecks of water collected in the twelfth month. Wait until spring equinox, gather 49 good peach kernels, with their skin and tips removed, and ten pounds of white wheat flour. Add the kernels and the flour to the flowers mentioned above to make a mould ferment, wrapped in paper for 49 days. When the time has come, give one pill of the ferment and one lump of flour into one bottle of clear water and keep it sealed for a long time until the wine is ready. If it is bland, add another pill of the ferment.

Purslane
Portulaca oleracea L. Vol. VI, 27-11

To avert and resolve epidemic qi. On the sixth day of the sixth month collect purslane and dry it in the sun. On New Year's day boil it until done, mix it with salt and vinegar, and eat this. This can resolve the qi of epidemics. *Tried and Proven Recipes of Tang Yao.*

Soapbean tree
Gleditsia sinensis Lam. Vol. VII, 35-21

To prevent sores and pimples. If a child every year on the sixth day of the sixth month swallows as many soapbean tree pod seeds as correspond to its years of life, this prevents suffering from ulcers and pimples. Adults, too, can swallow seven seeds, or 21 seeds. This is a recipe transmitted by Lin Jingzhai. Wu Min, *Recipes for Supporting Long Life.*

Paper mulberry tree fruit
Vol. VII, 36-04-01

Pharmaceutical Preparation. After collecting them soak them in water for three days. Then stir the liquid to let the water whirl, and remove those that float on the surface. Dry them in the sun and then soak them in wine for a full day. Steam them from 9.00 – 11.00 to 21.00 – 23.00, bake them over a slow fire until they are dry, and use them for therapeutic purposes. The method to boil paper mulberry tree fruits recommended in the *Tried and Proven Later Recipes*: On the sixth day of the sixth month boil five pints of paper mulberry tree seeds in one peck of water down to five pints, remove the dregs, and boil the liquid until it has assumed a consistency of malt sugar. Then it can be used.

Water collected on the fifth day of the fifth month during *wu* hours
(11:00 –13:00). Vol. II, 05-16-04

Suitable for preparing all types of elixirs and pills for malaria and free-flux illness, sores, ulcers, and wounds resulting from metal objects/weapons, as well as poison of the hundreds of worms/bugs and *gu*.

Tinder fire
Vol. II, 06-02

Li Shizhen: The sequence of the great fires seen in heaven is based on the movement of the stars. In the third month of spring, when the dragon was seen at the cardinal direction East-South-East, the Sacrificial Fire Manager came forward with the fire, and this was the beginning of the season with summerheat. In the third month of autumn, the dragon hid in the cardinal direction West-West-North and the Sacrificial Fire Manager took in the fire. This was the beginning of the season with cold. In their being active and resting, all the workers followed the DAO of heaven and thereby they prevented widespread occurrences of flooding and drought disasters. In later times, on the day of Cold Food all fires were forbidden. This was to mark the change of fire from being taken in to being brought forth, but it is commonly assumed that this day is to mark the Jie Tui affair.[21] That is wrong.

Soil removed from the ground in relation to the position
of the major yang constellation in the nine mansions diagram
Vol. II, 07-06

If a taboo is violated when people move soil, this will cause their children to suffer from panting. According to the "nine mansions diagram," examine in which mansion the sun happened to be during the taboo violation, remove soil from this mansion, boil it in water and drink this. This will settle the panting. Li Shizhen, quoted from the *The Orthodox Transmission of Medical Studies.*

Soil taken from a location in the North-West on a clear day.[22]
Vol. II, 07-06-A04

Li Shizhen: A plaster prepared from this soil and dog hair, and smeared into the holes of one's home will forever bar snakes, mice/rats, and all types of worms/bug from entering.

---

21 Jie Zitui 介子推 served King Wen of the State of Jin, 5th c. BCE. Eventually he withdrew with his mother to the forests. King Wen summoned him to his court to show his gratitude. When Jie Zitui refused to appear, the king had the forest set on fire to force him to leave his abode. Jie and his mother died in the fire in 476 BCE. The king ordered that no fires were allowed on that day in future, and food was to be consumed cold. Hence the name of that day, *han shi* 寒食, "cold food." BCGM Dict III, 224-225.

22 *Qing ming ri* 清明日 could refer to the *qing ming* festival, 清明節, celebrated on the 15th day after spring equinox, or to any bright and clear day. As the first of these alternatives would limit the gathering of soil to only one day in a year, the second alternative may be more practical.

Soil of the Spirit Sovereign. Soil taken on the second day of a year
Vol. II, 07-06-A05

Li Shizhen: Every month on the first day take this soil, plaster with it the four corners of your home, and stuff the holes opened by mice/rats. Within one year all traces of mice/rats will have been eliminated. This is a method to get rid of mice/rats devised by Reclusive Scholar Li. The "Spirit Sovereign" time is the time twelve double hours after the beginning of counting hours on the first day of the first month of a year.

Verdigris
Vol. II, 08-09

Suddenly being struck by wind and phlegm. The "bluish jade elixir" serves to treat a profuse emergence of phlegm and saliva, sudden stroke, and an inability to speak with all types of paralysis caused by wind. Grind two ounces of verdigris to a fine powder. Dissolve it in water and remove any stones that remain undissolved. Heat the liquid over a mild fire until it is dry. The processing and mixing is to be conducted on a *chen* day, at *chen* hours (07:00 – 09:00), at a *chen* location.[23] Add one tenth of an ounce of musk, and form, with glutinous rice powder, pills the size of bullets. Dry them in a shady place. When someone is suddenly struck, each time let him ingest two such pills, to be sent down ground in mint wine. For wind that remains, send the pills down dissolved in cinnabar wine. This leads to a vomiting of greenish-bluish saliva, and an outflow discharge of malign items. Very effective.

Arsenic. Arsenic trioxide
Vol. II, 10-17

Lei Xiao: For all medicinal applications, place the raw arsenic into a small porcelain jar and add the two substances purple back *malva* herb and *ranunculus sceleratus* herb. Calcine it with fire from 09:00 – 11:00 to 15:00 – 17:00, and then soak it in water in which *glycyrrhiza* root was cooked from 15:00 – 17:00 to 23:00 – 01:00. Remove it and wipe it dry. Give it into a jar and calcine it again. Then grind it three times ten thousand times before making therapeutic use of it.

---

23 *Chen* is the fifth in the sequence of the earthly branches. It is associated with the two hours 7.00 to 9.00, and with the cardinal direction SEE.

Chinese water chestnut root
Eleocharis dulcis (Burm. f.) Trin. ex Henschel. Vol. VI, 33-14-01

Red and white discharge with free-flux illness. On a *wu* 午 day at *wu* 午 hours (midday) take complete, good Chinese water chestnuts, wash them clean and rub them dry. They must not be damaged or broken. Soak them in a jar in good brandy, tightly close it with yellow mud, and store this. When you happen to meet a patient suffering from this disease, take two of these Chinese water chestnuts, let the patient chew them finely and send them down, on an empty stomach, with the wine sed to soak the chestnuts before. *Tried and Proven Recipes of Tang Yao.*

Poplar tree bark
Populus davidiana Dode. Vol. VII, 35-32-01

Pharmaceutical Preparation. Lei Xiao: For all therapeutic applications remove the coarse bark with a copper knife. Steam the remaining bark from 9.00 – 11.00 to 13.00 – 15.00. Wrap it with a piece of cloth and hang it at the eastern corner of the house. Wait until it has dried and then use it for therapeutic ends.

White bark of silkworm thorn tree roots extending East
Maclura tricuspidata Carr. Vol. VII, 36-02-01

To clear the eyes by washing them. Wash the eyes with a warm silkworm thorn wood decoction on specific days from 3.00 – 5.00 to 21.00 – 23.00, and stop. This is always effective. The days are: First month, second day. Second month, second day. Third month: no washing. Fourth month, fifth day. Fifth month, fifteenth day. Sixth month, eleventh day. Seventh month, seventh day. Eighth month, second day. Ninth month, second day. Tenth month, nineteenth day. Eleventh month, no washing. Twelfth month, fourteenth day. A recipe of Xu Shenweng. *Recipes from Abroad.*

Human qi
Vol. IX, 52-23

Ge Hong in his *Bao pu zi* states: "Man exists within qi, and the qi are within man. All the creatures under heaven and on earth require qi to live. Those who are experts in maintaining the passage of qi, they internally nourish their body, and externally ward off the malign. However, to make the qi pass requires a certain technique. The hours from 23.00 – 1.00 to 9.00 – 11.00 are those of living qi; the hours 11.00 – 13.00 to 21.00 – 23.00

are those of dead qi. The experts always inhale qi, through the nose, during the hours of living qi. They let much in, and let only a little out. They close nose and mouth and start counting: From nine times nine, through eight times eight, seven times seven, six times six, and five times five, and then they stop and gently spit out the breath again. The ears must not hear a sound. If one through repeated practice gets used to this, he may increase the numbers counted to one thousand. This is the fetal breathing. Or, in spring one may consume the greenish qi from the East. In summer one may consume the red qi from the South. In autumn one may consume the white qi from the West, and in winter one may consume the black qi from the North. During the last month of each season one may consume the yellow qi of the center. This, too, is very effective. Hence, those who are good at maintaining the passage of qi, they are able to ward off hunger and thirst, and they can extend the years of their life, they can walk on water, they can reside in water, they can cure the hundreds of diseases, and they can enter warmth epidemics without fear of falling ill themselves.

Fortune's *chloranthus*
Chloranthus fortunei (A. Gray) Solms-Lamb. Vol V, 18-41

Xu Xueshi in his *Recipes Based on Facts* states: "*Jian cao* serves to cure exhaustion consumption with blood spitting and injured lung, and wild blood movement. This is treated with the 'paste transmitted by spirits.' The method is as follows: Each time clean one pound, dry it in the sun, and grind it into powder. Add two pounds of fresh honey, prepare a paste, and fill it into a vessel. It must not be offended by iron vessels. Steam this once per day. End it after nine times steaming and nine times drying in the sun. The patient rises in the early morning hours and sits down facing East. He must not speak. Take the pharmaceutical drug with a spoon and let the patient eat four spoons. After a long time the ointment is pressed down with a thin millet or rice beverage. The pharmaceutical drug must only be ingested cold. The rice beverage must not be too hot, either. If this results in vomiting or discharge, this is of no concern. In the case of a long-lasting disease with a lung injury and blood spitting, a cure is achieved after only one ingestion. In the case of continuing cough with a wild movement of blood, it is appropriate to ingest one spoon each time.

There was a noble woman who suffered from consumption. It took nine days to prepare this medication. The night before the medication was supposed to be taken for the first time, the patient had a dream. Some person warned her of an imminent chaos and that she should not ingest the medication. The next day when she was just ready to ingest the medication, soil from the roof fell into the vessel and the medication was no longer usable. It was prepared again and when she was ready to ingest it the vessel was overturned by a cat and once again she could not eat the paste. When it was prepared anew, the woman had died. This medication is associated with such strange occurrences. If the blood moves only a little wildly, just one sip is enough to cause healing." This pharmaceutical drug is so wondrous, but its transmission in the world is lost. What a pity!

Dried ginger
Zingiber officinale L. Vol. VI, 26-17-01

Alternating sensations of cold and heat associated with a malaria illness. A collection on phlegm in spleen and stomach effuses as alternating sensations of cold and heat. Pound four ounces of fresh ginger and let the natural juice remain with one cup of wine in the open for one night. Early in the next morning drink it standing facing North, and the disease will stop. If it does not stop, ingest the liquid a second time. *Mirror of Medicine.*

Rat/mouse seal
Vol. IX, 51-39-04

Li Shizhen: Nan Gongcun in his *Spirit Book of Gou lou Mountain* has a story of "rat/mouse seal and sex," and comments: "The external kidneys of male rats/mice have a décor that is reminiscent of a seal. When the two kidneys/testes that form a pair are completely covered by seals in vermillion script, then they are particularly good. On any day of the eleventh or second month, on the fifth day of the fifth month, on the seventh day of the seventh month, and at daybreak of the first day of the first month, assume a position facing North. Scrape the 'seal' to obtain fine pieces that are to be dried in the shade. Write down a character resembling the seal on the rat's/mouse's testes on a piece of cloth, wrap the scraped off pieces with it, and carry them with you in a greenish pouch. Males on the left, females on the right, tied to the arm. All those who see this will be happy, and the person wearing this will be sought after by others with their heart's intensity."

5. Demons and spirits, shamans and exorcism

Since remote, prehistoric times, perhaps no other area of Chinese culture has seen such a flourishing creativity of concepts, activities, and literary output as that concerned with the many types of spirits known to exist together with and within humans. In pre-imperial China, during the Shang era, mediums known as *wu* occupied a leading role in their clans. They conducted rituals to the Supreme Deified Ancestor and other ancestral spirits as these were assumed to send misfortune, including illness, to their descendants if they failed to behave according to long-established norms.

With the political turmoil during the Warring States period beginning in the 8th century BCE, a belief in the principally benevolent attitude of ancestral spirits waned; the image of the *wu* weakened. When the new concept of "bearing false witness" required generating a meaningful character, a combination of two available characters was chosen: "to speak" and "*wu* medium." At least to those responsible for the development of Chinese script, *wu* mediums had lost credibility. The previously used character for "healing" showed a *wu* medium with a quiver filled with an arrow and holding a weapon in his hand. Obviously, this character no longer did justice to the faded image of *wu* mediums. The component "*wu* medium" was replaced by a component reminiscent of "wine" and thus corresponded to the increasing claim of a healing science based on herbs prepared with wine.

All this coincided with the emergence of a concept of *gui*, demons. Ancestors could be related to living individuals. In contrast, demons were anonymous spirits driven in their behavior by hatred for the living. They might emerge from the corpse of someone who died an unjust death, or from corpses left unburied. The reasons of their malevolence could be many. The *wu* mediums now claimed to be able to restrain minor spirits and violent demons harmful to man. Exorcism became their chief responsibility. A new expertise involving "invoking the origin of disease" emerged. As late as during the second millennium, it was for a while granted the status of one of the officially recognized medical specialties. Its practitioners focussed on defense against all kinds of evil spirits.

Documented in great detail, since the Han era, mediums, shamans, diviners, exorcists, magicians, and others appealed in imperial China not only to the illiterate masses but also to the educated, the ruling class. Their services proved indispensable. Early Daoism has been seen as an attempt to transform a chaotic diversity of beliefs and practices into the orderly coexistence of man and the spiritual world, with Daoist priests assuming the role of intermediaries. In the late Han era, they were joined by Buddhist priests. They, too, claimed to influence the behavior of spirits and gods with their recitations and rituals. Local and ethnic traditions added their own views and practices to ward off evil qi, to exorcise demons and to protect mankind. Over the centuries enormous creative energy identified apotropaic substances and devised material amulets with magic potential; oral and written spells, often resonating with legal orders, were cast, and various new symbolic characters were devised to ensure human dominance over the ever-present demonic adversaries.

Apparently, the results of all these practices were sufficiently convincing, and the arguments casting doubts on the underlying concepts found only marginal acceptance. The belief in demons as causative factors for misfortune and disease never waned. The diversity of strategies employed is impressive. Henry Doré, French missionary to China and sinologist, beginning in 1911 published his *Researches into Chinese Superstitions* in 13 volumes. He left a most detailed documentation of their ability to survive throughout millenia.[24]

Li Shizhen took the *Ben cao gang mu* as a platform to offer all authors of the past two millennia a chance to present their views. The *Ben cao gang mu*, as the following limited anthology may indicate, contains numerous examples of different concepts and activities for coping with demonic health threats. They were part of an indisputable reality acknowledged as such by Li Shizhen, even if he occasionally added a comment denying their validity. His generosity in presenting views with which he may have not agreed is unique.

Peach seed kernels
Amygdalus persica L. Vol. VI, 29-06-03

Corpse qi attachment-illness and demon attachment-illness. This is one of five types of corpse qi transmission. Also, a ghost affliction caused by a demon's evil qi. The disease changes constantly and may appear in 36, up to 39 types. Generally speaking, it causes alternating sensations of cold and heat, and urinary dripping. The disease is located in the depth and

---

24 Additional reading: Kenneth J. DeWoskin, *Doctors, Diviners and Magicians of Ancient China: Biographies of Fang-shi.* Columbia University Press. New York, 1983. Michel Strickmann, edited by Bernard Faure, *Chinese Magical Medicine.* Stanford University Press. Stanford CA, 2002.

makes no sounds. Patients do not know what they suffer from and they feel highly uncomfortable all over their body. This continues for months or years and eventually ends in death. After a patient has died, the disease is transmitted to a bystander. Quickly grind 50 peach kernels into a mud, boil it in four pints of water and let the patient ingest it to induce vomiting. If the vomiting fails to end the disease, induce vomiting again three to four days later. *Recipes to be Kept Close at Hand.*

Transmitted corpse and demon qi. Coughing and string-illness and aggregation-illness. This is a qi influx. Blocked blood and qi movement. Emaciation increases every day. Remove the skin and the pointed ends of one ounce of peach kernels. Grind them into small pieces, boil them in one pint of water to obtain a juice. Add husked rice and cook a congee. Eat it on an empty stomach. ... Demon attachment-illness with heart pain. Pound one tenth of a pint of peach kernels into a pulpy mass, boil it in water and ingest the decoction. *Recipes for Emergency Rescue.*

Peachwood talisman
Vol. VI, 29-06-10

Being struck by the malign. For essence goblins and evil qi, boil it in water and ingest the resulting juice. Meng Shen.

Li Shizhen: The *Classic Erudition* states: "Peachwood is a wood of the West. It is the essence of the five woods. It is the wood of the hermits/immortals. It has an acrid flavor and malign qi and, therefore, is able to press down evil qi and to check the hundreds of demons. For this reason, people nowadays attach peachwood talismans above the door."

The *Treasury of the Jade Candle* states: "Peachwood boards attached above a door keep away the evil. This is based on the meaning implicit in a record in the *Classic of Mountains and Seas* of the immortal brothers Shen Tu and Yu lei. They resided under a twisted peach tree from where they exerted control over all demons."

Xu Shen states: "Yi was killed with a peach stick. ... Therefore demons fear peachwood. Today, people use peachwood stalks to make short wooden posts to keep away demons."

The *Record of Rites* states: "When the King mourns the death of his officials, shamans use peach tree twig brooms to clear his way. This serves to ward off the inauspicious."

The *Monograph on a Wide Range of Things* states: "A peach tree root can be made into a seal to summon demons."

The *Notes on Discerning Extraordinary Things* states: "Demons are only afraid of twigs on the South-Eastern side of peach trees."

All these records suggest that the twigs, leaves, root, kernels, peaches remaining on the tree throughout winter, and peachwood pegs can keep away trouble caused by demons and ghosts. The fact is, they are the origin of disease. Qian Yi in his *Recipes for Children* uses *croton* seeds, sal ammoniac and mercury as pharmaceutical drugs on various occasions to cure heat qi accumulation and qi nodes in the chest, and sends them down in the body with a peachwood talisman decoction. This, too, is based on the understanding that they suppress demons and evil qi.

Sweet gum
Liquidambar formosana Hance. Vol. VII, 34-21

Su Gong: Sweet gum trees are everywhere in the great mountains.

Su Song: Today, there are especially many in the South and in Guan shaan. The trees are very tall and big; they resemble poplars. The leaves are round with bifurcations. Some have three corners and are fragrant. The trees have flowers in the second month, white in color. The fruits are attached; they are as big as duck eggs. When they have ripened in the eighth or ninth month, they are dried in the sun and can be burned as incense.

The *Forms of Herbs and Trees from the Southern Regions* states: "Sweet gum fruits are found only in Jiu zhen. Their use yields divine effects, but they are difficult to obtain. The resin is 'white glue aromatic.' To collect it cut a notch in the trees in the fifth month and collect the resin in the eleventh month."

The *Explaining Single and Analysing Compound Characters* states: "Sweet gum trees have thick leaves and weak twigs that tend to wave in the wind." During the Han, they were often planted in the palace gardens where after frost the leaves turned into a lovely cinnabar-red. Hence, they spoke of "palace grounds of sweet gum trees."

Ren Fang in his *Records Narrating the Extraordinary* states: "In the South are trees called 'sweet gum demons.' When they grow old they assume the shape of humans. They are also called 'numinous sweet gum trees'." The fact is, these are tumors and goiters covering the trees. To this day, shamans in Yue obtain them to cut them in the shape of demon spirits to achieve numinous, strange effects.

Han Baosheng: Wang Guan in his *Basic Annals of Xuanyuan* states: "Huang Di killed Chi You on Mount Lishan. Then he threw his weapons into the wasteland, where they turned into a forest of Formosan storax trees."

A comment to the *Examples of Refined Usage* states: "When the resin enters the ground, within one thousand years it becomes amber."

Li Shizhen: The twigs and trunk of sweet gum trees are tall and towering. Big ones reach a circumference of several arm-spans. Their wood is very hard. It may be red or white. The white wood is fine and oily. The fruits are spherical, with soft thorns. When Ji Han says that "sweet gum fruits come only from Jiu zhen," it is not clear whether they are the sweet gum fruits discussed here or not.

Sun Yan in his *Correct Meanings in the Examples of Refined Usage* states: "'Sweet gum demons' are parasitic twigs on sweet gum trees. They are three to four feet tall. Put mud on them in times of drought and it will rain."

Xun Bozi in his *Records of Linchuan* states: "Old sweet gum trees in Lingnan develop tumors in the shape of humans. Exposed to a thunderstorm and rain shower they extend to a length of three to five *chi*. They are called 'sweet gum wood people'."

Song Qiqiu in his *Book of Transformations* states: "Old sweet gum trees transform into feathered persons."

These are many different statements. Basically, only what they say about tumors and goiters growing on these trees appears to make sense.

Zhi-bird
Vol. IX, 49-29

Li Shizhen: According to Gan Bao's *Records of Searching for the Supernatural*, "in Yue di, deep in the forests, there are *zhi* birds. They are as big as turtledoves, and of greenish color. They pierce holes into trees to build their nests the size of a vessel holding five to six pints. The holes to the nests are several inches in diameter, and they are decorated with soil and chalk to create red and white parallels, and they look like the targets of archers. When woodcutters see such trees, they avoid them. If they were to go against them, the *zhi* birds were to send tigers to harm these persons, and they will burn down their houses. When they are seen during daylight, they appear as birds. If one hears their cries during nighttime, it is the sound of birds. At times they assume the physical appearance of humans, and are three fathoms long. They enter into ravines to remove crabs, and they roast them over fire and eat them among humans. The people living in the mountains call them 'ancestors of the shamans/exorcists of Yue'."

Also, in Duan Chengshi's *A Miscellany from Za zu* it is said: "Legend has it that in an earlier time, a man was caught in a flooding. He ate the skin of the *du* trees, but eventually starved to death and was transformed into this item. Those who stay in the root of a *du*-tree, they are called pig-*du*. Those who stay in the middle of the tree, they are called man-*du* 都. Those who stay at the tail end of the tree, they are called bird-*du*. The bird-*du* below their ribs on the left side have a mirror-like seal, 2.1 inches wide. The people in the South eat their nests; they taste like *ganoderma* fungus."

I personally say: Among wild animals, there are *shan du*, *shan sao*, and *mu ke*, and among the birds, too, there are *zhi niao*, *shan xiao*, and *mu ke* birds. Perhaps it is such that they all were bestowed with an identical vicious qi but have assumed different physical appearances?

Honeysuckle
Lonicera japonica Thunb. Vol. V, 18-61

The five types of corpse qi influx.

Flying corpse qi. They race through the skin, and penetrate the long-term depots and short-term repositories. Each outbreak is accompanied by a piercing pain, with movements occurring at irregular intervals.

Run-away corpse qi. They are attached to the bones and have entered the flesh. They attack the blood vessels. Each outbreak is initiated by an invisible corpse whose wailing sounds can be heard.

Wind type corpse qi. They jump around in the four limbs making it impossible to exactly locate the pain. Each outbreak results in absent-mindedness of the patient and is initiated by an exposure to wind and snow.

Sunken corpse qi. They entangle the long-term depots and short-term repositories, with each outbreak initiated by an exposure to cold and accompanied by a twisting and cutting pain pulling on the heart and the flanks.

Corpse qi attachment-illness. The body feels very heavy, with a jumbled essence spirit and frequent loss of consciousness. Every exposure to seasonal qi results in a massive outbreak.

All these are conditions of external evil qi drawn in by corpse demons residing in the body. For a therapy it is appropriate to cut several bushels of honeysuckle stems and leaves into fine pieces, boil them to obtain a thick juice, and boil the juice again to obtain a paste. Each time ingest a piece as big as a chicken egg, to be sent down dissolved in warm wine. To be ingested two or three times a day. *Recipes to be Kept Close at Hand.*

A greenish body following a demon attack. Painful. Boil one ounce of honeysuckle in water and drink it. Li Lou, *Exceptional Recipes for Strange Diseases.*

Cynanchum root
Cynanchum thesinides (Freyn) K. Schum. Vol. IV, 16-34-01

To keep away, by means of exorcism, warmth epidemics. On the first *yin*-day of the first month pound *cynanchum* root into a powder, fill it into a triangular deep red bag, and attach it to a curtain. Very auspicious. *Recipes to be Kept Close at Hand.*

Prayer bead tree
Abrus precatorius L. Vol. VII, 35-50

Cat demons in the wild on roads. The eyes see cat leopard cats, and the ears hear their sounds. Prepare a mixture of one prayer bead, one castor bean and one *croton* seed, and four scruples each of cinnabar and beeswax. Pound them, prepare pills the size of hemp seeds, and ingest them. Then lay an ash circle around the patient and place one peck of an ash fire in front of him. He is to spit the medication into the fire. Once it boils write the character 十 above the fire. All the cat demons die. *Recipes Worth a Thousand in Gold.*

Wine made in Dongyang
Vol. V, 25-24-07

Warts on the face and the body. Steal sour wine from a libation pot, wash the affected region, and recite the following incantations: "Warts-illness, warts-illness that knows no shame. With sour wine from a libation pot I wash your head. Quick, quick. This is equivalent to an order." Recite this incantation seven times and a cure will be achieved. Arcane Essential Recipes from the Outer Censorate.

Soybean relish produced in Puzhou
Vol. V, 25-01-02

Alternating sensations of cold and heat of children, when malign qi have struck one. Grind moist soybean relish and form pills the size of a chicken egg. Use this pill to rub the child's cheeks, palms, and soles six to seven times. Also, rub the heart/central region and the navel and repeatedly recite an exorcistic incantation. Then break open the soybean relish pill and see whether there is fine hair in it. Throw it away along the road, and a cure will be achieved. *Heart Mirror of Diet Physicians.*

Least mallow
Malva parviflora L. Vol. IV, 16-12

Also, according to Nan Gongcong's *Spirit Book of Gou lou Mountains*, "purple back least mallow comes from Shuzhong; it is a magic herb. It grows close to waters. When mercury is boiled with its natural juice it hardens. It can also be boiled together with the eight stones/minerals to make them resistant to fire."

Furthermore, according to Chu Yushi's *Proven Recipes Recorded in Ancient and Modern Times*, "start a vegetarian diet and fasting prior to the fifth day of the fifth month and watch out for least mallow growing under mulberry trees. On the fifth day at noon proceed to below a mulberry tree and recite the following incantation: *Jilihujudansupoke.* Following this incantation, rub your hands on the yin/shady side of the mulberry tree and chew in your mouth least mallow and common crowfoot to a paste. Spit it into your hands and rub them to distribute it all over your hands. Then, again, continue a vegetarian diet for seven days. Do not wash the hands. Thereafter, you will heal those who have been hurt by snake bites, and worm/bug and scorpion stings by stroking them with your hands."

I, Li Shizhen say: In ancient times there was a discipline "to exorcise the origin of a disease." The action just outlined is part of this. However, I do not know what sense it makes to specifically resort to least mallow for it. If one were to say that this is a case of mutual checking, then one should add that there are many herbs serving to cure the poison of worms/bugs.

The core of the wood enclosed by the *poria* sclerotium
Vol. VII, 37-01-04

Sun the Perfected One in his *Records Kept in one's Headrest* states: If *poria* is ingested for a long time, within one hundred days it eliminates your diseases. After two hundred days you will not fall asleep during day and night. After two years you will be able to let demons and spirits work for you. After four years the Jade Girl comes to serve you.

Kite's tail iris
Iris tectorum Maxim. Vol. IV, 17-30

Demonic seduction-specters and evil qi. The "powder with four items, including kite's tail iris." Grind one tenth of an inch each of kite's tail iris from Dong hai, native gold (referred to here as "yellow tooth, i.e., gold tooth"), henbane seeds, and *peucedanum* root into powder and ingest with wine the amount held by a square inch spoon. If it is intended to let the patient have visions of demons, add an additional one tenth of a pint of *peucedanum* root. If he is supposed to meet a demon, again add one more tenth of a pint. Immediately effective. An overdose is to be avoided. Chen Yanzhi, *Recipes from the Small Essays*.

Calabash
Lagenaria siceraria (Molina) Standl. var. *microcarpa* (Naud.) Hara
Vol. VI, 28-04

Suspended obstruction-illness in the lower body parts. Choose a day when the body's spirit is not present in the affected body part.[25] Boil ferment prepared from Chinese nutgalls, dry it, and grind it into a powder. Mix it with well splendor water and let the patient ingest one bowl on an empty stomach. After a slight free flow take autumn calabashs, also called "suffering from not getting old," those that have grown on a rack and are bitter, cut them into pieces, and place them on the sore. Perform two times seven cauterizations on them. Xiao Duanshi suffered from this illness for several years. One cauterization resulted in a cure. *Eternal Key Recipes*.

---

25 Chapter 39 of the *Arcane Essential Recipes from the Outer Censorate* offers a detailed record of the regions in the human body passed through by the body's spirit at specific times. To apply acupuncture or cauterization at a place at the time of its being visited would offend and harm the spirit, with severe negative consequences. The therapy by means of cauterization of a suspended obstruction-illness in the "lower body parts," that is, the perineum, requires that the physician inform himself of the days the body's spirit is not present there.

Madder
Rubia cordifolia L. Vol. V, 18-40

To resolve being struck by *gu*-poison. With vomiting and a discharge of blood similar to pig liver. Boil three-tenths of a pint each of madder roots and Japanese ginger leaves in four pints of water down to two pints. Ingest this and the disease is healed. It is essential to call the name of the person acting as host of the *gu* spirit. Chen Yanzhi, *Recipes from the Small Essays*.

Indian turnip
Arisaema thunbergii Bl. Vol. IV, 17-23

Phlegm confusion with the orifices of the heart obstructed. The "pills of the Heavenly Body/God of Longevity." They serve to cure fright affecting heart and gallbladder, with their spirits no longer guarding their ordinary residence. Also, phlegm confusion with the orifices of the heart obstructed resulting in absent-mindedness and forgetfulness, absurd speaking, and absurd visions. Prepare one pound of Indian turnip. First dig a pit, one foot deep, into the soil and with a fire lit by 30 pounds of charcoal heat it until it turns red. Then pour five pints of wine into it, and wait until it has seeped in and the pit is dry. Then place the Indian turnip into the pit, cover it with an overturned bowl, and close the edges with ashes so that no qi will escape. The next day remove the Indian turnip and grind it into powder. Grind one ounce of amber and two ounces of cinnabar into powder, and with fresh ginger juice and wheat flour prepare a paste to form pills the size of *firmiana* seeds. Each time ingest 30 to 50 pills, to be sent down with a ginseng root and *acorus* decoction. To be ingested three times a day. *Recipes from the Pharmaceutical Bureau*.

Croton tree
Croton tiglium L. Vol. VII, 35-47

Harm caused by cold, warm malaria, alternating sensations of cold and heat. *Croton* seeds break up concretion-illness and conglomeration-illness, and qi nodes, accumulations, and collections with hardening. Abiding rheum and phlegm aggretation-illness. Water swelling of the abdomen. They drain the five long-term depots and six short-term repositories. They open closures and blockages. They free the pathways of water and grain. They remove malign flesh. They eliminate evil items such as demon poison and *gu*-attachment-illness. *Original Classic*.

They heal blocked female menstruation and a festering fetus; purulent and bleeding wounds caused by metal objects/weapons. They do not benefit husbands, and kill the poison of blister beetles, snakes, and venomous vipers. It is possible to heat process them for consumption to boost blood and vessels. They improve your complexion, and support change and transformation to enable communication with demons and spirits. *Supplementary Records by Famous Physicians.*

They serve to cure ten kinds of water swelling, dysfunction of limbs, and blockage of vessels. They cause miscarriage/abortion. *Discourse on the Properties of Pharmaceutical Substances.*

They disperse all types of disease qi, drain obstructing, stagnant qi, eliminate wind, supplement exhaustion, strengthen the spleen and open the stomach, dissolve phlegm, break up blood accumulation, eliminate pus, dissolve swelling with poison, kill worm/bugs in the abdominal long-term depots, and serve to cure malign sores, tumorous flesh growth, as well as *jie*-illness, repudiation-illness, and pin-illness swelling. *Rihua.*

Love apple root
Paris polyphylla Smith var. *chinensis* (Franch.) Hara. Vol. IV, 15-17-01

Use a bamboo knife to remove the skin of a love apple root and cut it to pieces the size of a dice. Cover them with wheat flour, give them into a porcelain jar, and boil them with water until they float on the surface. Filter the liquid to remove the root and let them harden while they cool. Then fill them into a new cloth bag and suspend them at a windy location until they have dried. Each time ingest three pills in that in the early morning hours at first you recite an exorcistic spell, and then send them down with well water. Ingest the three pills one after another. This enables you to end the consumption of food. If you feel a desire to drink and eat, drink a soybean decoction first. Then boil the medicinal pills in a watery gruel, and slowly eat it. The spell is: "Under a golden sky with clear qi the cocks crow. Today, I ingest this medication with the wish to have a long life. Today, to feel neither thirst nor hunger, I rely on a magic strength obtained with this divine herb of the immortals."

Japanese raisin tree wood juice
Hovenia dulcis Th. Vol. VI, 31-31-02

Fox odor qi from under the armpits. Cut a hole in a Japanese raisin tree and obtain one or two bowls of its juice. Boil it together with *aristolochia* root, peach tree twigs stretching eastwards, willow tree twigs stretching westwards, and the nursing milk of seven women once or twice to bubbling and then use the decoction to wash the armpits on the fifth day of the fifth month in the morning when the cocks crow. Place the water at a crossroad and quickly return home without looking back. That results in a cure. The first person who comes across the water on the crossroad must carry the odor qi with him. Hu Ying, *Easy and Simple Recipes for Protecting Life*.

Red mung bean
Vigna umbellata (Thunb.) Ohwi et Ohashi. Vol. V, 24-04

Some say that "Mr. Gonggong had an untalented son. He died on Winter Solstice day. He became an epidemic demon who fears red mung beans. This is why on that day they prepare a red mung bean congee to suppress a demon epidemic." That is one of those fictitious, absurd stories.

Water flowing against a sloping terrain
Vol. II, 05-14-04

Chen Cangqi: Both water that has flowed a thousand *li* and water flowing eastward are suitable for washing away evil and dirt. When used to boil a medication, they will ban and exorcise spirits and demons. Turbid water flowing into puddles can still be offered as provision to kings and dukes. How much more does this apply to water that is quick in its movements and has come a long way?

Mercury
Vol. II, 09-02

Spirit seduction-specter demon disease. Boil one ounce of mercury with one ounce of fermented water of foxtail millet over a charcoal fire down to three parts of ten. Remove about a soybean size amount of the mercury, wrap it in an exorcistic talisman, and swallow this. To be ingested again at night. After one or two days the disease will end. *Recipes for Extensive Assistance*.

Realgar
Arsenic disulphide. Vol. II, 09-07

Evil qi in a house. Give three maces of realgar into a bowl of water, recite an exorcistic prayer, and with peach twigs that have grown toward the

South-East spray the liquid throughout the entire house. This will eliminate all traces of the evil qi. Do not allow women to observe and get to know this. *Simple Recipes from the Collection of Li Binhu.*

Spider spec
Aranea ventricosa (L.) Koch. Vol. VIII, 40-10

Zheng Xiao in his *Compilation of My Studies* states: "In Sai lan, in the Western regions, in summer and autumn, small, black spiders develop on herbs that are very poisonous. People bitten by them will cry loudly because of pain. The local people recite exorcistic prayers and stroke the location of the bite with mint twigs. Or they rub their entire body with goat/sheep liver. After one day and one night the pain will end, and following the cure, patients will shed their skin like a slough. Oxen and horses wounded by such spiders will die abruptly."

Yuan Zhen in his *Collection from the Reign Period "Long-lasting Favor Accorded by Our Association with Heaven"* states: "Spiders in Bazhong are big and poisonous. The body of some may be several inches wide, and their shins may even be several times longer. Where they weave their webs, bamboo and trees will all die. When they strike humans, this causes abnormal sores, bruises, pain, and itch. The only way to cure such persons is to apply a mixture of bitter wine and realgar to the location of the bite, and also to let pill bugs eat the threads. If no immediate assistance is provided, the poison will reach the victim's heart and this may kill him."

Duan Chengshi in his *A Miscellany from Youyang* states: "Deep in the mountains there are spiders as big as cart wheels. They are able to devour human beings."

All these many reports must be known. The chapter *All the Ten-thousand Arts of Huainan* states: "Feed a red dot spider with pig fat for one hundred days, kill it, and apply it to a fabric. This will make it waterproof. If it is killed and applied to one's feet, he can walk on water."

The *Master Embracing Simplicity* states: "To ingest spiders, sea horses, and 'Feng Yi's pills of water hermits' enables one to live in water." All these are fantasy sayings of recipe specialists that cannot be believed.

The beetle that kowtows
Pleonomus canaliculatus Faldermann. Vol. VIII, 41-28-A04

Li Shizhen: These are black bugs of the size of blister beetles. When one presses their behind, they knock their head on the ground and make sounds. They are able to enter one's ears. Drip fresh oil into the affected ear and they will come out. According to Liu Jingshu in his *Garden of Extraordinary Things*, "the physical appearance and the color of kowtow beetles resemble those of soybeans. An exorcistic prayer stimulates them to 'knock their head' and also to 'spit out blood'. They can be taught all this. To kill them brings misfortune. To wear them on one's garments lets people give and seek love." During the Jin era, Fu Xian composed a prose poem on this.

Meat of white roosters
Vol. IX, 48-01-03

Chen Cangqi: After a white rooster is raised for three years, it may be used for demon spirit services.

Li Shizhen: In Tao Hongjing's *Declarations of the Perfected* it is stated: "When someone studies the WAY in the mountains, he should raise white chicken and white dogs. They are able to ward off evil." Nowadays, all specialists of Daoist techniques use white chicken when praying for exorcism. This goes back to that report in T'ao Hongjing's *Declarations of the Perfected*. It is one of those reports based on strange principles. How could chicken be in the service of spirits or goblins?

The head of a pig obtained during the twelfth month
Vol. IX, 50-01-03

The *Illustrated Compilation To Benefit the People* states: "On the fifth day of the fifth month, offer a pig's head as a sacrifice to the God of the kitchen furnace, and ask to have your wishes granted. Hang the ear of a pig obtained during the twelfth month from a beam above. This will make you rich." That is, the head of a pig obtained during the twelfth month is something that can also be used for exorcism.

All types of copper utensils
Vol. II, 08-19

Li Shizhen: Zhao Xihu in his *Records of Entering Heaven* states: Mountain spirits and water goblins have existed for many years. Hence they can exert evil influences. Vessels and sacrificial utensils handed down by at least three generations are older than mountain spirits and water goblins. Hence they are able to repudiate such influences.

Stone crabs
Telphura sp. Vol VIII, 45-16-03

Tang Shenwei: Crabs live only in the caves of snakes and eels. Hence those patients who have eaten eels and are struck by their poison will resolve it by eating crabs. Their natures are in fear of each other.

Shen Gua in his *Brush talks* states: "There are no crabs in Guanzhong. The local people consider their physical appearance and shape as something strange. They collect and dry them and hang them above the door gate to ward off malaria. It is not so that only the people do not know what this is all about; the demons, too, do not know it."

Donkey trough
Vol. IX, 50-07-19

Unending obstinate crying of children. Have the women of three different families hold the child and place it into a donkey trough. The crying will end immediately. Do not let other people become aware of this treatment. Chen Cangqi.

Li Shizhen: The *Poetry from the Brocade Bag* states: "Fasten a crab and hang it on the door to ward off demonic illness. Draw a picture of a donkey and hang it on the wall to end the crying of children." It is said that the people of Guan xi hang a crab shell on the door to repudiate evil malaria. And the people of Jiang zuo draw a donkey upside down and hang the drawing on the wall to end the crying of a child during the night. This is identical with the idea of ending a child's crying by placing it in a donkey trough. All these are exorcistic methods to escape misfortune.

Wang liang
Vol. IX, 51-56

Li Shizhen: The "Gentleman Who Sees Four Directions," mentioned in the *Rites of Zhou*, "who held a dagger-ax in his hands when he entered a tomb to drive out the *fang liang*," he dealt with exactly these creatures. The *wang liang* love to eat the livers of the dead. Hence they are driven out from the tombs. By their nature, they fear tigers and *platycladus* trees. Hence one erects on tombs stone tigers and plants cypresses.

The *Records Narrating the Extraordinary* states: During Qin times, in Chen cang a hunter caught an animal that resembled both a pig and a goat/sheep. He then met two boys who told him: "The name of this animal is *fo shu* and it is also called *yun*. It eats the brain of dead people below the ground. One needs to stick a cypress wood into its head to kill it." This was a *wang liang*. It is of no interest as a pharmaceutical substance, but it is of relevance to the dead. Hence this is recorded here. They have four eyes. Those with two eyes, they are the qi. They all alike are demonic creatures. In ancient times, the people designed human effigies to portray them. Formerly, Fei Zhangfang got to know from Li E medicinal pills with *fang xiang* brain as an ingredient. So, this creature has been added as a pharmaceutical substance to exorcistic recipes. But this tradition has been lost in the meantime.

Human qi
Vol. IX, 52-23

Ge Hong in his *Bao pu zi*: In Wu and Yue, they have a method to exorcise demons and maintain the passage of qi. If they encounter a massive epidemic, they can go to bed together with a patient of this epidemic and there will be no transmission of the disease from one to another. When they encounter essence goblins in that they may hear a certain sound, or they see a certain physical appearance, which may throw a stone or light a fire, they ban them with their qi, and such apparitions are interrupted as a result. Or, when they are injured by a poisonous snake, they blow qi to the affected region and they are cured. Such cures will even be achieved from a distance of one hundred miles, if the healer waves his own hand – for males the left hand, for females the right hand – blows his breath qi, and voices an exorcistic curse. Now, the qi come from what has no physical appearance, but their therapeutic application may have such effects. How much more will one's years of life be extended if he stops to eat grain?

Li Shizhen's comment: This applies to the vastness of spiritual qi that we all grow inside of ourselves. The experts of amulet exorcism act on the basis of the qi of their ancestors here. However, the qi of their modern adepts are all putrid, and these are just mediocre persons who try to imitate the ancients. How could they obtain any good results?!

6. Involvement of Buddhists and Daoists

Three rather distinct world views found followers in ancient China. Confucianism, Daoism, and Legalism. In their understanding of humankind's position in the universe, of man's relationship with numinous forces and of the most desirable social structure, they represented clearly discernible ideologies, with implications for health care. Nevertheless, many individuals were able to combine in one way or other Confucianism, Legalism, and Daoism in their personal daily life. Buddhism, however, introduced to China from India in the late Han era, offered an alternative that left little room for compromises with the autochthonous doctrines.

In terms of health care and therapeutic approaches, no explicit Confucianist program was ever formulated. The *Yellow Emperor's Inner Classic* of the early Han era was compiled by authors primarily influenced by a belief in the ubiquitous validity of natural law. The message delivered may have received approval by Legalists and Confucianists, but it survived the first millennium in only a weak tradition. Neo-Confucianism of the Song-Jin-Yuan era gained it more attention when linking it to a more realistic attitude towards health and disease.

In the *Yellow Emperor's Inner Classic*, several chapters with contents of unknown origin, focusing on purely medical issues, appear to have been extended at their beginning or end to include socio-political statements. Other such statements are found embedded in a more general context. For example, chapter 68 of "Pure Questions" says: "Correspondence (with the law) is compliance. If there is no correspondence with the law, this is opposition. Opposition gives rise to changes. Changes result in disease." That is, a social program requires that people abide by the law lest their behavior result in disease.

The reward for abiding by the law is health. Personal and social well-being are affected alike. Near the end of chapter 2, the rewards for law-abiding behavior and the penalties for unlawful behavior are restated: "To follow yin and yang results in life. To oppose them results in death. To follow them results in order. To oppose them results in disorder." Social and personal well-being are closely tied to a life in agreement with natural and social law. The promise of law-abidance, social order, and personal health is even more clearly expressed in the final lines of chapter 3: "If the WAY is carefully observed as the law demands, the mandate of heaven will last long." And in chapter 1, to cite a final example, it is pointed out:

"When essence and spirit are guarded internally, where could a disease come from?"

The Yellow Thearch's medicine required no substance-based therapy; a law-abiding way of life was recommended as sufficient for remaining healthy as long as the heavenly mandate allowed. Diet change and needle stimuli were advocated to correct slight deviations from the normal state of health. In an introduction to his *Classic on Interdictions*, the Tang physician Sun Simiao (581 – 682?), an eclectic author, quotes a saying by Lao zi: "That I have to suffer is because I have a body. If I had no body, what cause would there be for suffering?" Sun Simiao added his comment: "That is, form and matter alone lead to disease. Only formlessness knows no suffering." This is in direct contradiction to the statement in the *Yellow Thearch's Classic*.

The Daoist view of life realistically acknowledges that suffering, i.e., disease, is unavoidable because the human body is part of an eternal cycle of birth, growth, decline, and death, with threats present at every stage. Daoists expanded a prehistorical knowledge of pharmaceutically active natural substances to generate an ever more complex pharmacotherapy. Eventually some of them assumed that there were ways to overcome the burdens of physical life and achieve longevity with the help of carefully crafted elixirs. Their *materia medica* was based on experience; for more than one millennium it remained virtually free of the doctrines of natural law, yin yang, and Five Phases.

The *Ben cao gang mu* at no place explicitly refers to the Confucian world view or to Confucians as a distinct group. Daoists as a group are difficult to define. Still, they are mentioned quite often as "Daoists." Apparently, they were known to carry out specific health care and curative activities characteristic of their overarching world view. This is different with Buddhists. They, too, are occasionally named as a group. But there is no distinct strategy of health care they could be associated with. The final aim of Buddhist teachings is to enable followers to leave an endless cycle of material existence, followed after death by a non-material existence resulting after rebirth in another material existence. The goal to be reached is Nirvana, translated into Chinese as *wu bing*, "free of disease." That is, human life, material life, is itself the disease that has to be prevented from endless repetition.

Buddhism cares about the quality of bodily life, and so it suggested a wide range of health care behaviors as well as disease related therapies. Still, these behaviors and therapies were not meant to maintain, in addition to individual bodily health, a preferred social order. Health care advice found in Buddhist scriptures was eclectic. It combined a wide range of different measures simply meant to make corporeal existence as comfortable as possible before it was left behind forever.

Like Daoists, Buddhists addressed spirits and gods and recommended reciting sutras and prayers. The male bodhisattva Avalokiteshvara reappeared in Chinese Buddhism as a female goddess Guan yin with a thousand eyes to look for all who need help and with a thousand arms to provide assistance. Buddhists brought with them from India ophthalmology. Cataract surgery was practiced for centuries, the success tied to recitations of spells. The Buddhists introduced the Four Elements theory in China. Sun Simiao integrated it in his recipe books, but it did not fall on fertile grounds. The underlying principles were poorly translated into Chinese and soon forgotten.

Li Shizhen repeatedly referred to "Buddhist experts," to Buddhist rituals and ceremonies, to a Buddhist aversion to plants considered pollutant, and to Buddhist views on other substances. He explained the foreign names of items originating in Buddhist and Sanskrit writings. Why the collection and processing of Manchurian catalpa tree leaves must not occur in the presence of Buddhists and Daoists, as well as women, sons in a state of filial piety, chicken, and dogs, remains unexplained.

Thunderball fungus
Polyporus mylittae Cook at Mass. Vol. VII, 37-05

Li Shizhen: According to Chen Zhengmin's *Idle Views from a Secluded Study*, "Yang Mian in his prime age got a strange illness. Whenever he said something, this was echoed by a low voice in his abdomen. Over a long time, the voices turned louder and louder. A Daoist heard of this and said: 'This is a case of "echo worms/bugs." You only need to read the names of pharmaceutical drugs listed in the *Ben cao*. Take the item that is not responded to with an echo and this serves to cure this disease.' Yang Mian read the drugs listed in the *Ben cao* and when he reached thunderball fungus, no echo followed. Hence, he ingested several grains of thunderbolt fungi and was cured."

Arborvitae tree leaf
Platycladus orientalis (L.) Franco. Vol. VII, 34-01-02

Li Shizhen: Arborvitae trees wither late in their life and persist for a long time. They are endowed with a hardening and congealing matter often providing the trees with longevity. It is for this reason that the leaves are ingested as daily food. Daoists put them into hot water and regularly ingest it. Wine in which arborvitae leaves are soaked on New Year's day wards off evil qi. All these usages take advantage of the characteristics of arborvitae leaves. Musk deer eat them and their body becomes fragrant. The hairy girl has eaten them and her body was relieved of its weight. This, too, is evidence of their effects.

Chinese white pine
Pinus armandi Franch. Vol. VII, 34-02

Tao Hongjing: Pines and arborvitae contain the moisture of resin and do not wither even in cold winter. For this reason the resin is considered an excellent item and it is often resorted to to be ingested as daily food. Still, many people consider it unimportant and ignore it.

Su Song: Daoists consume the resin as daily food, others mix it with *poria*, the fruits of pines and arborvitae and *chrysanthemum* flowers and prepare pills, or they ingest it as an individual substance.

Li Shizhen: Pine leaves and pine fruits are required if one intends to eat pharmaceutical drugs as daily food. Pine nodes and pine heartwood last long without decay. Pine resin is the liquid essence splendor of the pine tree. Lying on the soil it does not decay; over a long time it transforms into amber. It is a suitable substance to avoid eating grain and prolong life.

Laurel *magnolia*
Magnolia amoena Cheng. Bd. VII, 34-08

Tao Hongjing: Laurel *magnolia* trees are present in Ling ling all over the place. They are shaped like nanmu trees. They have a very thin bark that is of acrid flavor and fragrant. Those found in Yizhou today have a thick bark, shaped like *magnolia* bark, and superior qi and flavor. People in the East today assume it to be mountain cassia bark, and they are related. Daoists also use it for making incense with good results.

White sandalwood
Santalum album L. Vol. VII, 34-13-01

Du Bao in his *Records of Retrieved Stories of the Reign Period "Great Inherit-ed Responsibility"* states: During the Sui dynasty a Buddhist master named Shou was wondrously competent in the medical arts. He prepared five aromatic beverages to help the people. The aloes wood beverage, the sandalwood beverage, the clove beverage, the shiny bugleweed beverage, and the *nardostachys* rhizome beverage, they all alike had an aromatic as their main ingredient, with further pharmaceutical drugs added. They had a delicious flavor and quenched thirst, and at the same time they supplemented and boosted your qi." Sandalwood is called "bath aromatic" in Daoist writings. It should not be burned to be offered in sacrificial ceremonies.

Fragrant rosewood
Dalbergia odorifera T. Chen. Vol. VII, 34-14

Li Xun: The *Recipes Transmitted by Immortals* states: "When it is mixed with other aromatics and burned, the smoke rises straight up. Cranes touched by the smoke are led to descend. It is the best incense to be used in Daoist ritual ceremonies aimed at the stars; its power of making predictions possible has proven extremely effective." The name "to make the true force of the stars/spirits descend" is based on this.

Sweet gum tree bark
Liquidambar formosana Hance. Vol. VII, 34-21-02

Massive wind sores. Mix equal amounts of sweet gum wood, burned with its nature retained and ground into a powder, and calomel with sesame oil and apply this to the affected region. Extremely wondrous. In Zhang gong, a horn blower had this disease. A Daoist gave him this recipe, and he was cured. *Tried and Proven Good Recipes*.

Phellodendron wood/tree
Phellodendron amurense Ruppr. Vol. VII, 35-01

Supplementary Records by Famous Physicians: *Phellodendron* wood grows in the mountain valleys of Hanzhong and in Yong chang. Tao Hongjing: That coming from Shao ling today, which is light, thin, and deep in color, it is superior. That coming from Dongshan is thick and light in color. The root is resorted to by Daoists as a "wooden ganoderma" item; but people today no longer know how to obtain and ingest it.

Magnolia tree bark
Magnolia officinalis Rehd. et Wils. Vol. VII, 35-05

Supplementary Records by Famous Physicians: *Magnolia* trees grow in Jiao zhi and Yuan ju. The bark is collected in the third, ninth, and tenth month. It is dried in the yin (i.e., shade).

Tao Hongjing: Today the bark comes from Jian ping and Yi du. Those specimens are good that are very thick with a meat purple in color. Those with a thin and white "shell" are not so good. *Magnolia* bark is often used in common recipes. Daoists do not condone its use.

Catalpa bungei C. A. Mey. Manchurian *catalpa* tree leaf. 35-10-02

Scrofula pervasion-illness and fistula sores. "Divine recipe of Manchurian *catalpa* tree decoction." Early in the morning or later in the evening around autumn equinox ask someone to take a bag, collect Manchurian *catalpa* tree leaves and put them into the bag. Weigh 15 pounds and boil them with one picul of water in a clean cauldron down to three pecks. Exchange the cauldron and boil the liquid down to seven or eight pints. Exchange the cauldron again and boil the liquid down to two pints. Then pour the liquid into a watertight vessel. Before this prepare one-twentieth of a pint of sesame oil, one-tenth of a mace of beeswax, and as little as the size of one millet seed of butter and let them dissolve to generate a paste. In addition, take seven apricot kernels, grind them together with a little fresh ginger into a powder and add it, together with two maces of rice powder, into the paste. Stir it to generate an even mixture. First, apply it to the surface of the sore. Two days later wipe it off. Then evenly apply the Manchurian *catalpa* tree leaf decoction with a comb on the entire sore and cover this with a soft piece of silk fabric. Continue to apply the paste and wipe it off once every day and apply new medication. After no more than five or six applications the sore breaks open and new muscles grow. If the sore fails to break open, it is dissolved from within. After a cure is achieved patients should be careful not to harm the affected region for half a year. Collecting the pharmaceutical drugs and the process of boiling them should not be observed by sons in a state of filial piety, women, Buddhist monks and Daoists, as well as chicken and dogs. *Recipes Kept in the Quiver*.

Chinese soapberry
Sapindus mukorossi Gaertn. Vol. VII, 35-23

Cui Bao in his *Notes on Things Old and New* states: "In ancient times a divine sorcerer lived named Yao Qu. With his talismans he was able to expose the misdeeds of the hundreds of demons. When he got hold of a demon he prepared a club with this wood, and with this club he killed it. Tradition has it that when this wood is used to make tools it suppresses demons and monsters. Hence, it is called 'frees from suffering'." People also distort this name to "wood causing suffering."

Li Shizhen: A common name is "demons worried by its sight." This is the idea underlying its use by Daoists in their recipes designed to avert misfortune. Buddhists use it to make beads. Hence, they call it "Bodhi seeds." This is also the name of Job's tears.

Croton tree
Croton tiglium L. Vol. VII, 35-47

Tao Hongjing: Daoists also apply methods to refine and eat *croton* seeds. To ingest them, they state, enables one to become an hermit/immortal. Someone swallowed one *croton* seed and died, while there was a mouse/rat that ingested them for three years and grew to a weight of 30 pounds. The nature of things allows for such differences in the tolerance of *croton* seeds.

Li Shizhen: During the Han era, recipe masters said that refining and eating *croton* seeds provides you with a good complexion and makes you a spirit immortal. The *Supplementary Records by Famous Physicians* included them into the *Ben cao*. Zhang Hua in his *Monograph on a Wide Range of Things* says: "A mouse/rat ate *croton* seeds and grew to a weight of 30 pounds." This is as absurd as it is false. But Mr. Tao Hongjing believed it to be a fact, and he was wrong. He also said that someone swallowed one *croton* seed and died. This, too, borders on exaggeration. So, both these statements are corrected here now.

Paper mulberry tree fruit
Broussonetia papyrifera (L.) Vent. Vol. VII, 36-04-01

Su Song: Recipes of the hermits/immortals recommend to ingest the fruits as a single substance. The fruits are collected when they have assumed a truly red color. Then they are dried in the yin (i.e., shade), pounded, and passed through a sieve to generate a powder. The amount held by a two maces spoon ingested with water over a long time has excellent effects.

The *Master Embracing Simplicity* states: "When red paper mulberry fruits are ingested by old people, they become young again. They let you see demon spirits."

The Daoist Liang Xu was 70 years old when he ate them and became even younger and stronger. At the age of 140 years he was still able to walk and to run as fast as a horse.

Slenderstyle *acanthopanax* root bark
Acanthopanax gracilistylus W.W. Smith. Vol. VII, 36-23-01

Tao Hongjing: The root and the stem are boiled in water, the liquid is used to brew wine and drunk boosts one's qi. Daoists burn them to ashes and boil them with minerals, and they have secret methods to process them with *sanguisorba* root.

Tang Shenwei: The *Method for Stone Cooking by the Perfected One Donghua*, "Method for Stone Cooking by the Perfected One Donghua," states: "In former times in the western regions lived a perfected man, hermit of Mount Wang wu. Wang often stated: 'How can a long life be achieved? Why not eat minerals with slenderstyle acanthopanax? How can a mother achieve longevity? Why not eat minerals with *sanguisorba* root? Both are made to medicinal drugs to be eaten boiled with minerals to reach longevity.

Li Shizhen: Slenderstyle *acanthopanax* root bark serves to cure dysfunction and blockage related to wind intrusion and the presence of moisture. It strengthens sinews and bones. Its therapeutic potential is good and reaches into the depth. What Daoists have to say may be overly emotional. The fact is, their sayings are excessive, but they include some common principles nevertheless.

Pear tree fruit
Pyrus bretschneideri Rehd. Vol. VI, 30-01-01

As the *Categorized Compilation* states: "A scholar appeared to have an illness. He was always in a bad mood and eventually went to Yang Jilao for an examination. Yang said: 'Sir, your condition of heat has reached an extreme. It dissolves and melts your qi and blood. Three years from now you will die of an impediment-illness.' Then the scholar heard of a Daoist on Mount Maoshan whose medical art was on a par with that of spirits. Not wanting to announce his condition, he dressed as a servant and went to the mountain to ask for a paid job. The Daoist accepted him as one of his disciples. After some time, the scholar told him the truth. The Daoist examined him and said with a laugh: 'You may as well leave the mountain. Just eat one good pear every day. If no fresh pears are obtainable any longer, take dry ones and soak them in hot water. Eat the dregs and drink the juice, and your illness will be healed as a result.' The scholar did as he was told and one year later he met Yang Jilao again. When the physician saw his fat and moist complexion and noticed the harmonious movement in his vessels, he was startled and said: 'Sir, you must have met an extraordinary person. If not, how could your health have been restored?' The scholar told Yang Jilao the entire story, and Yang Jilao dressed formally, paid a visit to Mount Maoshan and regretted his own insufficient learning."

Polygonum multiflorum
Thunb. Vol. IV, 18-24

Li Ao wrote the *Notes on Polygonum*. It states: He Shouwu was a man of Nan hexian in Shunzhou. His grandfather was named He "who can have offspring." his father was named He Yanxiu. Earlier, He "who can offspring" was named He "child in a field." He was impotent and weak all his life. He had no wife. He found pleasure in Daoist techniques and followed his teacher into the mountains. One day he was drunk and lay down in the wilderness of the mountains. Suddenly he saw two vines growing separate from each other in a distance of more than three feet. Their creeping seedlings interacted with each other and separated again after some time. Eventually they interacted again. "Child in a field" was amazed by this strange behavior. The next morning he unearthed the roots of the vines and returned home. He asked all sorts of people, but nobody knew what it was. Later the Old Man of the Mountain happened to come by and "Child in a field" showed him the roots. The Old Man responded: "You have no offspring. This vine is strange. Perhaps it is a pharmaceutical drug of spirits and hermits/immortals. Why don't you ingest it?" So he ground it into powder and ingested one mace on an empty stomach with wine. After seven days he understood the WAY of humankind. After several months he was strong and healthy. Hence, he ingested it regularly and increased the dosage to two maces. Over the years all his former illnesses were healed. His hair remained black and he kept a youthful appearance. Within ten years he fathered several sons and changed his name to "Can have offspring." Also, he gave the substance to his son Yanxiu to ingest it. Both reached a long life of 160 years. Yanxiu is the father of Shouwu. When Shouwu ingested this pharmaceutical drug, he, too, fathered several sons. At an age of 130 years, his hair was still black. There was a Mr. Li Anqi who lived in the same village and was on good terms with Shouwu. He stole the recipe, ingested it, and he, too, achieved a long life. Eventually, he spread the message and made it widely known.

Kernels/seeds of Job's tears
Coix lacryma L. Vol. V, 23-16-01

Also, the *History of the Later Han* states: "When Ma Yuan was stationed in Jiao zhi, he regularly consumed Job's tears fruits, and he claimed that 'they relieve the weight of the body, curb sexual desire, and overcome miasma qi'."

Also, Zhang Shizheng in his *Records of Weary Wanderings* states: "Xin Jiaxuan suddenly suffered from an elevation-illness ailment, with a segment of his intestine as big as a cup falling from the loin. A Daoist monk taught him to stir-fry Job's tears pearls in yellow soil from an eastern wall, boil them in water to generate a paste, and ingest it. When he had ingested this several times, the elevation-illness dissolved." When Cheng Shasui suffered from the same disease, Xin Jiaxuan gave him the recipe and it was effective for him, too. In the *Materia Medica*, Job's tears is recorded as an upper rank pharmaceutical drug that nourishes the heart. Hence it has such a therapeutic potential.

Red mung bean
Vigna umbellata (Th unb.) Ohwi et Ohashi. Vol. V, 24.04

Also, the *Mr. Zhu's collected and Proven Recipes* states: "When Song Emperor Ren zong was a prince he suffered from mumps. Zan Ning, a Daoist, was ordered to cure him. He ground seven times seven grains of red mung beans into powder, applied it to the affected region and the prince was cured.

Rice boiled with the shoots of Asiatic bilberry
vaccinium bracteatum Thunb. Vol. V, 25-06

The *Precious Classic of the Highest Origin* states: "When you ingest herbs and trees of royal quality, your qi communicate with the spirits. When you consume the fluids of Greenish Candle, your life will never end." That is a reference to the item discussed here. Today, Daoists on Mount Maoshan prepare these cooked rice meals; some send them to places far away. The recipients steam them a second time and eat them. They are very fragrant and sweet.

Leek. *Allium tuberosum*
Rottl. ex Spreng. Vol. VI, 26-01

Li Shizhen: Leek has hot leaves and a warm root. Their therapeutic potentials and applications are the same. As long as they are fresh, they are acrid and disperse blood. Once they are heat prepared, they are sweet and supplement the qi in the center. They enter the foot ceasing yin conduits; they are a vegetable for the liver.

The *Basic Questions* says: "In the case of a heart disease it is advisable to eat leek."

The *Materia Medica of the Food Mirror* states: "It turns to the kidneys."

These are different wordings, but they are based on related principles. The fact is, the heart is the child phase of the liver, while the kidneys are the mother phase of the liver. A mother can cause repletion in its child. "In the case of a depletion of the child supplement the qi of the mother." Daoists view leek as one of the strong-odored vegetables. They say, it can confuse one's spirit and excites depleted yang qi.

Stem and leaf of oil rape
Brassica campestris L. Vol. VI, 26-11-01

Meng Shen: Those who previously have suffered from illnesses affecting their lower back and legs should not eat large amounts of them; if they eat large amounts of them, their problem would get worse. Also, this would harm their yang qi and induce sores and mouth and tooth diseases. Persons with a barbarian stench must not eat them. Also, they can generate all types of worms/bugs in the abdomen. The Daoists, in particular, avoid stem and leaves of oil rape. They regard oil rape as one of the five strong-odored/pollutant items.

Seed kernels in the pits of dates that have been stored for three years
Vol. VI, 29-09-03.

Li Shizhen: According to the *Supplementary Biography of Liu Gen*, "the Daoist Chen Zi behaved like a fool. Still, in Jiang xia, Yuan Zhongyang respected him and took him into service. Chen Zi said: 'This coming spring you will be affected by an illness. You should ingest 27 seed kernels from within dates.' Later, Yuan Zhongyang indeed had a severe disease. He ingested the seed kernels and was cured. He also stated: 'If you constantly ingest date seed kernels, not one of the hundreds of evils will affect you again'. Yuan Zhongyang ingested them and that proved to be effective." Henceforth it was said that "Chinese dates are capable of curing evil qi attacks."

Also, a Daoist book states: "To always hold a date kernel in the mouth serves to cure qi disorder and lets the mouth develop fluids. To swallow them is excellent."

Xie Cheng in the *History of the Later Han* also states: "Mengjie was able to hold date kernels in his mouth and to eat nothing for up to ten years." All these reports are evidence of the idea to generate, by means of Chinese dates, body fluids and obtain their qi. And when these fluids are swallowed they reach the Yellow Mansion (i.e., the crown of the head) to keep yang and yin in mutual exchange.

Pear
Pyrus bretschneideri Rehd. Vol. V, 30-01

Only a kind named "mulberry pears" is worth to be eaten boiled with honey as it ends oral dryness. Eaten fresh, mulberry pears are not good for humans as they cool their center. There are also the "purple flower pears." They heal heart heat. The Tang Emperor Wu zong had this illness. None of the hundreds of pharmaceutical drugs proved to be effective. A Daoist named Xing from Mount Qing chengshan took these purple flower pears, squeezed them to obtain a juice and offered it to the Emperor. The illness of the Emperor was cured.

Common quince
Cydonia sinensis Thouin Koehne. Vol. VI, 30-07

Su Song: The wood, the leaves, the flowers, and the fruits of common quince are very closely related to those of quince. However, common quince fruits are bigger than those of quince, and they are yellow in color. When their fruit bases are compared, the only difference seen is that quince has a second fruit base similar to a teat. If there is no such second fruit base, it is common quince. It can be added to wine and serves to eliminate phlegm. Daoists press the fresh fruits to obtain their juice. They mix it with *nardostachys* rhizome and *scrophularia* root powder to prepare a moist type of incense, and they state that burning it greatly clears the spirit.

Firefly

Luciola vitticolis Kies. Vol. VI, II, 41-28

The *Divine Immortal's Text on Interactions* states: Wu Chengzi's "pills with fireflies" serve to ward off illnesses and disease, malign qi and the hundred demons, all kinds of poison by tigers, wolves, and snakes, by bees/wasps and scorpions, the naked swords of the five kinds of soldiers, and the ferocious injuries caused by robbers and other enemies. In ancient times, during the Han era, Liu Zinan, general and procurator of Wu wei, obtained the recipe of these pills from a Daoist named Yin gong. In the twelfth year of the reign period "Eternal Peace" (58 – 75) he fought a battle with the foreign devils at the northern frontier and lost all his fighters. He himself was surrounded, and arrows descended upon him like rain. However, when the arrows came close to Liu Zinan's horse, in a distance of several feet they suddenly dropped on the ground. The Lu thought he was a spirit, and withdrew. Liu Zinan taught the recipe to his followers, and henceforth none of them was ever harmed again. At the end of the Han era, the Daoist Qingniu obtained it. He passed it on to Huangfu Long of An ding, and Huangfu Long in turn passed it on to Emperor Wu of the Wei dynasty. So that some people came into its possession.

Silverfish

Lepisma saccharina L. Vol. VIII, 41-22

Supplementary Records by Famous Physicians: Silverfish live in the plains and marshlands of Xian yang.

Su Song: Nowadays, they are everywhere. There are few of them in garments, but very many of them in book scrolls. Their body is white; it is covered with a thick layer of powder that falls off when touched by one's hand.

Duan Chengshi states: "Zhang Zhoufeng, Rectifyer of Omissions, witnessed melon seeds on a wall transforming to 'wall fish'. Hence, one knows that the dictum in *Lie zi*, 'rotten melons transform to fish', was by no means meaningless. Legend has it that when silverfish enter the Daoist scriptures, they eat the characters symbolizing 'divine' and 'hermit/immortal', and their body, as a result, assumes the five colors. When a human person manages to swallow them, this person will become a divine hermit/immortal. During the Tang era, the younger son of Zhang Xi wrote down many times the characters 'divine hermit/immortal'. Then he cut them out and gave them into a jar. He also put silverfish into it, hoping that these woodborers would eat the characters. But this did not happen. Eventually, he developed a heart illness. I have recorded this here to warn against being misled by such legends."

Toad
Bufo bufo gargarizans Cantor. Vol. VIII, 42-01

The *Discourse on Nature* states: "Toads give birth by spitting out their young ones, and they defecate from their mouth." *The Master Embracing Simplicity* states: "Toads of 1,000 years have a horn on their head, and a cinnabar-red writing underneath their abdomen. They are called '*ganoderma* fungus consisting of meat'. People who obtain one and eat it can become immortals. The specialists in Daoist arts resort to them to let fog rise and to pray for rain, to keep soldiers away, and to free themselves out of a binding." Nowadays, those with the necessary skills collect toads and use them in shows as they are able to listen to the instructions of their masters. The nature of the items is mysterious, as can be inferred from this example.

Small toad
Rana limnocharia Boie. Vol. VIII, 42-02

According to the *Picking up the Green Fragmentary Writings* cited in Zhang Gao's *Medical Anecdotes*, "there was a man who suffered from sores on his legs. They were not present in winter and he was alright. But in summer, they were malodorous and festered, and they were painful beyond words. He met a Daoist and was told: 'This is because the disease hides in winter and comes out in summer. Pound living small toads to a paste and apply this to the affected region. Replace the paste with new paste three to four times per day.' After three days had passed, a small snake came out of the sore, and was picked up with iron pincers. After that, the disease was cured."

Earthworm
Pheretima aspergillum E. Perrier. Vol. VIII, 42-11

Supplementary Records by Famous Physicians: Earthworms with a white neck live in the soil of the plains. They are gathered in the third month, and they are dried in the sun.

Tao Hongjing: Those with a white neck are added to medication; they are the old ones. When they are collected, remove the soil from them, add salt, and dry them in the sun. After a short while they will generate water that is often resorted to by specialists in the Daoist arts of longevity. Their excrements are called "an earthworm's mound," and also "six and one mud."[26] Because they eat fine mud, without sand and stones, they lend themselves to seal cauldrons used for preparing cinnabar-elixirs.

Snakehead fish
Ophiocephalus argus Cantor. Vol. VIII, 44-32

Li Shizhen: They are of a long physical appearance, and they have a round body. They are of equal size from head to tail. Their fine scales are of dark color, with dots and a flowery pattern design. They somewhat resemble pit vipers. They have a tongue, they have teeth, and they have a belly. On their back and on their abdomen they have fins reaching to their tail. The tail is not forked. Their physical appearance and shape are simply abominable, and they emit qi with a fishy, malodorous stench. It is a food of low rank. Among the Southerners are some who value them; especially the people in the North abstain from them. Daoists consider them to be among the "detestables in the waters," and they are not recommended as part of a vegetarian diet.

Meat of the three-footed turtle
Vol. VIII, 45-12-01

Fracture harm. It ends the pain and transforms stagnant blood. Pound raw/unprepared meat to a pulp and apply this to the affected region. To ward off all kinds of detestable, filthy, and dead qi, Daoists may draw an image of a soft-shell tortoise with three feet to end an affection by such qi. Su Song.

---

26 "Six and one" refers to the heaven and earth numbers associated with the cardinal direction "North" in ancient Chinese alchemy.

Dog meat
Canis familiaris L. Vol. IX, 50-02-01

Li Shizhen: The Daoists consider dogs as detested creatures living on the ground, and hence they do not eat them. Dog meat of all kinds must not be eaten roasted lest it cause melting with thirst. When pregnant women eat it, their children will be mute. If eaten after a heat disease, it will kill one. Those who ingest life-prolonging elixirs must not eat it. During the ninth month, dogs must not be eaten; this would harm one's spirit. Emaciated dogs have a disease. Frenzied dogs cause madness. Dogs that have died without apparent cause are poisonous. The meat of dogs with trotters will harm one. Those with red legs, and showing restlessness, they emit a foul qi. Dogs with red eyes. They all must not be eaten.

Deer meat
Cervus elaphus L. Vol. IX, 51-15

Tao Hongjing: Among the wild animals, the meat of Pére David's deer and (common) deer can be eaten. As long as it is fresh, it does not have the rank odor of other wild animals. Also, Pére David's deer and (common) deer are not associated with the twelve celestial bodies, and they are not controlled by the eight trigrams. Furthermore, their meat is warm and supplementing, and has no specific effect on human life or death. Daoists permit it to be prepared as dried/preserved food, because its flavor surpasses all the other animals' meat. However, even though the meat of chicken, dogs, oxen, and goats/sheep is supplementing and boosting too, eating it is a transgression against the departed *hun*-souls of these animals. Hence it must not be eaten.

Kou Zongshi: The fact that dried deer meat is resorted to in the performance of the three sacrifices to the gods is based on the same idea. Also, the flavor of deer meat is superior to that of other kinds of meat.

Li Shizhen: Mr. Shao states: "The entire body of deer boosts the qi of humans. Regardless of whether it is boiled, or steamed, or prepared as preserved food, it is good when eaten together with wine." Basically, the deer is an animal of the hermits. It is an item of pure yang and many years of life. Its meat can pass through the supervisor vessel. Also, since it eats good herbs, its meat and horns do only have a boosting but no harming effects. What Tao Hongjing said was unfounded.

Roebuck meat
Capreolus pygargus Pall. Vol. IX, 51-19-01

Tao Hongjing: The so-called "white meat" refers to roebucks. Its bile is white, and it is easily frightened and alarmed.

Meng Shen: If the meat is brewed together with the meat of Pére David's deer to a wine, this is good. The Daoists use this meat to make offerings, and they call it "white preserve." They say, "it is associated with the twelve celestial bodies, does not have a bad odor or greasy nature, and is not burdened with any taboo."

Li Shizhen: Roebucks have a white bile, and they are timid by nature. When they drink water and see their own reflection they will run away. The Daoist texts say that "Pére David deer and common deer have no *hun*-soul."

Chen Cangqi: For a person with a bold character, dry heart and liver of a roebuck under the sun, powder them, and have that person ingest this with wine all at once. As a result he will be less daring. If a timid person eats this, then he will be even more timid and he will not know how to act.

Refined white human urine sediments
Vol. IX, 51-12

Effusion of heat following the ingestion of an elixir. There once was a man who ingested large amounts of elixir drugs with dormant fire. Eventually, he developed sores at the back of his brain with slowly ascending heat qi. A Daoist taught him to apply cauterization at the "windy market" needle insertion hole (GB-31) several tens of times and the patient was cured. However, after some time the disease was active again. This time he taught the patient how to produce "autumn minerals" by yin refinement, and had him ingest them with a decoction of dried soybean sprouts. He was cured as a result. This was a combination of yin and yang. Wang Mingqing, *Yu hua fang.*

Human saliva
Vol. IX, 52-19

Li Shizhen: Underneath the human tongue there are four openings. Two of these openings are passed by the heart qi, and two of them are passed by the kidney liquids. The heart qi flow into the downside of the tongue and become "divine water." The kidney liquids flow into the downside of the tongue and become "spiritual fluid." The Daoists name it "golden syrup" and "jade sweet wine." Where it overflows, this is the "spring of sweet wine." Where it collects, this is the "pond of splendor." That which dissipates constitutes the body fluids. That which descends is the "sweet dew." It is through this that the long-term depots and short-term repositories are supplied with moisture, and that the extremities and the body are provided with humidity. Hence those experts who seek to cultivate and nourish their body, they swallow body fluid and ingest qi, and they call this "irrigation of the spiritual root with clear water." Such people are able to refrain from spitting all day long. Hence, their essence qi is sustained forever, and their facial complexion does not wither. If one spits for a long time, then this will harm his essence qi and generate a lung disease. His skin will be dried up. Hence the saying goes: "Spitting into a distance is not as good as spitting nearby. Spitting nearby is not as good as not spitting at all." When one has a disease, his heart and kidneys fail to communicate and the kidney water fails to rise. Hence, his body fluids dry up and his true qi are used up. As Qin Yueren in his *Classic of Difficult Issues* states: "The kidneys control the five body fluids. Those that enter the liver, they become tears. Those that enter the lung, they become snivel. Those that enter the spleen, they become saliva. Those that enter the heart, they become sweat. Those entering the tongue itself, they become spittle."

Cinnabar
Vol. II, 09-01

The *Categorized Compilation* states: "Vice Minister Qian Pi at night had many malign dreams, and he was unable to sleep throughout the night. He was worried that such dreams might signal bad luck. Eventually, he met Hu Yongzhi, a prefectural judge in Dengzhou, who told him: 'Long ago I continuously suffered from the same problem. Then a Daoist told me to wear on my body cinnabar shaped like metal arrowheads. After only ten days this proved effective. For four, five years now I have had no such dreams again'. Then he took a red bag from the tuft of hair on his head and handed it to the Vice Minister to wear it himself. That night the Vice Minister had no dreams, his spirit and *hun*-soul were pacified and calm." Daoist texts claim that cinnabar wards off the malign and pacifies the *hun*-soul. These two events may serve as evidence.

Golden thread

Coptis chinensis Franch. Vol. III, 13-01

Li Shizhen: Neither the *Original Classic* nor the *Supplementary Records by Famous Physicians* have records of a long-term ingestion of Golden Thread to prolong life. Only Tao Hongjing speaks of "Daoist recipes advising one to ingest Golden Thread to prolong life." According to the *Biographies of Divine Immortals*, "Feng Junda and Hei xue gong ingested Golden Thread for 50 years and became immortals." I dare to say, Golden Thread is a pharmaceutical drug with a massively bitter flavor and a massively cold nature. It is applied to let fire descend and to dry moisture. When it has struck a disease, its ingestion must end. How could it be ingested for a long time, which would mean that its stern command of killing is perpetuated, resulting in an elimination of the qi responsible for generation and harmonization? ... Cold and bitter medication is not only unable to prolong life. Ingested for a long time, it increases qi to a unilateral dominance, and this is the origin of a sudden early death. ... The statements by Mr. Tao Hongjing and those of Daoist books are all erroneous chats.

Love apple

Paris polyphylla Smith var. *chinensis* (Franch.) Hara. Vol. IV, 17-27

Li Shizhen: Love apple is a pharmaceutical substance for the foot ceasing yin conduits. For all conditions of fright epilepsy, malaria ailment, scrofula pervasion-illness, and obstruction-illness swelling the *Original Classic* recommends it as suitable. The Daoists have included it in their approaches to ingesting medicinal substances for food. But it is not known whether it is beneficial or not.

Fire lit with common mugwort leaves

Vol. II, 06-06

The *History of Southern Qi* records the following incident. "During the time of Emperor Wu di, a Buddhist monk from North Qi came with a red fire. The red color of this fire was more intense than that of ordinary fire, and it was smaller. He claimed that it served to heal illness. Patients of noble rank and commoners, they all strove to make use of it. The monk cauterized using seven sticks and this often proved effective. In Wu xing, Yang Daoching had suffered from a depletion illness for 20 years. When he was cauterized by the monk, he was cured. Everybody said that it was a 'Fire of the Sages'. An imperial order prohibited its further application, but it could not be stopped." It remains unknown what kind of an item was burned to produce such a fire.

Ancient mirror
Vol. II, 08-16

The *Records of the Immortals of the Clouds* states: Mr. Wang in the capital city had a mirror with six handles. It was always surrounded by clouds and fumes. When he illuminated them with his mirror, everything in the three directions to the left, to the right, and in front of him became apparent. When the army of Huang Chao approached the capital, he illuminated them with his mirror and the mirror reflected the soldiers and their armor as if they were right in front of him.

The *Brush talks* states: A Buddhist monk Wu had a mirror illuminating and reflecting locations from where auspicious and inauspicious events were to originate in future. Also, there are "fire mirrors" to obtain fire, and "water mirrors" to obtain water. All these are examples of the astonishing potentials of mirrors.

Large-leaved senna
Cassia sophora L. Vol. IV, 16-23-A01

Tao Hongjing states: "Fetid *cassia* leaves are similar to large-leaved senna leaves." Now, large-leaved senna grows at the roadside. The leaves are smaller than those of fetic *cassia*. Its nature is balanced; it is nonpoisonous. Roasted in fire it can be prepared to a most fragrant beverage. It dispels phlegm and ends thirst. It does not let one sleep. It regulates the center. During the Sui dynasty, a Buddhist master Chou collected an herb and prepared a five-color beverage that he submitted to Emperor Yang di. That is the item discussed here.

Job's tears
Coix lacryma L. Vol. V, 23-16.

Li Shizhen: People often plant Job's tears. They grow by themselves from a perennial root in the second and third month. The leaves are similar to those of woolly beard grass. A stem rises in the fifth and sixth month and opens flowers that form fruits. Job's tears has two kinds of grains. One kind sticks to the teeth. They are pointed and have a thin shell. They are Job's tears. Their husked grains are as white as those of husked rice. They can be cooked as congees and meals, and they are ground to obtain a flour for consumption. Furthermore, together/identical with husked rice they can be brewed into wine. The other kind of grains is round and has a thick, hard shell/husk. These are the bodhi-seeds. ... The grains are only pierced and several pearls are strung together as beads which go through the fingers of Buddhist monks when they recite sutras. Hence people also call them "sutra recitation pearls/beads." The roots of both kinds are white and as big as a spoon handle. They band together and their flavor is sweet.

Rice boiled with the shoots of Asiatic bilberry,
vaccinium bracteatum Thunb. Vol. V. 25-06.

Li Shizhen: This cooked rice meal is prepared in accordance with the methods used by hermits/immortals who ingest pharmaceutical drugs as food. Also, nowadays Buddhists prepare it in the fourth and eighth month as an offer to Buddha. When they prepare it, they add several tens of branches with persimmon leaves and poplar leaves to intensify its color. Or they add a lump of raw iron. They only know how to adopt the color of these additives; they do not know that the experts who ingest pharmaceutical drugs as food warn against such additives.

Dried malt-sugar wine brewing residue/sediment
Vol. V, 25-27-03.

A wealthy man in Chang shu suffered from turned over stomach. He travelled to the Sweet Dew Temple in Jing kou to sponsor a Buddhist ceremony. Upon his arrival, he had his boat moored at the bank of the lake. That night he dreamed of a monk holding a decoction that he gave him. He drank it and sensed a comfortable feeling in his chest. The next morning he went into the temple and the priest serving the decoction was the monk he had seen in his dream. He gave him this decoction just as he usually treated visitors. Hence, he changed the name and henceforth called it "sweet dew decoction." I myself once treated a low ranking official with it and achieved a cure. It is something that should definitely not be neglected.

Capsella bursa-pastoris (L.) Medic. Shepherd's purse
Vol. VI, 27-05.

Explanation of Name. "Life saving herb." Li Shizhen: Shepherd's purse (Chinese: *Ji*) grows abundantly (Chinese: *ji ji*). Hence, it is named *Ji*. Buddhists use its stem to prop up the wick of an oil lamp. It can repel mosquitoes and moths. When it is called "life saving herb," that is to say: it can save many lives.

Indian lotus rootstock
Nelumbo nucifera Gaertn. Vol. VI, 33-10.

Li Shizhen: Lotus grows in the mud, but it is not soiled by the mud. It resides in the water but it does not vanish in the water. The root, the stem, the flowers, and the fruits are different from all other such items. Lotus is clean and it offers beneficial applications; it is beautiful in all respects. From the various nodes of its stalk, the stem, the leaves, the flowers, and the rootstock develop. From the flowers the filaments, the fruits, the seeds, and the plumules develop. The seeds are yellow in the beginning. Then they turn from yellow to greenish, from greenish to green, and from green to black. Inside they have white meat, with a greenish core hidden in its center. The stone-hard lotus seeds are hard; they survive a long time. The plumule (Chinese: *Yi* 薏) contains the idea (Chinese: *Yi* 意) of life. The root includes the sprouts. They spread and are reborn in incarnation. An endless process of creation and transformation. Hence, the Buddhists use it for analogies as it contains all the wondrous principles. Physicians use it as something to be ingested or eaten as it is able to eliminate the hundreds of diseases.

"Loving bamboo" juice
Vol. VII, 37-13-14

Li Shizhen: Bamboo juice is by its nature cold and smoothing. In general, it is suited for those who because of wind intrusion, fire, and dryness have phlegm. If those with cold, a presence of moisture, stomach qi depletion, and a smooth intestinal passage ingest it, contrary to their expectations they harm their intestines and their stomach. Bamboo shoots smoothen and clear a passage. Eaten in large amounts they drain you. When Buddhists call them a "a fine-toothed comb scraping the intestines," then this is this understanding.

Sea snail
Rapana venosa Valenciennes. Vol. VIII, 46-21

Su Song: The group of sea snails in the sea includes very big specimens. "Pearl sea snails" are lustrous and clean like genuine pearls. The physical appearance of "parrot sea snails" resembles the head of parrots. They all can be made to cups. "Shuttle sea snails" have the physical appearance of shuttles. They are used today by Buddhists as a wind instrument. None of them are added to medication.

Decayed shell of a water snail
Bellamya quadrata Benson. Vol. VIII, 46-24-02

Roaring ailment of children. Grind water snails that have been in a wall facing south for years to powder. Mix it by late afternoon with water and by sunset have the patient raise his hands and put his palms together as required in Buddhist rituals and then swallow the powder. This will be effective. Mr. Ye, *Selected Profound Recipes*.

Asian particolored bat droppings
Vespertilio superans Thomas. Vol. IX, 48-21-04

Li Shizhen: Bat droppings and bats are medications for the blood section of the receding yin liver conduit. They can quicken the flow of blood and dissolve accumulations. Hence they are able to cure eyeshades and blindness, malaria, drought demon diseases, *gan*-illness and fright, as well as dripping and diseases of women below the belt, scrofula pervasion-illness, and obstruction-illness with swelling, as all these are diseases of the ceasing yin conduits.

According to the *Categorized Stories*, "Mr. Xu Daoheng of Ding hai suffered from red eyes. Once he ate crabs, and this resulted in an inner obstructive shade. Five years later, he suddenly dreamed of a Buddhist monk who gave a medication to him to rinse his eyes, and he advised him to ingest the 'pills with lamb liver'. When Mr. Xu Daoheng enquired about the recipe, the monk told him: 'To rinse the eyes use one ounce each of bats droppings, *angelica* root, cicada sloughs, and *equisetum* herb with the nodes removed, and grind them to powder. Then boil four ounces of black lamb liver in water until it becomes a pappy substance and mix it with the afore mentioned powder to prepare pills of the size of *firmiana* seeds. Ingest 50 such pills with hot water after a meal.' Mr. Xu Daohong ingested the pills according to the rules, and his eyes became clear again."

Fine cream
Vol. IX, 50-12

Tao Hongjing: Buddhist scriptures say that milk is made to yogurt, yogurt is made to butter, and butter is made to fine cream. Its color is yellow-white, and it is used to make cakes. It is very sweet and fat. That is correct.

Animal gall stone
Vol. IX, 50-17

Li Shizhen: Animal gall stone grows between liver and gallbladder of all domestic animals, as are running animals, oxen, and horses. It is wrapped in meat, and may reach a weight of up to one ounce. Big ones are like chicken eggs. Small ones are like millet grains or hazelnuts. They have a white color and resemble stones, but they are not stones. They resemble bones, but they are not bones. When they are broken, several layers appear. In 1540, a man named Hou in Qizhou slaughtered a yellow ox and found this item. Nobody knew what it might be. A foreign Buddhist monk stated: "This is extremely precious. Domestic animals, as are oxen, horses, and pigs, they all have them. They may serve to pray for rain. In Western regions a secret incantation is practiced. As a result a continuous rain will begin immediately. Those who do not know this incantation, they simply soak it in water and play with it. This, too, may result in rain." Later, Tao Jiucheng's *Records Taken while Stopping from Field Work* was consulted, and the animal gall stone listed there was the object found by Mr. Hou.

The *Records Taken while Stopping from Field Work* says: "When the people in Mongolia pray for rain, they soak several such stones in a basin filled with clean water. They wash them, filter the liquid and play with them with their hands, and fervently say incantations. After an extended period of time, there is always rain. The stones are called *zha da*. Big ones are as large as chicken eggs; small ones are of various sizes. They grow in the stomach/abdomen of running animals. But only those of oxen and horses are especially wondrous. Actually, they are in one group with ox yellow/ bezoar and 'dog gems'."

Also, according to the *Jing Fang's Divination by the Classic of Changes*, "in regions with strong soldiers who are actively engaged in warfare, oxen grow such stones in their stomach/abdomen." Based on this, animal gall stones are of the same group as "dog gems." However, only those growing in a dog's stomach/abdomen are "dog gems."

Stomach and gallstones of dogs
Vol. IX, 50-18

The *Posthumous Works of the Cheng Brothers* records the story of "a man from Persia who opened a tomb in Min. There was nothing left in the coffin except for the heart that was as hard as a stone. When it was sawed open, it contained a landscape of greenish-bluish color, like a painting. To the side there was a beautiful woman leaning on a fence. The fact is, this woman in her love was addicted to mountains. From morning to evening, she thought of nothing else. Hence, the interior of her heart and the mountains she looked at fused and formed concretions like this."

Also, the *Literary Collection of Song Qianxi* records the following story. "In Linchuan, there was a Buddhist who acted in accordance with the Buddhist doctrines. In particular, he practiced the precepts outlined in the Pratyutpanna Samādhi Sūtra. After he had passed away, he was cremated, and only his heart did not transform. It emitted rays of five colors, and it contained a three inches high image of Buddha that was neither a bone nor a stone. All parts of the body were present in perfect detail. Also, in Hui shui there was nun named You who practiced Zen meditation. When she had died she was cremated. Her heart contained a Guan yin image that looked as if carved."

All these events result from one's mind concentrating on something with undivided attention. Eventually, one's essence and spirit qi and liquids will, because of such emotions, congeal and assume a physical appearance. This is the same as when a pregnant woman's emotions are affected by some extraordinary appearance which then transforms into a demon fetus. Such occurrences are not auspicious. They are disease. They are signs of something without emotions existing within those who have emotions.

7. The human body: Its organs and paths of entrance

The *Ben cao gang mu* was not written to impart hitherto undisclosed and inaccessible information on the location, size, capacity, nature, and functions of the individual parts of the human body. Li Shizhen could be sure that readers of his encyclopedia were well aware of the body's morphology and of the functions and connections attributed to it. When the *Inner Classic of the Yellow Thearch* appeared during the Han era, the situation appears to have been different. The fact is, for the most part in the earliest texts of Chinese medicine, the so-called Yellow Thearch is not the creator of a new medicine, as he is often depicted in later times. His role is that of someone being introduced to a new medicine. Much of the content of the ancient classics of Chinese medicine leaves the reader with the impression that it was compiled to answer questions on a corpus of information brought in from afar.

There is no doubt that from pre-historical times on people who dissect animals for food or sacrifices, those who kill other people in battles or as sacrifices, and those who are involved in funeral rituals, all are quite knowledgable regarding the morphological facts of the human body. This would certainly be true for China, and the texts propagating the new medicine are full of data on those inner organs and other structural elements that appeared relevant to the new concepts of physiology and pathology. This is also where problems arise for the historiographer. On the one hand, a system of bodily functions is presented that nicely agrees with the underlying doctrines designed to explain normal and abnormal conditions in the human organism. Let us assume that the yin yang and Five Phases doctrines are a product of ancient Chinese intellectual reasoning, regardless of remote, perhaps non-Chinese stimuli to seeing all phenomena in the universe as interrelated. On the other hand, the morphological-anatomical facts presented in the ancient classics do not always fit into a system designed to give all body parts an appropriate place and function.

The three classic texts of Chinese medicine, *Basic Questions*, *Classic of the Numinous Pivot*, and *Classic of Difficult Issues*, presumably compiled during the Han era, at some time between the 2nd c. BCE and the 2nd c. CE refer to many tangible structural elements forming the inner and outer body. Why, one might ask, were five yang organs, open for fast flow, contrasted with six yin organs meant to store things a bit longer, when this failed to fit into the new theories. A sixth yang organ, a so-called "network enclosing the heart" was identified to jump in when theory required this. Why did a notion of "three sources of heat," usually translated today as "Triple Burner," remain enigmatic from the beginning, with countless experts of later times trying to make sense of the term *san jiao*? Could it be that this was a foreign idea that was somehow introduced to China, where its origins and meaning were soon forgotten?

The term *xu li* is used only once in the *Yellow Thearch's Inner Classic*; it is even more enigmatic than the "three sources of heat." Its literal meaning in ancient times remains uncertain; the characters suggest a "structure/texture" of a hill or abandoned place. In the *Inner Classic* it is given a definition apparently unrelated to the meaning of the characters, that is, "network vessel of the stomach." It is a concept never resorted to again in subsequent writings.

Several such incompatibilities and terms no longer used in later times make one wonder if some anatomic-morphological knowledge was present in ancient China, perhaps introduced from outside, that was initially acknowledged but remained marginal and was forgotten later on. Other data were kept and further developed as part of a theoretical system that was superimposed on them with inconsistencies apparent to this day.

When the *Ben cao gang mu* was written, anatomical and morphological knowledge had been stabilized for a long time. For a long time, authors preceding Li Shizhen had rarely engaged in relevant discussions. There were some who wondered why the brain and the uterus were omitted from the theoretical body. And there had been disputes for some time as to the roles played, for instance, by the stomach, the kidneys, and the heart. Nevertheless, the body parts themselves were known and their material existence was acknowledged. The body, inside and out, offered terrain and inroads for a very diverse spectrum of manipulations and therapeutic interventions.

In the *Ben cao gang mu* numerous applications of liquid, solid, and vaporous medications are referred to in the thousands of recipes. The location of the inner organs, their various connections through vessels, sinews, and membranes required well-designed strategies if the effects of a pharmaceutical substance were to reach the assumed exact whereabouts of a disease. The entire body from the top of the skull to the soles of the feet offered paths of entry for affecting the inner organs and their processing of solid and liquid food as well as for influencing the different qi that the body accepted from outside or formed by itself within. The bregma, the eyes, the ears, the mouth, the lips, the tongue, the gums, the teeth, the throat, the nape, the nipples of the female breasts, the armpits, the navel, the penis, the testicles and the vagina, the anus, a prolapsed uterus and a prolapsed rectum, the pores in general, and last but not least the palms of the hands and the soles of the feet, they all were regarded as more or less open entries for introducing the pharmaceutical effects of herbs, plants and minerals, as well as of heat, cold, fire, and dampness into the human body.

Since antiquity, blood and qi were known to pass through the entire human body. Vessels penetrated all its regions and an endloss flow of blood and qi occurred as if "in a ring." Ideas of a network of vessels included those seen as part of the circulatory system and others with separate functions. The ailments and diseases to be treated that are listed in the *Ben cao gang mu* speak of contorted bladders related to blocked urination, of liver problems responsible for the incorrect position of the pupils in the eyes. The stomach duct, one of those enigmatic relics of past times, may be blocked by blood; blood and qi in general may be dirty, turbid, and stagnant; they may congeal to lumps, and suitable measures are recommended to stimulate their flow. Worms may eat the lung, which is described as a hollow organ in contrast to the liver which is said to be solid. A woman's infertility may be caused by bent intestines; another problem may be related to a shriveled womb, and the fact that a child is tied by its navel cord to the placenta was widely known. Internal piles were distinguished from external piles and required different therapies.

Aloes wood containing resin
Aquilaria agallocha (Lour.) Roxb. Vol. VII, 34-10

A contorted bladder with blocked urination. This is not a disease of the small intestine, or the urinary bladder or the ceasing yin conduits. It results from forcibly resisting an urge to have sexual intercourse, or by overly restraining urination. The resulting qi disorder must be cured, and the problem will be healed. The passage of the restrained qi cannot be opened by means of medication serving to free a passage. Grind two maces each of aloes wood and *costus* root into a powder and ingest it with clear, boiled water on an empty stomach until the passage is freed. *Supreme Commanders of the Medical Ramparts.*

Dried ginger
Zingiber officinale L. Vol. VI, 26-17-01

Someone asked: "Fresh ginger is acrid and warm and enters the lung. Why is it said that it enters the stomach orifice?" The answer is: "It is commonly assumed that the stomach orifice is situated below the heart. That is wrong. The lower end of the pharynx, where items with a material shape are received, and where it is linked to the stomach unit, that is the stomach orifice. It is on the same pathway as the lung unit. This is why ginger can enter the lung and open the stomach orifice."

Pollen of cattail,
typha spp. Vol. V, 19-08-02

Blocked urination because of a twisted urinary bladder. Wrap cattail pollen with a piece of cloth and attach it to the patient's lower back and kidneys. Then let the patient bend his head down to the ground. He is to repeat this several times and the passage of his urine will be freed. *Recipes to be Kept Close at Hand.*

Pain in the central and abdominal region
Vol. I, 03-67

Black bone chicken. Rubbed above the location of the heart.

Blood spitting, nosebleed
Vol. I, 03-38

Leek juice. To stop blood spitting. Mixed with boys' urine and ingested, it serves to dissolve blood stagnating in the stomach duct.

Aloes wood containing resin
Aquilaria agallocha (Lour.) Roxb. Vol. VII, 34-10

Depletion constipation of the large intestine, when because of perfuse sweating the body fluids are exhausted. Grind one ounce of aloes wood containing resin and two ounces of desert broomrape, soaked in wine and baked over a slow fire, into a powder. Form a paste with the juice obtained by grinding hemp seeds in water, and with the juice and the powder make pills the size of *firmiana* seeds. Each time ingest 100 pills, to be sent down with a honey decoction. Yan Zili, *Recipes to Benefit Life.*

Gardenia
Gardenia jasminoides Ellis. Vol. VII, 36-07

A fiery pain in the stomach duct. Stir-fry seven or nine big mountain *gardenia* fruits until scorched, boil the residue in one cup of water down to 70%, add fresh ginger juice, and drink this. The pain ends immediately. If a relapse occurs, it will not be effective. Use one mace of thenardite instead, and the pain ends immediately. *Edited Essentials of Zhu Danxi.*

Castor oil plant seeds
Ricinus communis L. Vol. IV, 17-13-01

Prolapsed uterus. Grind equal amounts of castor oil plant seed kernels and processed alum into powder, spread it on a piece of paper and use it to push the uterus back into the abdomen. In addition, grind 14 castor oil plant seed kernels to an ointment and apply it to the center of the woman's head. This will let the uterus enter the body again. *Selected Profound Recipes.*

Chinese sumac gallnuts
Rhus chinensis Mill. Vol. VI, 32-10

Li Shizhen: The kernels of Chinese sumac gallnuts are pale green; they are shaped like kidneys.

Borneo camphor
Dryobalanops aromatica Gaertn. f. Vol. VII, 34-30-02

Li Shizhen: Ancient recipes in the specialties concerned with the eye and children say that Borneo camphor is acrid and cool, and can enter the heart conduits. Therefore, it is often used in recipes designed to cure eye diseases and fright wind. For smallpox sores with heart heat and blood stagnation with inverted moles, it is resorted to to lead pig blood directly into the heart orifices, and thereby to send the poison qi to disperse toward the outside. As a result, the movement of blood is accelerated and the pox papules are stimulated to develop. All such sayings appear to be correct, but in fact they are not.

Hardy rubber tree
Eucommia ulmoides Oliv. Vol. VII, 35-06

Li Shizhen: The fact is, the liver controls the sinews; the kidneys control the bones. When the kidney qi are sufficient, the bones are firm. When the liver qi are sufficient, the sinews are strong. Bending, stretching and free use of the limbs, all this depends on the sinews.

Bitter orange fruit
Citrus aurantium L. Vol. VII, 36-05-01

Zhu Zhenheng: Bitter oranges drain phlegm; they are able to dash against walls and push down ramparts. They are a pharmaceutical drug that smoothes passage through the orifices and breaks up qi accumulation.

Zhang Yuansu: For obstacle-illness below the heart and food remaining in the body undissolved overnight, it is appropriate to use bitter oranges and *coptis* rhizome.

Li Gao: Applied roasted with honey they break up water accumulation and drain qi. They eliminate internal heat. Zhang Jiegu uses them to eliminate accumulated blood in the spleen conduits. If there is no accumulated blood in the spleen, there is no obstacle-illness below the heart.

Varnish tree leaf
Ailanthus altissima (Mill.) Swingle. Vol. VII, 35-07-01.

Meng Shen: Varnish tree sprouts eaten in large amounts excite wind; they send steam into the twelve conduit vessels, five long-term depots and six short-term repositories. They confuse your spirit and diminish blood and qi. Regularly eaten with pork and hot pasta they cause a sensation of fullness in the center. The fact is, they obstruct the conduits and network vessels.

Bitter orange fruit
Citrus aurantium L. Vol. VII, 36-05-02

An obstacle-illness resulting from too early a discharge therapy. If yin conditions related to harm caused by cold are treated with a discharge therapy too early, an obstacle illness forms with a sensation of fullness below the heart, and no pain. If pressed it feels spongy and soft. Grind equal amounts of bitter orange fruits and *areca* seeds into a powder. Each time ingest three maces, to be sent down mixed with a *coptis* rhizome decoction. *Recipes of Illumination.*

Chinese *photinia* leaf
Photinia serrulata Lindl. Vol. VII, 36-27-01

Open eyeball of children. When a child has accidentally fallen, or was hit on the head, or its brain is affected by fright, the liver connection has received wind and this results in an improper position of its pupils. When it looks east and looks west, when it looks west and looks east, it is appropriate to blow the "powder with Chinese *photinia*" into its nose from where it penetrates to the top of its head. *Recipes of Universal Benefit.*

Wind intrusion and phlegm
Vol. I, 04-11-02

Kaya nut. For corpse throat with pain and itch, and inability to speak, with worms/bugs eating away the throat, form pills together with big fruit elm fruit, apricot kernels, and cinnamon bark and hold them in the mouth.

The eyes
Vol. I, 04-04

Gypsum. For sparrow eyes with nocturnal clouding boil it with lard and eat this. When wind and cold have entered the brain connection and decayed blood congeals and stagnates causing cold in the eyes, grind it with Sichuan lovage and Chinese liquorice root into powder and ingest it.

Chinese redbud wood and bark
Cercis chinensis Bge. Vol. VII, 36-32-01

Li Shizhen: Chinese redbud has cold qi and a bitter flavor. It is purple in color and by its nature it is descending. It enters the blood section on the hand and foot ceasing yin conduits. Cold overcomes heat; bitter flavor runs into the bones. Purple color enters the camp qi. Hence, Chinese redbud can quicken blood and dissolve swelling, clear the passage of urine and resolve poison.

Yang Qingsou in his *Recipes Transmitted by Immortals* has a "paste to harmonize with vigor" with Chinese redbud as its ruler ingredient. The fact is, this, too, is based on this therapeutic purpose. This recipe serves to cure all types of obstruction-illness and impediment-illness with an effusion on the back and poison influx causing all types of swelling and undistinguishable sensations of cold and heat. Grind three ounces of stir-fried Chinese redbud, three ounces of stir-fried *angelica biserrata* root, with nodes removed, two ounces of stir-fried red *paeonia* root, one ounce of fresh *angelica dahurica* root, and one ounce of stir-fried Japanese sweet flag/*acorus* into a powder. Mix it with an onion decoction and apply this hot to the affected region. When blood is exposed to heat it moves. The onion can disperse qi. If the sores are not very hot, mix the powder with wine. In the case of extreme pain, add frankincense. If patients are unable to stretch their sinews, add frankincense, too.

Generally speaking, obstruction-illness and impediment-illness, as well as disease episodes of influx are always caused by congealing and stagnating blood. This recipe has a warming and balanced effect. Chinese redbud bark is the essence of wood. It breaks up blood accumulation and dissolves swelling. *Angelica biserrata* root is the essence of soil. It ends wind intrusion and stimulates the movement of blood, thereby pulling out and leading off the poison in the bones. It removes the moisture and evil qi responsible for a blockage. *Paeonia* root is the essence of fire. It generates blood and ends pain. *Mu la* 木蠟 is the essence of water. It dissolves swelling and disperses stagnating blood. Combined with *angelica diserrata* it is capable of breaking up stone-hard swelling. *Angelica dahurica* root is the essence of metal. It removes wind intrusion, stimulates the growth of muscles, and ends pain.

The fact is, as long as blood is produced, death cannot occur. As long as blood moves it flows and penetrates everywhere. When muscles grow they do not rot. When the pain ends, heat no longer radiates. When the wind is removed, stagnating blood disperses as a result. When stagnating qi are broken up, hardenings can dissolve and the poison leaves as a result. When these five items are combined in a therapy, which disease could remain uncured?

Stagnant blood.
Vol. I, 03-63.

Chinese liquorice root stimulates the passage of dirty, turbid blood through the two ceasing yin and yang brilliance conduits. Yellow vetch drives away malign blood in the five long-term depots. Largehead *atractylodes* rhizome serves to free the passage of blood in the lower back and navel region.

Unidentified. "Brown tree bark."
Gan tuo mu pi. Vol. VII, 37-A10

Li Xun: According to the *Record on the Western Territories*, "it grows in western countries. People there use it to dye the robes of monks brown. Hence the name. ... The trees are big and their bark is thick. The leaves are similar to cherry leaves." The trees are also present in Annan. Their qi are warm, balanced, and nonpoisonous. The bark controls concretion-illness and conglomeration-illness with qi congealed to lumps. It warms the abdomen and relaxes the stomach. It ends vomiting with qi counterflow. It is equally good for all these issues. To break up abiding blood, blocked menstrual bleeding of women, and intraabdominal blood lumps, boil the bark in wine and ingest it.

Top of Chinese licorice root
Glycyrrhiza uralensis Fisch. Vol. III, 12-01-03

Used raw it is able to free the movement of foul blood stagnating in the two conduits foot ceasing yin and yang brilliance. It dissolves swelling and leads away poison. Zhu Zhenheng.

It controls swelling associated with obstruction-illness. It is a suitable additive to medication stimulating vomiting. Li Shizhen.

Wounds caused by flogging
Vol. I, 04-26-05

Pseudoginseng. Ingest with wine three maces so that the blood does not rush against the heart. Also, chew it and apply it to the wounds.

Large recipes.
Vol. I, 01-08-01.

Zhang Congzheng: There are two types of "large" recipes. Some large recipes have one ruler, three ministers, and nine assistants. If a disease results in various pathological signs and is caused by more than one type of evil qi, it is not appropriate to cure it with only one or two substances. Then there are large recipes with a large amount of components that are ingested all at once. They are suitable for diseases in the liver and the kidneys, and the lower body parts, and have to go a long way to these far away regions.

Grand Servant Wang defined the heart and the lung as being "near", the kidneys and the liver as being "far away," and the spleen and the stomach as being in the "center."

Liu Hejian identified the body's exterior as "far away," and the body's interior as "near."

As I see it, the three qi in the upper half of the body are the section on heaven. The three qi in the lower half of the body are the section on the earth. The stomach duct in the center, that is the section on man.

Oily walnut
Juglans regia L. Vol. VI, 30-28-02

Li Shizhen: The Triple Burner is a messenger, divided into three parts, of original qi. The Gate of Life is the source of the Triple Burner. The fact is, one of them (i.e., the Gate of Life) is the source of original qi and the other one (i.e., the Triple Burner) is a unit the original qi are entrusted to. The name "Gate of Life" is to indicate the short-term repository where the original qi reside. It is the item to store the essence that is tied to the bladder. The name "Triple Burner" refers to separate locations where the original qi and the essence are processed. The Triple Burner oversees the receiving and giving out of what is decomposed. The fact is, one (i.e., the Gate of Life) is named for its physical body; the other (i.e., the Triple Burner) is named for its function. The physical body of the Gate of Life is neither composed of fat nor of flesh; it is enclosed by a white membrane and is situated next to the seventh vertebra, between the two kidneys. Two strings tie it to the spine. Downward it is connected to the two kidneys; upward it is connected to the heart and the lung, with a further attachment to the brain. It is the source of life and controls the minister fire. It is the short-term repository of essence qi. All humans have it. That humans come to life and that individual items come to life always has its origin in the Triple Burner.

The *Classic of the Numinous Pivot* in its treatise "To consider the long-term depots as foundation" already described the shape of the short term repositories as "thick or thin, relaxed or curved," while Bian Que's *Classic of Difficult Issues* was unaware of the distinction between "origin/source of qi," and "the unit the qi are entrusted to," between a unit that has a "physical body" (i.e., the Gate of Life) and another that has only a "function." It identifies the right kidney as Gate of Life, and it says that "the Triple

Burner has a name but no physical shape." Gao Yangsheng who allegedly compiled the *Rhymed Instructions on the Movements in the Vessels* accepted such erroneous sayings and transmitted this error to people in later times. Only when Zhu Gong wrote his *The Book from Nanyang for Saving People's Lives*, when Chen Yan wrote his *On Recipes for the Three Causes*, and when Dai Qizong wrote his *Correction of Errors in the Rhymed Instructions on the Movements in the Vessels*, the ancient errors were rejected for the first time, but those who are aware of them remain few.

Walnut kernels are quite similar in shape. As their outer skin and watery juice are greenish and black, they are able to enter the North, to penetrate the Gate of Life and to free the passage through the Triple Burner, to supplement the qi and to nourish the blood, and together with scurfy pea fruits they are a medication supplementing the qi of the lower section on the Triple Burner, the kidneys, and the Gate of Life. Now, the qi of the Gate of Life communicate with the kidneys; both store essence and blood and abhor dryness. When the kidneys and the Gate of Life are not dry, and when essence qi abound internally, beverages and food provide one with strength, the muscles and the skin are glossy, the intestines and the short-term repositories are moist, and the blood vessels are passable.

These walnut kernels serve to assist supplementing medication. They have a function to let one become strong and have appetite. They moisten the muscles and blacken the hair. They solidify the essence, serve to cure dryness and regulate the blood. Once the Gate of Life is passable, the passage through the Triple Burner is free. Hence, a communication with the lung above is established and patients with depletion cold, panting, and coughing should benefit from walnut kernels. A communication with the kidneys in the lower body parts is established and patients with a painful depletion in the lower back and the legs should benefit from walnut kernels.

> Whenever beeswax is used in pills, melt it, add a little honey,
> stir this, and add the other pharmaceutical drugs
> Vol. I, 01-06-17

Li Gao: Beeswax is used in pills with pharmaceutical drugs to take advantage of its strength to stabilize the qi and flavor of the other pharmaceutical drugs, enabling them to overcome barriers and exert their effects. When honey is added, the pills more easily disperse and transform when they move down in the throat. How else could they reach the five long-term depots? But if the pills include poisonous drugs, contrary to one's intentions they harm the five long-term depots. So, this cannot be the meaning underlying the use of beeswax.

The voice
Vol. I, 04-11

Muteness may be related to lung heat, or lung dysfunction. It happens that wind poison has entered the lung, or that worms/bugs eat the lung.

Floating stone/mineral. Pumice
Porous lava. Vol. II, 09-31

According to Yu Yan's *Dogmatic Conversations Among the Learned*, the liver is associated with the phase wood. It should float on the surface but, on the contrary, it sinks into the depth. The lung is associated with the phase metal. It should sink into the depth but, on the contrary, floats on the surface. Why is this so? The liver is solid and the lung is hollow. Hence when a stone is given into water it will sink into the depth, but in the Nanhai there are stones that float on the surface. When wood is given into water it will float on the surface, but in the Nanhai they have aromatic wood that sinks in water into the depth. Such are behaviors of hollow and solid items that are contrary to normal.

Garlic
Allium sativum L. Vol. VI, 26-07

When someone is struck by poison in the water, this is also called "struck by rivulet poison," also "struck by moisture," and also "water disease." It is similar to being struck by the archer, but nothing material is involved. At the beginning of this ailment patients develop an aversion to cold, and a mild pain in the head and the eyes. They recover in the morning, and the ailment turns to the worse in the evening. Hands and feet are cold because of yang qi counterflow. On the third day, worms/bugs develop. They eat the lower body section, (i.e., the rectum) but patients feel neither itch nor pain there. After six or seven days, the worms eat the five long-term depots, with an unending downpour. Boil three pints of garlic until they are slightly done – if they were massively done, they would lose their strength – and bathe the entire body in the liquid. If the body develops red macule lines do not regard this as another disease that should be cured with an additional treatment.

Cerasus japonica (Thunb.) Lois
Vol. VII, 36-14

The *Biography of Qian Yi* states: "A nursing woman was frightened and fell ill. After she was cured her eyes remained wide open and she could not close them. Qian Yi said: 'Boil Chinese dwarf cherries and let her drink them in wine until she is drunk. This results in a cure. The reason is, the eye connection is linked within the human body with the liver and the gallbladder. When a person is in fear, the qi are bound. The gallbladder lies horizontally and cannot move down. Chinese dwarf cherries can remove the bound qi. They follow the wine into the gallbladder. Once the bound qi are removed, the gallbladder descends. As a result, the eyes can be closed. This is a wondrous result of hitting the crucial point.'"

Chinese scholar tree
Sophora japonica L. Vol. VII, 35-16

The "pills with the tips of Chinese scholar tree leaves." They serve to cure the five types of blood outflow related to intestinal wind. If the bleeding occurs prior to defecation, this is called "external piles." If a bleeding follows defecation, this is called "internal piles." If the large intestine is not drawn in, this is called "prolapsed rectum." If the pathway of grain/the colon has tumorous flesh growth on four sides similar to female breasts, this is called "raised piles." If they have a hole in their tip, they are called fistula sores. If there are worms/bugs inside, they are called "worm/bug piles." These pills cure all these conditions. *Recipes from the Pharmaceutical Bureau.*

Daphne flower
Daphne Genkwa Sieb. et Zucc. Vol. IV, 17-36

Li Shizhen: Now, there are five kinds of rheum. All of them result from an intake of water or soup inside, or from the absorption of moisture qi from outside. They are stored pent-up and become stagnant rheums. When they flow into the lung, this is a "propping rheum." It lets one pant or cough with alternating sensations of cold and heat. Patients spit foam and feel cold in the back. When they flow into the lung, this results in a "suspended rheum." It lets one cough with spitting, with a pain pulling on the "empty basin" (acupuncture needle insertion hole ST-12). When they flow into the area below the heart, this results in a "hidden rheum." It lets one vomit with a feeling of fullness in the chest, alternating sensations of cold and heat, dizziness, and blood induced brain movement. When they flow into the intestines and the stomach, this results in "phlegm rheum." It lets one have abdominal sounds and spit water, with a propping fullness in the chest and the flanks, and occasionally with outflow, or a sudden gain of weight or sudden emaciation. When they flow into the conduits and network vessels, this results in a "spilling rheum." It lets one have a feeling of extreme heaviness and influx pain, sometimes with a surface swelling caused by water qi.

Daphne flower, Peking spurge, and kansai root by their nature drive out water and let moisture flow off. They are able to directly proceed to the location of a hidden pouch of water rheum. When they are used in moderate amounts, their effects show very fast. They must not be overdosed, lest they drain the original qi.

Worms/bugs and hidden worms/bugs
Vol. I, 04-12-03

Croton seeds. For toothache caused by wind intrusion and worms/bugs, wrap them in silk floss and bite on this. Burn them and with the smoke fumigate the affected teeth. Together with garlic inserted into the ears.

Asafetida. *Ferula assa foetida* L
Vol. VII, 34-32

Toothache related to the presence of worms/bugs. Grind equal amounts of asafetida and realgar into a powder and with a wheat flour paste form pills the size of mung beans. For each application, wrap one pill in silk floss and depending on where the toothache is situated insert it into the left or right ear. Immediately effective. *Sagely and Benevolent Recipes.*

Silverfish. *Lepisma saccharina* L
Vol. VIII, 41-22

Urination with blood of women. Insert twenty silverfish, obtained from within garments, into the yin orifice (i.e., vagina) of the patient. *Secret Records About Children and Mothers.*

Trumpet flower
Campsis grandifl ora (Thunb.) Loisel ex K. Schum. Vol. V, 18-15

Sores running through the skin, with the cheeks and the top of the head filled with moisture and assuming a pulpy consistency, eventually reaching both ears. The affected region itches and releases water, with irregular periods of activity and dormancy. People in the wild call this "grieved sheep sores." Prepare a decoction with trumpet flowers and leaves and wash the affected region every day. Yang Renzhai, *Straightforward Guide to Recipes*.

The Hu people's *coptis* rhizome
Picrorhiza scrophulariifl ora Pennell. Vol. III, 13-02-01

It strengthens the walls of the intestines and the stomach, and boosts the complexion. Soaked in human milk sap and the liquid dripped into the eyes it has very good effects. Zhu Zhenheng.

White bark and root bark of varnish trees
Ailanthus altissima (Mill.) Swingle. Vol. VII, 35-07-02

Intestinal wind related to poison in the spleen. Wind qi have availed themselves of a depletion weakness of camp and guardian qi and assailed them. Heat qi have occupied their place and blood has seeped into the intestines, resulting in defecation with blood discharge. *Recipes Based on Facts*.

Carp gall bladder/bile
Vol. VIII, 44-01-03

Painful red eyes with heat. Green blindness. It clears the eyes. Ingested over a long time it lets one become strong and brave, and boosts the mental qi. *Original Classic*.

Dripped into the eyes it serves to cure painful swollen red eyes with shades. It is smeared on swellings with heat of children. Zhen Quan.

When dripped into sparrow eyes with painful dryness, it will clear the eyes. *Recipes to be Kept Close at Hand*.

Dripped into the ears, it serves to cure deafness. Chen Cangqi.

Ink/soot from the center of a cauldron's bottom
Vol. II, 07-52

Ears shedding pus and blood. Blow the ashes from below a cauldron into the affected ears. They should enter deeply into the ears and this will not cause additional discomfort. The blood and the pus will leave the ears as a result. *Recipes to be Kept Close at Hand*.

Sneezeweed
Centipeda minima (L.) A.Br. et Ascher. Vol. V, 20-10

It frees the passage of nasal breathing qi, opens the nine orifices, and stimulates spitting out of wind phlegm. Xiao Bing.

To remove films in the eyes rub it to pieces and insert them into the nose. The membrane screens will fall off as a result. Meng Shen.

Dog skull
Vol. IX, 50-02-18

Tumorous flesh growth in the nose. The amount of ashes of a dog head held by a square inch spoon, and one half mace of bitter cloves are ground to powder. When this is blown into the nose, the flesh growth will transform into water. One may also add a small amount of sal ammoniac. Especially wondrous. *Mr. Zhu's Collected and Proven Recipes.*

Sudden qi recession. Cures from the outside
Vol. I, 03-05-01

Cockscomb blood. For death during sleep and sudden death because of being struck by the malign, apply it to the patient's face and heart, and insert it into the mouth and the nose.

Hemp
Cannabis sativa L. Vol. V, 22-03

A festering pharynx related to wine drinking, with sores in the mouth and on the tongue. Grind one ounce of hemp seed kernels and two ounces of *scutellaria* root into powder, form it with honey to pills and hold them in the mouth. *Recipes Worth a Thousand in Gold.*

Throat blockage with nipple moth. Grind equal amounts of "black dragon's tail," prepared alum, and small *gleditsia* seed, roasted with salt until they have turned yellow, to a powder and either blow this into the throat or apply this to the affected region. The effects are always wondrous. *Mr. Sun's Collected Efficacious Recipes.*

Snakehead fish bile
Ophiocephalus argus Cantor. 44-32-03

Throat blockage with impending death. Drip a small amount into the throat and a cure is achieved. If the disease is located deeper, mix it with water and pour it into the throat. *Recipes from the Numinous Garden.*

The snuff of a lamp wick
Vol. II, 06-10

When children incessantly cry at night because of evil heat in their heart, give two or three pieces of snuff into a decoction of common rushes and smear this on the teats of its nursing mother for the child to suck. Li Shizhen.

White bark of mulberry tree roots
Morus alba L. Vol. VII, 36-01-01

Doubled tongue of children. Boil white mulberrry root bark in water, apply the resulting juice to the nursing mother's teats, and let the children drink from it. *Secret Records About Children and Mothers.*

Wild turmeric root
Curcuma longa L. Vol. III, 14-27-01.

Li Shizhen: Wild turmeric root enters the heart and the heart enclosure. It serves to cure blood diseases. ... Unending spontaneous sweating. Mix wild tumeric powder with a liquid and apply this to the female breast when going to bed. *Simple Recipes from the Collection of Li Binhu.*

Polygonum multiflorum, Vol. V, 18-24.

Unending, spontaneous sweating. Mix *polygonum* powder with the patient's saliva, i.e., body liquid and seal the navel with it. *Simple Recipes from the Collection of Li Binhu.*

All types of copper utensils
Vol. II, 08-19

For cholera with contorted sinews, and for painful attachment illness affecting the kidney region and the region below the navel, roast such utensils and press them hot, separated by the patient's clothes, on the region of the navel, the abdomen, and the kidneys. Li Shizhen.

Uniflower swisscentaury
Stemmacantha unifl orum (L.) Dittrich. Vol. IV, 15-33

It penetrates the small intestine and serves to cure outflow of sperm, urination with blood, intestinal wind, red eyes caused by wind, strong heat of children, and injuries caused by an attack. It reconnects sinews and bones. It serves to cure breast obstruction-illness, scrofula pervasion-illness, wounds caused by metal objects/weapons, and ends bleeding and festering. It supplements blood and stimulates the growth of flesh. It penetrates the conduit-vessels. Da Ming.

Persian lilac tree fruits
Melia azedarach L. 35-15-01

Li Shizhen: Persian lilac tree fruits lead off heat in the small intestine and urinary bladder, and they lead down the minister fire in the heart enclosing network. For this reason they are an important pharmaceutical drug for pain in the central and abdominal region and elevation-illness qi.

To boost the qi and nourish the blood
Vol. I, 04-33-02.

Heat processed Chinese foxglove. For harmed center with a shriveled womb, irregular menstruation, and heat hidden in the thoroughfare and controlling vessels, resulting from a long time in childlessness, make it together with Chinese *angelica* and *coptis* rhizome into pills and let the woman ingest them.

Human placenta
Vol. IX, 52-29

A child in the uterus is tied by its navel to the placenta, and the placenta is tied to the mother's spine. It is nourished by the mother, and receives its father's essence/sperm, and its mother's blood. It gets its form from a blending of father's essence/sperm and mother's blood. The placenta is where the true original qi concentrate.

Stalactite. Calcium carbonate
Vol. II, 09-21

Cold in the large intestine resulting in an unending smooth passage of defecation. Grind one ounce of stalactite powder and half an ounce of nutmeg, cooked over a slow fire, to a powder and form with boiled date meat pills the size of *firmiana* seeds. Each time ingest 70 pills, on an empty stomach, to be sent down with a rice beverage. *Recipes to Benefit Life*.

Yellow tangerine peel
Citrus reticulata Blanco. 30-17-02

When Mr. Zhang Jiegu states: "Long-stored tangerine skin and bitter orange skin free the flow of qi, and phlegm is sent down/discharged as a result," then this is based on the meaning outlined here. Combined with apricot kernels it serves to cure qi blockage in the large intestine. Combined with peach kernels it serves to cure blood blockage in the large intestine. This is always based on its ability to free the passage of stagnant/sluggish qi and blood. For details, see under "apricot kernels."

According to Fang Shao's *Compilation from Bozhai*, "tangerine skin widens the passage through the diaphragm and sends down qi. It dissolves phlegm rheum, and has an extraordinary therapeutic potential. All other pharmaceutical drugs are valued when they are fresh; this one is valued when it has been stored for a long time."

Chinese clematis
Clematis chinensis Osbeck. Vol. V, 18-39

It penetrates the five long-term depots. It removes stagnating cold from within the abdomen, phlegm and water from the heart and the diaphragm region, long-lasting accumulation, concretion-illness and conglomeration-illness, string-illness and aggregation-illness with qi lumps, pus and malign water staying in the urinary bladder overnight, and painful cold in the lower back and knees. It heals fracture harm. *Materia Medica of the Reign Period "Opening Treasures"*.

Catechu
Vol. II, 07-40

Control. It serves to cool heat rising to the diaphragm. It transforms phlegm and generates body fluid. It is applied to wounds caused by metal objects/weapons, and all types of sores. It engenders the growth of muscles and ends pain. It stops bleeding and withdraws moisture. Li Shizhen.

Ashes from the furnace of a forge
Vol. I, 07-59

Uterus prolapse following delivery. Evenly mix purple dust/ashes from a furnace of an iron forge with sheep fat, wrap this in a piece of fabric, roast it until it is hot, and press it on the prolapsed uterus to push it back upward. *Mr. Xu's Recipes for Pregnancy and Birth.*

Red spider lily
Lycoris radiata L'Herit. Vol. IV, 13-17-01

Prolapse of the birth intestine. Boil one handful of red spider lily in three bowls of water down to one and a half bowls. Remove the dregs and steam and wash the affected region with the liquid. Divinely effective. *Mr. Wei's Recipes to Obtain Good Results.*

Vervain seedling
Verbena offi cinalis L. Vol. IV, 16-32-01

Women with blocked menstruation, forming conglomeration-illness lumps and a distension of the ribs so large that the patient wishes to die. Finely chop five pounds of vervain root and seedling and boil them in five pecks of water down to one peck. Discard the dregs and simmer the liquid to generate a paste. Each time let the woman ingest a spoonful, to be sent down prior to a meal dissolved in warm wine. *Sagely and Benevolent Recipes.*

Pig iron
Vol. II, 08-20-02

Stagnant blood caused by a blow. When it is in the joints and outside the ribs and fails to go away, boil one pound of pig iron in three pints of wine down to one ounce and ingest this. *Recipes to be Kept Close at Hand.*

Piper nigrum. Pepper fruit
Vol. VI, 32-06-01

Accumulation and aggregation-illness related to a depletion with the presence of cold qi, located outside of the membrane on the back and flowing into the two flanks, with qi countermovement and hectic panting. If this lasts for a long time, the camp and the guardian qi congeal and stagnate, and break out as obstruction-illness and impediment-illness. Often this ends in a state in which no help is possible. Recipes to Assist Life.

Native nitrokalite
Vol. II, 11-11-02

For blood dripping, with no urine being released whatsoever, but an occasional discharge of blood, with pain, a sensation of fullness and tension, and also for heat dripping, when the urine is hot and of red color, with a tense pain below the navel, send the powder down mixed with cold water. For qi dripping with a sensation of fullness and tension in the lower abdomen and continued trickling following urination, send the powder down with an *akebia* herb decoction. For stone dripping, with pain in the penis and an inability to release urine, causing a bloating of the lower abdomen with tension and pain, or with a release of sand, with the urine causing heart-pressure and the flow of qi threatened to be cut off, give the medication powder into a kettle separated by a sheet of paper and fry the kettle until the paper is scorched. Then grind the powder again and have the patient send it down mixed with warm water. If urination is blocked, send it down with a wheat decoction. Shen Cunren, *Recipes from the Numinous Garden*.

Common *cnidium* seeds
Cnidium monnieri (L.) Cuss. Vol. III, 14-04

Red and white discharge from below the belt, with no menstruation. Grind equal amounts of *common cnidium* seeds and prepared alum to powder and form with vinegar and flour a paste to prepare pills the size of bullets. Coat them with rouge, wrap them in silk floss, and insert them into the yin gate (i.e., vagina). When the heat (in the vagina) has reached a maxium, exchange it. To be applied once a day. *How Scholars Should Serve Their Parents* recipe.

Wood whitlow grass
Lepidium apetalum Willd. Vol. IV, 16-29

Blocked menstruation. Grind one ounce of wood whitlow grass into powder and with honey form pills the size of a bullet. Wrap one pill in silk floss and insert it two *cun* deep into the yin gate (i.e., vagina). Replace it after one night. When a sap leaves end the treatment. *Recipes Worth a Thousand in Gold*.

Ox/buffalo/cow gallbladder/bile
Vol. IX, 50-05-18

Coldness of a male's yin member (i.e., penis). Place *evodia* fruits into ox bile and let them dry for one hundred days. Each time take two times seven of the fruits, chew them and insert them into the yin member (i.e. penis). After an extended period of time it feels like fire. *Recipes Worth a Thousand in Gold.*

Lycium seeds/root bark
Lycium chinense Mill. Vol. VII, 36-24

It controls the five internal evil qi, a hot center with melting and thirst, encompassing blockage associated with wind intrusion and the presence of moisture. Ingested for a long time, it hardens sinews and bones, relieves the body of its weight, prevents aging, and helps to endure cold and summerheat. *Original Classic.*

It serves to discharge qi in the chest and flanks, and to cure visitor heat and headache. It supplements qi in the case of internal harm with loud exhaling and inhaling. It stiffens the yin member (i.e., penis) and frees the passage through the large and small intestine. *Supplementary Records by Famous Physicians.*

The human penis
Vol. IX, 52-32.

Li Shizhen: A man's penis is not a pharmaceutical substance. As Tao Jiucheng in his *Records Taken while Stopping from Field Work* records, "when a Mr. Shen's adultery was revealed, he took a knife and cut off his own penis. The bleeding continued for months, and the wound did not close. Someone let him search for the severed penis, and when he found it had him grind it to powder and ingest this with wine. After only a few days he was cured." In view of this, all those who have lost their "silkworm chamber" (i.e., genital member) through castration must know this method. Hence it is attached here.

Harm caused by metal objects/weapons, arrowheads, bamboo and wood
Vol. I, 04-25

Human penis. For castrated men whose wound opening fails to close take their own severed penis, burn it with its nature retained, grind it into a powder, and let them ingest it with water.

Trichosanthes kirilowii Maxim. Vol V, 18-18-02

Swollen scrotum of a child. Boil in water one ounce of trichosanthes root and one and a half mace of roasted *glycyrrhiza* roots. Add some wine and let the child ingest this. *Heart Mirror of Healing the Young.*

Willow catkin alum
Vol. II, 11-17-02

Recurrence of a disease because of exhaustion during sexual intercourse, with a swelling of the testicles, or their shrinkage and withdrawal into the abdomen, and abdominal pain letting one wish to die. Prepare a barley gruel from one part of alum and three parts of nitrokalite and ingest as much as is held by a one square inch spoon. To be ingested three times a day. The heat poison will be released with both urination and defecation relief. *Recipes to be Kept Close at Hand.*

Persian lilac tree
Melia azedarach L. Vol. VII, 35-15

Longworms (i.e., roundworms) in the abdomen. Soak Persian lilac tree fruits in unmixed, bitter wine for one night. Wrap them in silk floss and insert this into the "grain pathway"/the anus about three inches deep. Exchange it twice a day. *Arcane Essential Recipes from the Outer Censorate.*

Croton seed shell
Croton tiglium L. Vol. VII, 35-47-03

Free-flux illness with a repeated prolapse of the rectum that is black in color and hard. Burn *croton* seed shells into ashes, boil them in the natural juice of bananas, add a little mirabilite, and wash the prolapsed rectum to soften it. Then light a fire with true sesame oil and let the oil drip on the prolapsed rectum. Grind alum and a small amount of dragon bones into a powder, apply this to the end of the rectum, and push it back into the anus with a banana leaf. *Mr. Wei's Recipes to Obtain Good Results.*

Dried Chinese dates
Zizyphus jujuba Mill. Vol. VI, 29-09-02

Itching lower body parts caused by the presence of worms/bugs. Steam big/dried Chinese dates to obtain a paste, mix it with mercury, and form a three inches long stick. Wrap it in silk floss and at night insert it into the lower body (i.e., rectum). The next day all the worms/bugs will have left. *Recipes to be Kept Close at Hand.*

Pink
arnebia. Arnebia euchroma (Royle) Johnst. Vol. III, 12-28

A hot body that is yellow because of an internal fire. In the afternoon the body cools down. When the body is covered with red dots or black dots, the disease is incurable. It is advisable to brand the palms of the patient's hands and the soles of the feet, the center of his back, and the "hundred convergences" (GV-20) and "lower ridge" (Li-8) acupuncture needle insertion holes.

Artemisia argyi Lèvl. et Vant. Common mugwort leaf
Vol. IV, 15-05-01

Cold shank sore openings that fail to close. Burn prepared mugwort leaves and steam the affected region with the smoke. *Tried and Proven Recipes.*

Cunninghamia lanceoloata (Lambt.) Hook
Chinese cedar. Vol. VII, 34-03-01

Shank sores that have turned black and fester. Burn many years old Chinese cedar wood and mix the ashes with sesame oil. Cover the sores with large-leaved bamboo leaves and apply the cedar wood ashes-sesame oil mixture separated by these leaves to the affected region. Bandage it with tough silk fabric. After several applications a cure is achieved. *Recipes for Rescue in Emergencies.*

8. Standing up to nature:
Cosmetics, body enhancement, anti-aging

Medicine is antithetical to the natural course of life. Empirical evidence suggests that humans can live up to the age of 80 or even 100. Medicine is based on the notion that to reach such an age is a human right, if not – religiously dressed up – an obligation. Early death is defined as unnatural and to be avoided. Mankind is the only biological species that has taken the initiative to liberate itself from many of the health problems that nature imposes. Pathogens, be they wind, cold and heat, or worms and bugs, have their legitimate place in nature. They may be identified as evil agents, that is as enemies, once they enter the human organism. Mankind has armed itself to effectively confront these enemies. Medicine is the perhaps most effective tool invented by humans to free themselves from the burdens of disease, disability and premature death. By the same token, however, medicine has also become a most effective tool leading to over-population, increasing demands for the exploitation of natural resources, with environmental disaster a foreseeable consequence. An end to this development is not in sight.

Chinese medicine is part of this world-wide defense of mankind against forces acting in their natural right when they threaten to end human life. The early Daoist philosopher *Zhuang zi* cites the story of three friends who believed in an eternal succession of bodily and non-bodily existence. Why care about death, they asked when one of them died. Death is transition from one state of existence to another. Eventually a deceased being will assume a bodily form again. Apparently, such a world view does not agree with most people's desire to live for as long as possible, and to do so in good health. Some Daoists responded to this desire. They were the first to seek means to extend the years of life and even to reach longevity, if not immortality. A search for longevity became one of their hallmarks.

Buddhism offered solace to those irritated by the prospect of an unavoidable death. The Buddhist doctrine claimed that while the human body was bound to be lost, the human spirit could survive and would even be reincarnated in another body at some later time. Still, Buddhist teachings included health care. If bodily death cannot be escaped, at least bodily suffering should be minimized during earthly life. In contrast, Zhu Xi (1120 – 1200), the Song era Neo-Confucian philosopher was very clear about life, death, and the question of immortality: "that which dies disappears and does not return!"[27]

The *Ben cao gang mu* bears visible witness not only to a wide range of therapies designed to prevent, cure, or at least mitigate bodily and, indirectly, mental suffering. Li Shizhen also included ample evidence of attempts at shifting the age limit, if not at deleting it altogether. Such are the excessive demands voiced in China since antiquity, and made on the minerals, herbs, and animal substances supplied by nature. Processed, they become new items that are to fulfill the longevity and immortality expectations propagated by their inventors.

From its very beginning, *materia medica* literature played an important role in spreading pertinent information. Li Shizhen did not often take sides on this issue. He quoted earlier authors making all sorts of promises as to the potentials of specific substances, and therapies based on their application, so as to achieve longevity and immortality. Every now and then he denounced a statement as unfounded and abstruse. Nevertheless, he did not entirely omit such claims. He must have been aware that many of his future readers believed in possible longevity and had longings for immortality. They obtained the information they were looking for, albeit in some cases with a judgment that was to discourage them from continuing to have such longings. This is particularly evident in Li Shizhen's detailed discussion of the effects of mercury. His descriptions of the fatal consequences of taking appropriate elixirs could not be more forceful warnings.

The *Ben cao gang mu* quoted a large number of earlier authors who had published schemes for enhancing the body and modifying the condition assigned to it by nature. Beauty standards required black hair and beards until old age. Many recipes were suggested as suitable formulas for dying grey or white hair, or for stimulating the body to grow black hair in the first place. Hair was supposed to be shiny like black lacquer; recipes promised to make dull hair turn glossy. Hair loss was a problem – a loss of eyebrows in particular worried not only females – and could be countered with appropriate measures.

The facial complexion deserved special attention. A whitish complexion was advocated by authors as a beauty ideal. The face and the skin in general were to have a pleasant appearance. They were to be free of moles, blemishes, heat pimples, and all sorts of dermal dark spots. Authors quoted by Li Shizhen demonstrated the way to remove these blemishes. Peeling by

---

27 Joseph Needham, *Science and Civilisation in China*. Vol. 2. History of Scientific Thought. Cambridge, Cambridge University Press, 1956: 490.

means of red ant poison was advocated for removing tattoos; rouge mixed with clam shell powder served to treat chapped breast nipples. Smelly armpits were considered "barbarian" and also required an effective treatment.

Similar to the many recommendations on how to "prevent aging" or at least "make aging tolerable," that is, "to enjoy a long life without aging," all of this therapeutic advice reflects a struggle with the body's natural endowments. Recommendations are included that might even be considered doping today. Relieving the body of its weight was a precondition for turning into an immortal, but it also helped those who simply wished to be "able to jump across banks and gorges" or "to run as fast as a galopping horse," "to climb high and to walk long distances," and "to feel like a child again." Even the condition of the corpse after death was of concern. Measures existed to keep a corpse from rotting; ingesting jade prior to death was advocated to prevent decay for at least three years – and here Li Shizhen voiced his opposition. Such practices serve, he wrote (probably imagining the value of the undigested jade available in the deceased body), "to attract grave robbers, and contrary to one's intentions, they cause violent destruction. Would it not be more meaningful to have a corpse quickly decompose and return to the void?"

Human essence/sperm
Vol. IX, 52-18

For black moles on the face, smear human essence/sperm mixed with the white parts of the droppings of goshawks, on them. After a few days a cure is achieved. *Recipes Worth a Thousand in Gold.*

Lard. Vol. IX, 50-01-05

It lets the skin appear pleasant. Prepared as a hand crème, it prevents the skin from chapping. Tao Hongjing.

When the placenta fails to be discharged, an ingestion, with wine, of large amounts is very good. Xu Zhicai.

"Horse mane crème" stimulates the growth of hair and lets the face appear pleasant. …Wart eyes on the body and on the face. Rub them with lard and let a little blood come out of them. Divinely effective; topped by nothing. *Recipes Worth a Thousand in Gold.*

Mulberry fruit
Morus alba L. Vol. VII, 36-01-03

Pull out white hair and change it to black hair. Put one pound of black mulberry fruits and one pound of tadpoles into a porcelain jar and firmly close it. Hang it at the eastern eaves of the house for 100 days. Then the contents of the jar have turned completely into black mud. White hair dyed with it turns as black as lacquer. *Chen Cangqi ben cao.*

Marking nut tree
Semecarpus anacardium L. Vol. VII, 35-27

To pull out white hair and stimulate the growth of black hair. Grind ten marking nut tree fruits, with their skin removed and the meat pressed to obtain a juice, two ounces of bear fat, one ounce of heat prepared fat from a white horse's mane, one ounce of fresh ginger, stir-fried, and half an ounce of cloves into a powder. Each time pull out the white hairs and drip the powder there. Let it enter the flesh and black hair grows. This is a recipe applied by Vice Censor-in-Chief Yan. Meng Shen, *Quick-Working Recipes.*

Tadpoles
Larvae of *Rana nigromaculata* Hallowell. Vol. VIII, 42-04

Fire flame heat sores and *jie*-illness sores. For both these ailments pound tadpoles to pieces and apply them to the affected region. Also, for dying beard and hair on the head, pound them together with the shells of greenish walnuts into pulp and dye the beard and the hair with it. Dyed once, they will never change their color. Chen Cangqi.

Red algae
Gloiopeltis furcata (Post. et Rupr.) J. Ag. Vol. VI, 28-15

Li Shizhen: Red algae grow amidst the rock cliffs in Donghai and Nanhai. They are three to four inches long, and as big as maidenhair fern. They are forked similar to antlers, and they are purple-yellow in color. The locals collect them, dry them in the sun, and market them as "sea jewelry." When they are washed with water and mixed with vinegar, they puff up and look like new. Their flavor is extremely smooth and delicious. Soaked in water for a long time they transform to a glue-like mass. Females use it when they comb their hair. The hair is set and not messy.

Wax gourd vine
Benincasa hispida (Thunb.) Cogn. Vol. VI, 28-06-06

Burned, the ashes enable one to eliminate tattoos applied as a punishment. Boiled in water, the decoction is used to wash dermal black spots and sores with *jie*-illness. Da Ming.

Pounded and the resulting juice ingested, it resolves the poison of tree ear fungi. The decoction is used to wash a prolapsed anus. Burned, the ashes can be used in liquids to temper copper and iron; they check the effects of arsenic. Li Shizhen.

Wax gourd seeds
Benincasa hispida (Thunb.) Cogn. 28-06-03

To make a facial complexion appear lustrous. Grind five ounces of white gourd kernels, four ounces of peach flowers, and two ounces of white willow bark into a powder. After meals ingest with a beverage the amount held by a square inch spoon. To be ingested three times a day. If you wish to have a white complexion, add additional gourd kernels. If you wish to have a red complexion, add additional peach flowers. After 30 days the face is white. After 50 days the hands and the feet are all white. Another recipe uses tangerine peels, and makes no use of willow bark. *Recipes to be Kept Close at Hand.*

The skin of sour pomegranates
Punica granatum L. Vol. VI, 30-16-03

To twirl the beard and let it turn black. Open a hole on the top of one big sour pomegranate that is forming on a twig extending toward South-East. Insert half an ounce of mercury, seal it with the original thick skin, and fasten it with a hemp string. Then cover and seal it with ox dung. After frost pick the fruit from the tree and pour out the water that has collected inside the shell. Wrap a finger with a fish bladder, dip it into the water, and twirl the beard. After a long time it will assume a black color. *Pu ji.*

Inner seed coat/tegmen of Chinese chestnuts
Castanea molissima L. Vol. VI, 29-07-03

Pound inner seed coats of Chinese chestnuts into a powder, mix it with honey, and apply this to the face. It gives the face a shine, tightens the skin, and removes wrinkles. Su Gong.

Castor oil plant seeds
Ricinus communis L. Vol. IV, 17-13-01

When the hair turns yellow and is no longer black. Fry castor oil plant seed kernels in sesame oil until they are scorched and remove the dregs. Three days later repeatedly brush the hair with the oil. *Selected Profound Recipes.*

Facial spots, (i.e.,) black moles. Grind rape turnip seeds into powder, add it to a facial crème, and night after night apply it to the affected region. It also serves to remove facial wrinkles. *Sagely and Benevolent Recipes.*

Wax gourd skin. *Benincasa hispida* (Thunb.) Cogn. 28-06-01

To make a black face white. Remove, with a bamboo knife, the skin of one wax gourd and cut it into slices. Boil them in one ounce of wine and one ounce of water until they have assumed a pulpy consistency. Pass this through a sieve and apply to the face every night. *General Records of Sagely Benefaction.*

Weeping willow leaf
Salix babylonica L. Vol. VII, 35-29-05

Loss of eyebrows. Dry drooping willow leaves in the yin (i.e., shade) and grind them into a powder. Each time mix it with ginger juice in an iron vessel and night after night rub the affected region with the liquid. *Sagely and Benevolent Recipes.*

Poplar twig
Populus davidiana Dode. Vol. VI, 35-32-02

When the face is not white. Grind 18 ounces of poplar twig bark, one ounce of peach flowers, and three ounces of white wax gourd seeds into a powder. Each time ingest the amount held by a square inch spoon. To be ingested three times a day. Within 50 days the face, the hands, and the feet are all white. *General Records of Sagely Benefaction.*

Verdigris
Vol. II, 08-09

Facial black moles. Lacerate the moles with some herb and apply verdigris powder to them. Do not wash them with water for three days, and they will fall off as a result. For those that are thick, add a second application. *General Records of Sagely Benefaction.*

Tin powder
Lead carbonate. Vol. II, 08-12

Facial skin injured by scratching. Apply lead carbonate mixed with sesame oil to it. A cure will be achieved after one night. *Simple Recipes from the Collection of Li Binhu.*

Muscovite
Vol. II, 08-39

The Master Embracing Simplicity: Methods to ingest muscovite. One is to dissolve muscovite with *cinnamomum cassia* bark, onions, and glass or crystal to a watery liquid. Or give it together with dew into an iron vessel and boil it with the original decoction water until it is dissolved to a watery liquid. Or fill it with nitrokalite into a bamboo tube and bury it until it has turned into a watery liquid. Or soak it in honey until it forms a junket. Or soak it in autumn dew for one hundred days, give it into a leather pouch, and squeeze it to crush its contents to a powder. Or eat it mixed it with *senecio* herb and *ailanthus* blood. If any of these preparations is ingested for one year, all the hundreds of diseases will be kept away. If ingested for three years, aging will be reverted to boyhood. After five years one will be able to take demons and spirits into his service.

Hu Yan: Method to refine a powder. Collect muscovite in the eighth or ninth month and mix it evenly with alum. Then give this into an earthenware pot, seal the opening and wait for three days and nights until the muscovite has softened. Remove the alum and the next day soak the muscovite in dew gathered from the tips of 100 herbs. After 100 days, give it into a leather pouch and squeeze it to form its contents to a powder.

To ingest muscovite as food. Break 20 pounds of best quality white muscovite to thin pieces and prepare a decoction of eight pecks of dew water. Divide this decoction into two halves and rinse the muscovite plates with them twice. Then take two pecks of dew water again to prepare another decoction. Add ten pounds of mirabilite and the muscovite and let them soak in a wooden vessel for 20 days. Then remove the muscovite, fill it into a silk pouch, and suspend the pouch from the top of a room. It must not be exposed to wind and the sun. When the muscovite has dried, fill it into a pouch made of deer hide and rub it from dawn to noon to eventually obtain a powder that is to be given through a sieve, only to be rubbed in the deer hide pouch again until five pecks of a good powder are obtained. Remainders are to be discarded. To one peck of muscovite powder add two pounds of cliff honey, stir this to a paste and fill it into a bamboo tube. Cut this tube into small sections, seal the openings with lacquer, and bury the tubes six feet deep in the ground and covered with soil at the bottom of a wall facing North, or of a cliff facing South. In spring and summer after 40 days, in autumn and winter after 30 days, dig them out again. The contents of the tube will have become a watery liquid. If not all the contents of the various tubes have dissolved, bury them again for 30 days. This watery liquid can cure myriad diseases, as well as qi exhaustion and wind pain. For each application ingest one *ge* mixed with warm water. To be ingested three times a day. After ten days, the urine should assume a yellow color. After 20 days, cold will be washed out of the abdomen. After 30 days, decayed teeth will be replaced by new teeth. After 40 days, one will fear neither wind nor cold. After 50 days, all diseases will be cured. One's complexion and facial appearance will look younger every day, and a long life of a spirit hermit/immortal results. *Recipes Worth a Thousand in Gold.*

Mercury
Vol. II, 09-02

Barbarian stench under the armpits. Mix equal amounts of mercury and lead carbonate with facial crème and repeatedly apply this to the armpits. *Recipes Worth a Thousand in Gold.*

Mercury powder
Calomel. Vol. II, 09-03

Facial crème for women. The "red jade ointment of highest sincerety." Grind equal amounts of calomel, talc, and peeled apricot seeds to a powder, steam it, add small amounts of borneol and musk, and mix this evenly with the clear contents of a chicken egg. Wash the face and apply this. After ten days, the face will have assumed the color of red jade. *Arrangements for the Ladies' Chambers.*

Mud from the bottom of a well
Vol. II, 07-39

Heat pimples of children. Apply mud from the bottom of a well to all four sides of the affected region. *Recipes of Tan Yeweng.*

Rouge
Vol. IV, 15-29

Chapped breast nipples. Grind rouge and clam shell powder into powder and apply it to the affected region. *Mr. Wei's Recipes to Obtain Good Results.*

Caper spurge. The white juice within the leaves and the stem
Euphorbia lathyris L. Vol. IV, 17-10-01

It serves to peel facial skin to remove dermal dark spots. *Materia Medica of the Reign Period "Opening Treasures."*

It is applied to white patches and pervasion-illness with ulcers. Da Ming.

Japanese *ampelopsis*
Ampelopsis japonica (Thunb.) Makino. Vol. V, 18-28-01

Facial acne. Grind two-tenths of a mace of Japanese ampelopsis root, one-fifth of a mace of apricot kernels, and one-tenth of a mace of the white parts in chicken droppings into powder. Mix it with honey and water and apply this to the face. *Recipes to be Kept Close at Hand.*

Red ant
Vol. VIII, 40-17

They are very poisonous. Where they come into contact with someone's skin and flesh, a swelling will emerge. They serve to peel a person's facial skin, and can completely remove tattoo characters down to the bones. They eat malign sores and tumorous flesh growths, and they kill the bugs of a *xuan*-illness. Chen Cangqi.

Oyster
Ostrea gigas Thunberg. Vol. VIII, 46-01

Dark facial complexion. Grind oyster powder to a fine powder and form, with honey, pills the size of *firmiana* seeds. Each time ingest 30 pills, to be sent down with clear hot water. To be ingested once a day. In addition, roast the meat of the oyster and eat this. *Recipes of Universal Benefit.*

Surf clam
Mactra chinensis Philippi. Vol. VIII, 46-18

To let a black facial complexion turn white. Grind equal amounts of surf clams, white *aconitum* accessory tuber, corals, and white parts from the droppings of hawks/eagles to powder. Every night apply this mixed with human milk to the face and wash it in the morning with fermented water of foxtail millet.

Sulphide of mercury
Vol. II, 09-06

The hundreds of diseases affecting the five long-term depots. It nourishes the spirit and pacifies the *hun*-soul and the *po*-soul. It boosts the qi and clears the eyes. It frees the passage through the blood vessels. It ends unrest and a feeling of fullness. It boosts the essence-spirit. It kills the qi of spirit seduction-specters and malign demons. Ingested over a long time, it lets one communicate with spirit-brilliance. It prevents aging, takes the weight of the body, and turns one into a spirit-immortal. It lets the heart acquire miraculous abilities. Tang Shenwei.

Orpiment
Arsenic trisulphide. Vol. II, 09-08

Malign sores, baldness on the head, crusts with *jie*-illness. It kills poisonous worms/bugs and lice, body itch, evil qi, and all types of poison. Refined with heat and ingested over a long time it takes the weight of the body, adds years of life, and prevents aging. *Original Classic.*

Erosions and tumorous flesh growths in the nose. Hidden worms/bugs sores in the lower body parts, white spots on body and face. It disperses dead muscles in the skin and serves to cure absent-mindedness with evil qi. It kills the poison of wasps/bees and snakes. Ingested over a long time, it extends the limits of one's brain. *Supplementary Records by Famous Physicians.*

Stalactite
Calcium carbonate. Vol. II, 09-21

Stalactites clear the eyes and boost the essence/sperm. They pacify the five long-term depots. They penetrate the hundreds of joints. They open the passage through the nine orifices. They serve to let down a nursing mother's milk sap. *Original Classic.*

They boost the qi, supplement depletion injuries, and heal weak, painful and cold legs, as well as harm and exhaustion affecting the Lower Burner. They strengthen the yin (i.e., genital) potential. Ingested over a long time, they extend one's years of life and boost longevity. They improve the complexion, prevent aging and let one have children. If one ingests them without prior refinement by heat, they cause urinary dripping. *Supplementary Records by Famous Physicians.*

Chalcanthite
Water soluble copper sulphate. Vol. II, 10-13

It clears the eyes and serves to cure pain in the eyes, wounds inflicted by metal objects, all types of epilepsy and spasm, painful erosion in the female yin (i.e., genital) region, urinary stone dripping, and alternating cold and heat sensations, collapsing center with a discharge of blood, and all types of evil and poison qi. It helps people to have children. Ingested processed with heat, it prevents aging. Ingested over a long time, it extends longevity and lets one become a spirit-hermit/immortal. *Original Classic.*

Fragrant Solomon's seal
Polygonatum odoratum (Mill.) Druce. Vol. III, 12-09

It controls being struck by wind with sudden heat, an inability to move, ruptured sinews and clotted flesh caused by a fall, and all kinds of insufficient qi. Ingested over a long time, it removes facial gloom, improves one's complexion, and generates a moist luster. It relieves the body of its weight and prevents aging. *Original Classic.*

Chen Cangqi: In addition to its therapeutic potential, it controls one's intelligence, regulates blood and qi, and lets one be strong and sturdy. Ingested as a powder mixed with the leaves of the lacquer tree, it controls the five long-term depots and boosts the essence/sperm. It removes the three worms/bugs, relieves the body of its weight, prevents aging, changes white hair to black, moistens muscles and skin, and warms up the lower back and the legs. Only patients with heat must not ingest it.

Virgate wormwood
Artemisia scoparia Waldst. et Kit. Vol. IV, 15-07

Wind, moisture, alternating sensations of cold and heat, evil qi. Heat accumulating to yellow *dan*-illness/jaundice. Ingested over a long time they relieve the body of its weight, boost the qi, and let one endure aging. The face remains white and joyful. They extend the years of life. White rabbits eating them turn into immortals. *Original Classic.*

They serve to cure jaundice covering the entire body and blocked urination. They remove heat from the head and eliminate deeply hidden conglomeration-illness. *Supplementary Records by Famous Physicians.*

Wormwood
Artemisia carvifolia Buch.-Ham.ex Roxb. Vol. IV, 15-08

The leaves supplement the center and boost the qi; they relieve the body of its weight, supplement exhaustion, maintain a youthful complexion, stimulate the growth of hair and keep it black, and prevent aging. At the same time, they remove gray hair. Da Ming.

Burn them to ashes, place the ashes on paper, let water trickle through the ashes and the paper, and boil the resulting juice with lime. The resulting liquid serves to cure malign sores, tumorous flesh-growth, and dermal black spots and wounds. Meng Shen.

Asiatic plantain seeds
Plantago asiatica L. Vol. IV, 16-30-01

Tao Hongjing: Asiatic plantain seeds by their nature are cold and free the flow of liquids. The classics of the hermits/immortals, too, recommend to consume them, stating "they relieve the human body of its weight, enabling one to jump across banks and gorges, and letting him enjoy a long life without aging."

Su Song: Asiatic plantain seeds are very often applied as pharmaceutical drug. The "pills to maintain one's condition" make use of the two items Asiatic plantain seeds and *cuscuta* seeds. These are pills prepared with honey that are ingested after a meal. They were regarded in the past as an outstanding recipe and are so still today.

Li Shizhen: According to the *The Divine Immortal's Classic of Ingesting Essences*, "Asiatic plantain is also named 'earth's garment'." It is the essence of thunder. To ingest it lets one's physical appearance transform.

Chinese *asparagus*
Asparagus cochinchinensis (Lour.) Merr. Vol. V, 18-22

Zhen Quan: Chinese *asparagus* is cold and can supplement qi. Persons suffering from any of the five kinds of depletion and heat should resort to it and add it to their medication. Ingested together with Chinese foxglove rhizome as its guiding substance it makes aging bearable and keeps the head from turning white.

Polygonum multiflorum Thunb. root
Vol. V, 18-24-01

It dissolves swelling related to obstruction-illness. It heals wind intrusion sores on the head and on the face. It serves to cure the five types of piles, ends heart pain, boosts blood and qi, blackens hair and beard, brightens the complexion, and ingested for a long time it stimulates the growth of sinews and bones, extends the years of life, and prevents aging. In addition, it serves to cure all types of illness of women following delivery and others below the belt. *Materia Medica of the Reign Period "Opening Treasures."*

Common clubmoss
Lycopodium clavatum Thunb. Vol. V, 21-14

Long-term suffering from blockage related to wind intrusion, with legs and knees experiencing a painful cold, a numb skin, and weakened qi strength. Ingested for a long time it eliminates blood disorder related to wind intrusion and wind itching (i.e., in changing places). It improves the complexion, changes white hair to black hair, and prevents aging. Soak it in wine and drink the liquid. Good. Chen Cangqi.

Kernel of hemp seeds
Cannabis sativa L. Hemp. Vol. V, 22-03-03

They supplement the center and boost the qi. Ingested for a long time they let one be fat and strong, they prevent aging and turn one into a spirit hermit/immortal. *Original Classic.*

They serve to cure wind stroke with sweating. They eliminate water qi, free urination, break through accumulated blood, restore blood vessels, and serve to cure illnesses following childbirth. When used to wash the hair, they stimulate its growth and let it appear moist. *Supplementary Records by Famous Physicians.*

White *ganoderma*
Vol. VI, 28-18-04

Cough with rising qi. It boosts the lung qi and penetrates and opens mouth and nose. It strengthens the mind, makes you courageous, and pacifies the *po*-soul. Ingested for a long time, it relieves the body of its weight and prevents aging; it extends the years of life and makes you a spirit immortal. *Original Classic.*

Indian lotus fruit
Nelumbo nucifera Gaertn. Vol. VI, 33-10-01

Chen Cangqi: After autumn, when they are really black, they are called "stone-hard lotus seeds." When they are placed in the water they sink. They can float only on a salt decoction/brine. When this item has remained in any remote region without decaying for hundreds of years, is then obtained by people who eat it, it keeps their hair black and prevents aging.

Meng Shen: All birds and monkeys that obtain them, they do not eat them but store them in their caves. When a person obtains them after 300 years and eats them, this prevents aging forever. Also, when wild geese eat the seeds and defecate them on fields in the wild and on mountain rocks, if these are shady places without rain, they do not rot for a long time. When humans obtain them and eat ten seeds every morning on an empty stomach, this relieves their body of its weight, and enables them to climb high and walk long distances.

Privet fruit
Ligustrum lucidum Ait. Vol. VII, 36-16-01

Hundreds of diseases related to depletion injury. Ingested for a long time the following recipe lets white hair turn black again. It reverses aging and makes you feel like a child again. Collect privet fruits in the tenth month on a first *si* 巳 day (i.e., the 6th day in the circle of 12 days associated with the earthly branches), dry them in the yin (i.e., shade), soak them in wine for one day, steam them until they are thoroughly penetrated, and dry them in the sun to obtain one pound, four ounces. Collect ink plants in the fifth month and dry them in the yin (i.e., shade) to obtain ten ounces, and grind them into a powder. Collect mulberry fruits in the third month and dry them in the yin (i.e., shade) to obtain ten ounces, and grind them into a powder. Mix all three pharmaceutical drugs and with heat refined honey form pills the size of *firmiana* seeds. Each time ingest 70 to 80 pills, to be sent down with a mild salt decoction. If the mulberry fruits are collected in the fourth month and pounded to obtain a juice that is mixed with the other two pharmaceutical drugs, and if the ink plants are collected in the seventh month and pounded to obtain a juice that is mixed with the other two pharmaceutical drugs, the honey is not required to make pills. *Simple and Convenient Recipes.*

The core of the wood enclosed by the *poria* sclerotium
Vol. VII, 37-01-04

The method for ingestion recommended in the *Tried and Proven Later Recipes*. Take a stick-size *poria* from Huashan and cut from it a piece the size of Chinese dates. Place it into a new earthen jar and soak it in good wine. Seal it with one layer of paper and open it after one hundred days. It will then have assumed a consistency of malt sugar. You may eat one such piece per day. After 100 days, your sinews and the body will be moist and glossy. After one year you can see things at night. After a very long time your intestines will have transformed to sinews. This extends the years of your life and helps to endure aging. Your facial complexion is that of a boy.

Jade. Nephrite
Vol. II, 08-29

Zhang Hua states: "When jade is ingested, if grain jade of white color from Lian tian is ingested regularly, it will let one become a spirit hermit/immortal. When people shortly before their death ingest five pounds, for three years after their death their color will not change. Since ancient times, when tombs were opened and the corpses appeared as if they were alive, without exception they were found with large pieces of gold and jade inside and outside their body and abdomen."

Han dynasty regulations required that all kings and dukes upon their death were to wear coats of pearls and to be equipped with small chests of jade so as to prevent the rotting of their corpse.

Li Shizhen: Han Emperor Wu di ingested jade fragments mixed with dew from golden stalks. It was said that this could extend the years of one's life, and this was the item discussed here. However, it is not for sure that jade will protect those who resort to it from dying. Its only effect is that it protects those who are dead from decaying. To nourish a corpse serves to attract robbers, and contrary to one's intentions, they contribute to a violent destruction. Would it not be more meaningful to quickly have a corpse decompose and return to the void?

Silverfish
Lepisma saccharina L. Vol. VIII, 41-22

Li Shizhen: Silverfish massively bore through garments, silk, books, and paintings. In the beginning, they are of yellow color. When they grow older, they have a white powder on them. When they are crushed to pieces, they are like silver and can be used to mark paper and letters.

According to Duan Chengshi, "He Feng in a book found a hair four *cun* long. It was rolled up for no reason. With some force he ruptured it, and water dripped from both ends. A recipe expert said: 'This is "one who watches from afar." When silverfish eat the characters "divine immortal" three times, they will transform into one. By holding one in the hand facing heaven, one can cause a star to fall, and this way acquire an elixir of immortality'."

This is even stranger than the legend of becoming an hermit/immortal by swallowing silver fish. It is entirely absurd nonsense. It is necessary to discuss and correct it.

Mercury
Vol. II, 09-02

Tao Hongjing: "When smelted and transformed, it returns to the state of cinnabar-elixir," is based on the classics of hermits/immortals. Ingested mixed with wine and dried in the sun it extends one's life.

Zhen Quan: Mercury is very poisonous. It is a liquid inside of cinnabar. It is the primordial mother of a return to the state of cinnabar-elixir – a pharmaceutical substance transforming one to an hermit/immortal who will never die. It is able to make, through a refinement with heat, the five metals succumb as a mud.

The Master Embracing Simplicity: When cinnabar is heated it becomes mercury. Through combined changes it can be made to cinnabar again, and this distances it greatly from herbs and woods. Hence it is able to extend human life. Gold and mercury in the nine orifices of a dead person will prevent its decomposition. How much more is this true for living persons who ingest it for food?!

Chen Cangqi: When mercury enters one's ears it will eat away this person's entire brain. When it enters his flesh it will let all his sinews contract and shrink. It turns the yin qi upside down and cuts off the flow of yang qi.

When people suffer from sores and *jie*-illness, they often apply mercury to the affected region. Its nature is smooth and heavy and hence it moves straight into the flesh. It should be applied only with great care. It must not be used for treating sores on the head lest it enter the conduits and network vessels and inevitably relax sinews and bones – problems none of the hundreds of medications are able to cure.

Kou Zongshi: When mercury is added to medication, this is always based on some well-defined method. But utmost circumspection is required nevertheless because of its poison. When women ingest much of it, it will interrupt their ability to become pregnant. When nowadays mercury is heated to generate cinnabar, physicians who are not entirely familiar with it may make mistakes in its therapeutic application. One must be very careful.

Han Yu of the Tang dynasty states: "Li Gan, a scholar at the Imperial Academy, met with Liu Mi, an expert of longevity recipes. He claimed to be able to heat mercury and prepare a pharmaceutical substance for eternal life. He filled a cauldron with lead, left an empty space in its center, and filled it in with mercury. Then he sealed it on all four sides and heated it to prepare cinnabar. When Li Gan ingested it, he discharged blood. Within four years his disease turned ever more acute. Eventually he died. I have no idea where the talk about ingesting cinnabar for food may have come from. It has killed innumerable people, and yet more and more people like it. They are truly deluded. The records in books and what they hear about such unfortunate outcomes are not discussed.

I have been a personal eyewitness. I have travelled to six or seven men who had been destroyed by such medication. They should serve as a warning for everyone. Gui Deng, Minister of Public Works, himself told of how he ingested mercury and fell ill. It was as if a hot iron cane had pierced him from the top of his head down. It broke in parts and caused a fire which eventually shot out of his orifices. He felt a maddening pain and screamed and was unable to weep. Mercury was found on his mat. Outbreaks of his disease alternated with periods of remission. For tens of years he spat saliva with blood until eventually he died.

Li Xuzhong, Palace Censor, had an impediment-illness that broke out on his back, and he died. Li Xun, Minister of Justice, told me: 'I mistakenly took cinnabar as a medication'. Then he died. Li Jian, Vice-Minister of Justice, died one morning without having been ill. Meng Jian, Minister of Commerce, invited me to Wanzhou and secretly informed me: 'I have acquired a secret medication. It is impossible that I am the only one to gain eternal life. Here now I give you one package, and you may use date pulp to prepare pills and ingest them'. The next year he fell ill. Later someone came and told me about this. He said: 'The medication you ingested some time ago was illusionary. Here is a recipe to discharge it. Once it is discharged, health will be restored'. Meng Jian died two years after he had fallen ill. Lu Tan, military commissioner in Dongchuan, discharged blood with his urine, and suffered from unbearable pain in his flesh. Eventually he died. Li Daogu, General of Jin wu, was accused because of his dealings with Liu Mi. He ate a secret medication and died, aged 54, at sea.

All these cases should serve as warnings. A saying is: 'When someone shielded from death dies soon, this is called wit'! Is this possible? The five types of grain and the three types of domestic animals, salt and vinegar, fruits and vegetables, they keep humans going. Nowadays, there are those who are misled, and they say: The five types of grain let humans die young. The three types of domestic animals kill humans. Their intake must be decreased. This way from an ordinary banquet, two or three elements out of ten are strictly forbidden. Such persons do not believe in the eternal WAY, and rather are engaged in demonic oddities. Only when they are close to dying, they regret their doings. Fans of such doings surviving them say: 'That they died is simply because they did not follow the right WAY. I am different'. When the elixir causes first reactions they say: 'This reaction is a medicinal effect on my diseases. Once the diseases are eliminated, and the medication works, I will not have to die'. Only when they are about to die, they regret. Alas! This is truly saddening!"

Li Shizhen: Mercury is the essence of utmost yin; it is endowed with a nature of sinking and adhering. When it is exposed to a fire for calcination and refinement, it flies upward and undergoes miraculous changes. When it is exposed to the steaming qi of humans, it enters their bones and pierces through their sinews. It cuts off the flow of yang qi and erodes the brain. Among all the items with yin poison, there is nothing that comes close to it. Still, Da Ming says it is nonpoisonous. The *Original Classic* says ingesting it for a long time lets one become a divine immortal. Zhen Quan says it is the primordial mother of a return to the cinnabar-elixir. And the *Master Embracing Simplicity* identifies it as a medication to extend life.

Those who since the six dynasties have been hungry for life and have ingested such elixirs for food, who were disabled as a result and eventually died, no one knows how many people these were. Of course, the experts of immortality recipes lack knowledge of the WAY, but how can it be that *materia medica* works include such absurd sayings! Mercury cannot be ingested for food, but its therapeutic effects must not be hidden. Cinnabar brought together with black lead and congealed to sand presses down phlegm and saliva. Cinnabar brought together with sulphur and congealed to sand offers emergency rescue from serious diseases. These are soldiers flexibly responding to changing requirements. When using them it is essential to get to the heart of the matter and to grasp the key to the problem at hand.

Henbane seeds
Hyoscyamus niger F.W.Schmidt. Vol. IV, 17-11-01

Toothache with an appearance of worms/bugs. Numbness, contraction and tension of flesh. Ingested for a long time they relieve the body of its weight. They let one walk forcefully, and enable one to run as fast as a horse. They strengthen the mind and boost one's strength. They enable communication with spirits and a vision of demons. Eaten in large amounts makes one run around like crazy. *Original Classic.*

Light colored sesame seeds
Sesamum indicum L. Vol. V, 22-01-02

To ingest sesame seeds as food. The *Master Embracing Simplicity* states: "Wash three pecks of sesame seeds from Shangdang in a pan and steam it to activate all their qi. Wash them again in water, remove the foam and steam them a second time. Do this nine times. Then soak them in hot water to remove the skin and winnow them to clean them of the chaff. Stir-fry them until they develop a fragrance and grind them into powder. With white honey or Chinese date pulp prepare pills the size of a bullet. Each time send down one pill dissolved in warm wine. To be ingested three times a day. While ingesting these pills poisonous fish, dog meat, and fresh vegetables should be avoided. When these pills are ingested for one hundred days, all ailments of obstinacy-illness are eliminated. After one year the body and the face are shiny and glossy, and the person feels no hunger. After two years, white hair has turned black again. After three years, where teeth have fallen out new teeth grow. After four years neither water nor fire can harm that person. After five years he will walk as fast as a horse runs. Ingested over long periods of time it grants longevity. If it is intended to cause a free flow discharge, send it down with a mallow juice beverage."

Paper mulberry tree fruit
Broussonetia papyrifera (L.) Vent. Vol. VII, 36-04-01

Tao Hongjing: Recipes of the hermits/immortals recommend to collect and pound them to obtain their juice and to use it mixed with some elixir. It can also be ingested dry. It lets you communicate with spirits and enables you to see demons.

The *Master Embracing Simplicity* states: "When red paper mulberry fruits are ingested by old people, they become young again. They let you see demon spirits."

The Daoist Liang Xu was 70 years old when he ate them and became even younger and stronger. At the age of 140 years he was still able to walk and to run as fast as a horse.

9. Social and natural conditioning: Gender and sex

To Li Shizhen the relationship between males and females, and hence the status of females in society, was clearly determined. Gendering, that is, the assignment of roles to the two sexes, was defined both by natural law and social convention. Ever since Confucian concepts of an ideal stratification had come to dominate social life in China, males were given the dominant status. Mainstream Han-Chinese society for the next two millennia was patriarchal, patrilocal, and – this is where an aspect of concern for medical intervention comes into play – patrilinear. A sequence, from generation to generation, of male descendants was required. Sacrifices addressed to the ancestors were performed to this end. In more concrete terms, in a marital union both males and females were responsible for generating the desired offspring. Men were expected to have sufficient sexual potency to contribute relevant "essence" to their female partner; females were considered interchangeable if they were unable to transmute their partner's essence into a male descendant. The status of a wife within her marriage family depended on the birth of sons.

Mencius (372 – 289), an early follower of Confucius and influential social philosopher, stated that the worst of unfilial acts was the failure to have male descendants. Families anxiously awaited the outcome of pregnancy and were disappointed when it resulted in a girl. Li Shizhen quotes the Tang physician Wang Bing (8th c.), who had made himself a name when he rescued the *Inner Classic of the Yellow Thearch* from possible oblivion. He collected, and compiled as a well-structured text, still extant fragments of that ancient classic. Wang Bing is quoted in the *Ben cao gang mu* with the statement: "When someone gives birth to three sons, the ruler of the country has achieved great peacefulness. When someone gives birth to three girls, the country is marked by licentiousness and the ruler neglects the government." The birth of girls was an unwelcome event, no matter whether the general condition of society or a mother's personal responsibility were the immediate cause.

Social conventions can be viewed as human constructs. When a changing environment demands it, such constructs can change as well. Natural laws, though, were supposed to be eternal. At least since the Han dynasty, the status of women in China became inextricably linked to the yin aspect of yin and yang duality. In yin and yang theory it may appear at first glance that two complementary forces interact. They have an equal share in shaping all phenomena and their functions. Winter is as necessary as summer;

darkness is as important as light. But there is a second level of assignments to yin and yang, and it is loaded with concepts that have an immediate bearing on culture in general and social structure in particular. Males were identified as yang, and this implied that they were the ones to represent hardness, assertiveness, action, and dominance. Women were understood as the opposite. Conceptualizing the differences between men and women in terms of yin and yang means that these differences are part of a natural, universal order. Nothing can and nothing should be altered about this.

The fact that there are two sexes, which have served the continuous reproduction of human, animal, and plant life since the beginning of a structured universe, was of course not discussed. As long as the yin and yang doctrine is accepted as a cosmogonic fact, there is no place for a third category, even if the assumed characteristics of the two sexes are not always clearly recognizable. The yin and yang doctrine allows gradations, however. Yin may include more or less of yang; yang may include more or less of yin. Spring is yin with a rising presence of yang; autumn is yang with a rising presence of yin.

Li Shizhen devoted a lengthy paragraph to this issue as if he had foreseen debates gaining momentum 500 years later. He cited ancient sources and offered his own view on males who may look like males but do not feel or act as males, and vice versa. He knew, of course, of hermaphrodites, "those whose body is both male and female. They are commonly called 'dual shape'. The *History of the Jin* holds that such persons are born from disorderly qi, and calls them 'human ailment'. There exist three groups of these. Those who are supposed to behave like males but act as females. Those who are supposed to behave like females but act as males. ... And those males who can act as a wife but not as a husband. All of them are equipped with a body, but cannot put it to appropriate use." Discussions relating to such "abnormalities" were part of an ongoing interest in sexual matters. Proper reproduction, it appears, was too important for society not to be concerned with openly.

The *Ben cao gang mu* bears witness to over two millennia of observations of the "proper" interaction of males and females as sexual partners in a relationship of mutual, albeit unequal, dependence. Li Shizhen offered suggestions on how to stimulate mutual love in marital partners and also on how to prevent undue lust while on travel far from home. He quoted earlier authors' advice on how to cure a male's inability to have sex and on how to stimulate a "lengthy, violent orgasm" in women. Just as pre-modern Chinese society was male dominated, Chinese medicine discriminated against women. Females were barred from observing some sensitive processes of pharmaceutical production. The *Ben cao gang mu* does not list a single example of processes that were not to be observed by males. Women are known to dream of sex; men are not. To avoid the disappointment of giving birth to a daughter, methods were recommended to identify a female fetus during pregnancy and to change it into a male fetus. There is not a single reference to the opposite. Violent or "excessive" sex, whatever may have been meant here, is mostly described as causing harm to the male partner, rarely to the female when, for example, her bladder is ruptured. Li Shizhen's *Ben cao gang mu* reflects these facets of historical Chinese society and medicine's compliance more clearly than does any earlier text.

Human abnormalities
Vol. IX, 52-37

Li Shizhen: At the absolute beginning, heaven and earth were not separate yet, forming one indistinct cloudy whole. As soon as the qi brought forth humans, there were males and females. These males and females joined their essence, and this way by themselves transformed to new life. Just like herbs and trees in the beginning generated seeds. Once they obtained qi, they had roots and seeds afterwards, resulting in a continuing growth of one after another. The changes and transformations of humans include phenomena that leave the regular order, and this is something those masters who take responsibility for human life/fate should be aware of, and learned men must know. Hence, writings on human abnormalities are attached here at the end of the section "man" to offer evidence of often heard impairments and faults.

The *Classic of Changes* states: "The entirety of yin and yang interaction is called DAO/The WAY. Males and females join their essence, and through their transformation the myriad things come to life. The DAO/WAY of *qian* 乾 brings forth males; the DAO/WAY of *kun* 坤 brings forth females."

This is a reference to the mechanism underlying the generation of life by the interaction of males and females, and to the spontaneous force of creation and transformation in the interaction of yin and yang.

Chu Cheng, minister of education of Qi, stated: "When the blood arrives first and wraps the essence, then a male will be born. When the essence arrives first and wraps the blood, then a female will be born. When yin and yang arrive together, this results in a body that is neither a male nor a female. When essence and blood disperse, this is a portend of twins and triplets."

The *Daoist Canon* states: "Conception on the first, third, and fifth day after the end of menstruation results in a male child; on the second, fourth, and sixth day results in a female child."

Dongyuan Li Gao states: "On the first, second, and third day, when the sea of blood is clean, conception results in a male child. On the third, fourth, and fifth day it results in a female child."

The *Classic of Sagely Benefaction* states: "When the qi move on the left and are supported by yang, then this generates a male child. When the qi move on the right and are supported by yin, then this generates a female child."

Danxi Zhu Zhenheng regarded Mr. Chu's statements as wrong, and agreed with Li Dongyuan. He condoned the doctrine of "left and right" in the *Classic of Sagely Benefaction* and based his own explication on it, tracing the generation of male and female children to whether the uterus is tied to the left or to the right side.

One may say that all these doctrines are based on good knowledge. I, Li Shizhen say: One cannot say that Mr. Chu was entirely wrong, and that Li Dongyuan was entirely right. Now, Mr. Chu spoke in terms of the earlier or later arrival of essence and blood. The *Daoist Canon* speaks in terms of the even and uneven number of days after the end of menstruation. Li Dongyuan spoke of the waxing and waning of blood in a woman. The *Sheng ji* and Zhu Danxi spoke of the attachment of the uterus to the left and right. Each of them held/holds their own view. When seen together, the underlying principle is grasped easily. Now, whether it is a single male or single female fetus, that can be discussed in terms of the number of days after menstruation. But how about the stimuli leading to twins and triplets? Are they, too, explained in terms of the number of days after menstruation? A survey of historical writings shows that there are very many records of one single birth episode bringing forth three or four children. It happens that half of them are males and half of them are females, or that there are many males and few females, or few males and many females.

The *Rural Records from the Western Watchtower* has a record from the reign period "Obedient to Heaven" (1457 – 1463) of our country's current dynasty. In Yangzhou, a woman among the common people at one time gave birth to five male children. All of them were successfully brought up. With a view on this, how could it be that conception on the first, third, and fifth day after menstruation results in a male, and on the second, fourth, and sixth day results in a female child? What principle could there be determining that a male child is conceived on the first, and a female child is conceived on the second day? Hence there is evidence justifying the emphasis by Mr. Chu, the *Classic of Sagely Benefaction*, and Danxi on the arrival of essence and blood, and the attachment to the left and right of the uterus, while the theory of the *Daoist Canon* and of Li Dongyuan on the significance of the number of days after menstruation can be doubted.

Wang Shuhe in his *The Classic of Movements in the Vessels* holds that the movement in the vessels, whether it is on the left or right, at the surface or in the depth, can be used to determine whether a male or female child was conceived.

Gao Yangsheng in his *Rhymed Instructions on the Movements in the Vessels* holds that it is possible to determine whether a woman is pregnant with twins or triplets on the basis of whether the movement in the vessels is longitudinal or sideways, contrary to or in agreement with the normal passage. Presumably, this is another personal opinion that cannot be considered as fact.

Wang Bing in his *Secret Conversations on the Mysterious Pearl* states: "When someone gives birth to three sons, the ruler of the country has achieved great peacefulness. When someone gives birth to three girls, the country is marked by licentiousness and the ruler neglegts the government. When someone gives birth to ten sons, all the dukes and princes compete for rank and position. When someone gives birth to a lump of flesh, the realm is hit by famine and starvation."

These are explications of the birth of numerous male and female children in terms of human affairs. But the transformations of qi are also linked to other phenomena. Now, the trigram *qian* 乾 stands for the father, and the trigram *kun* 坤 stands for the mother. That is the general principle. But there are five kinds of apparent males that are not real males and cannot become fathers, and there are five kinds of apparent females that are not real females and cannot become mothers. Why is that so? Is this not because those apparent males who are not real males have a deficit of yang qi, and that those apparent females who are not real females have their supply of yin qi blocked?

The five kinds of apparent females who are not females are the following. Snail kinds, line kinds, drum kinds, horn kinds, and vessel kinds. Snail kinds are those who in their vaginal opening have something like a snail. Line kinds are those whose vaginal opening is small like a line. These are "replete women." Drum kinds are those whose vaginal opening resembles a drum. Horn kinds are those who at their vaginal opening have something like a horn. This is what in ancient times was called "yin erection." Vessel kinds are those whose menstruation is irregular all their life, including those suffering from collapsing blood from below the belt.

The five kinds of apparent males who are not males are the following: Heaven type, bullock type, leakage type, coward type, and change type. The heaven type includes those with a dysfunction of their yang force. These are those called "eunuchs by heavenly fate" in ancient times. Bullock kinds are those who lost their yang force because of castration, and persons living in temples. Leakage kinds are those whose essence/sperm is cold and unstable and therefore regularly flows off and is lost involuntarily. Coward kinds are those with an incomplete erection. It may be that they encounter their match and their yang member fails to rise. Change kinds are those whose body is both male and female. They are commonly called "dual shape."

The *History of the Jin* holds that such persons are born from disorderly qi, and calls them "human ailment." There exist three groups of these. Those who are supposed to behave like males but act as females. Those who are supposed to behave like females but act as males. Those who are yin/female for one half of a month, and yang/male for the other half of a month. And those males who can act as a wife but not as a husband. All of them are equipped with a body, but cannot bring it to use appropriately.

Realgar
Arsenic disulphide. Vol. II, 09-07

To turn a female fetus into a male fetus. When a woman senses that she is pregnant fill a deep-red pouch with one ounce of realgar. When this is used to nourish the fetus, this will turn a female into a male. This is to avail oneself of yang essence entirely brought forth by the earth. *Recipes Worth a Thousand in Gold.*

Chinese tea
Camellia sinensis L. Vol. VI, 32-12

Aggregation-illness resulting from an addiction to tea leaves. A person suffered from this disease. A recipe master let the patient fill a new shoe with tea leaves and had the patient eat them whenever he wanted. Then he filled another shoe, and this was done three times. As a result, that person refrained from eating tea leaves. For males use the shoes of a female; for females use the shoes of a male. Their application results in a cure. *Simple Recipes from the Collection of Li Binhu.*

Ink plant
Eclipta prostrata(L.) L. Vol. IV, 16-38

Attaching medication to the arm to stop malaria. Pound ink plant to a pulp and attach it above the inch opening on the wrist, for males on the left and for females on the right side. Then press it with with an ancient coin and fasten it with a piece of silk. After quite some time this will draw small blisters. This is called "heavenly cauterization." The malaria will be stopped. Very effective. Wang Zhizhong, *Classic of Supporting Life.*

Croton tree
Croton tiglium L. Vol. VII, 35-47-01

Phlegm and panting of children. Pound a *croton* seed into a pulpy mass, wrap it in silk floss, and insert it into the child's nose. Into the left nostril of male children and into the right nostril of female children. The phlegm is discharged as a result. Gong shi, *Mirror of Medicine.*

Comb and fine-toothed comb
Vol. VIII, 38-48

Painful urinary dripping. Heat up a many years old wooden comb by retaining its nature and ingest it on an empty stomach with cold water. Males resort to a comb of a female; females resort to a comb of a male. *Recipes for Rescue in Emergencies*

Arsenic
Arsenic trioxide. Vol. II, 10-17

Malaria illness with alternating cold and heat sensations. Sun Zhenzong in his *Secret and Precious Recipes* recommends to proceed as follows. Grind two ounces of arsenic to a powder and separately grind three ounces of calcite to a powder. Then take a new iron kettle and spread a layer of calcite powder in it. Spread a layer of arsenic powder on it, and cover it with another layer of the calcite powder. Then firmly close the kettle with a thick cup and tightly seal it with ten layers of vinegar-paste paper. Calcine this with the fire of one pound of charcoal. Once the paper has turned black remove the kettle from the fire, wait until it has cooled down, scrape the arsenic powder from the inside of the cup, and grind it in a mortar to a fine powder. Prepare with millet and/or cooked rice pills the size of mung beans and coat them with cinnabar. Each time use three to four pills; children one or two pills. On a day of an outbreak of malaria let the patient send it down early in the morning with cool tea gathered in the twelfth month. He must not consume any hot item for the entire day. If the patient is a male, a woman is to place the medication into his mouth. If the patient is a woman, a male is to place the medication into her mouth.

Carpel of red prickly-ash from Shu
Zanthoxylum bungeanum Maxim. Vol. VI, 32-02-01

The "pills with red prickly-ash carpels." They serve to cure harm and fatigue affecting the original long-term depot (i.e., the kidneys), unclear vision and deafness. Ingesting them for 100 days the effects of these pills include a sensation of a body relieved of its weight and requiring little sleep. The feet are strengthened. Ingested for three years, your wisdom is realized and vision is several times clearer than normal. The complexion is red and joyful, the beard and the hair are shiny and black. Each time ingest with warm wine 30 pills. When this medication is prepared neither women nor chicken or dogs should observe this.

Peach
Amygdalus persica L. Vol. VI, 29-06

Yellow *dan*-illness/jaundice letting a patient's body and eyes appear like gold. In the early morning of a clear day – do not let chicken, dogs or women see this – collect a handful of Eastward extending peach tree roots as fine as a chopstick or similar to a hairpin, cut them into fine pieces, boil them in one generous *sheng* of water down to a small *sheng*, and ingest this on an empty abdomen all at once. Three to five days later, the yellow color dissipates like a thin cloud. After 100 days you will be healed as before. Chu Yushi, *Certainly Effective Recipes*.

Malaria illness with alternating sensations of cold and heat. Remove the skin and the pointed ends of 100 peach kernels. Grind them in a mortar into a paste. It must not come into contact with fresh water. Add three maces of minium and make pills the size of *firmiana* seeds. Each time ingest three pills. Swallow them, facing North, with warm wine on the day of an expected outbreak. The pills are prepared on the fifth day of the fifth month at noon. This should not occur in the presence of chicken, dogs, and/or women. *Materia Medica of Tang Shenwei.*

Chinese white pine
Vol. VII, 34-02

The "anti-aging elixir of four sages." Boil one pound of clear pine resin in ash-free wine several times to bubbling in an earthenware cauldron heated by a mulberry twig fire. Stir the liquid with a bamboo twig and stop the fire when it has become viscous. Pour it into water where it congeals to lumps. Then these lumps are boiled in wine nine times. The resin will appear like jade. End the process when it is no longer bitter and astringent and grind it into a fine powder. Take 12 *liang* and add half a pound of white *poria* powder, half a pound of yellow *chrysanthemum* flower powder, and half a pound of arborvitae seed kernels, with their oil discarded and only the pulp used, and form pills the size of *firmiana* seeds. Each time send down on an empty stomach 72 pills with good wine. To prepare this elixir an auspicious day should be chosen, and the preparation itself should not be done in the presence of women, chicken, and dogs.

Excrements of second generation silkworms
Vol. VIII, 39-17-02

Injuries received from a fall or a blow. With symptoms such as sprains and bones laying bare. Four ounces of silkworm excrements, fried until they have assumed a yellow color, four ounces of green bean powder fried until it has assumed a yellow color, and two ounces, four maces of calcined alum are ground to powder to be applied, mixed with vinegar, to the affected region. This is firmly wrapped with tough silk, with the bandage exchanged three or four times, until a cure is achieved. Pregnant women must not be permitted to get near such a treatment. *Tried and Proven Good Recipes of Shao, the Perfected one.*

Chinese scholar tree
Sophora japonica L. Vol. VII, 35-16

An effusion on the back with dissipated blood. Stir-fry one ounce each of Chinese scholar tree flowers and mung bean powder until they have assumed the color of ivory, and grind them into a powder. Boil one ounce of fine tea leaves in one bowl of water, let it remain in the open for one night, mix the liquid with three maces of the powder, and apply this to the affected region leaving the tip of the effusion uncovered. The medication should not be offended by the hands of married or unmarried females. *Miraculous Recipes to Conserve Life*.

Thunderball fungus
Polyporus mylittae Cook at Mass. Vol. VII, 37-05

Tao Hongjing: The *Original Classic* states: "It benefits husbands."

The *Supplementary Records by Famous Physicians* states: "Ingested for a long time it causes yin member (i.e., penis) dysfunction."

These statements contradict each other. Ma Zhi: The classic says that "it benefits husbands and does not benefit females." That is, it stimulates the movement of the original qi of males, and it does not stimulate the movement of the qi of long-term depots of females. Hence, it says that "ingesting it for a long time results in yin qi, (i.e., a female's qi) dysfunction."

Gekko
Gekko swinhonis Gunther. Vol. VIII, 43-07

Navel wind of children. Sever the back half of a gekko, bake it over a slow fire, and grind it to a powder. For a boy mix it with the milk produced by a nursing mother for a girl, and for a girl mix it with the milk for a boy. Add a small amount of chicken droppings and rub this on the root of the patient's tongue and his teeth. Also, dip your hand into the powder and massage the child until it sweats. Very wondrous. *Bifeng's Impromptu Poem Recipes*.

Human placenta
Vol. IX, 52-29

Placentas extend the years of life and benefit longevity. They have the power to enforce creating and transforming. Hence, one speaks of "great creation pills." When using a placenta, males use one from a female fetus, and females use one from a male fetus. Those of first born children are washed with the slop from rinsing rice. They are baked on a tile until they are dry, and then they are ground to powder. Or they are steamed with bland wine, pounded, dried in the sun, and ground to powder. This way, the strength of their qi is complete, and they have no fire poison. *Distinguishing Doubtful Points about All Disease Signs.*

The white section of onion stems
Allium fistulosum L. Vol. VI, 26-03-01

Sudden death following being struck by the malign. It may be that the patient had a disease before, or that a healthy person was at home lying in bed, with death occurring quickly. All these are cases of being struck by the malign. Quickly take a yellow onion heart and insert it into the patient's nose. For males on the left; for females on the right. Insert it seven to eight *cun* deep. Once blood is released from the nose and the eyes, the patient will regain consciousness.

Chinese *photinia* leaf
Photinia serrulata Lindl. Vol. VII, 36-27-01

The leaves nourish kidney qi, and serve to cure internal harm and yin qi weakness. They free the movement of sinews and bones and benefit skin and hair. *Original Classic.*

They heal weak legs, eliminate evil qi in the five long-term depots and remove heat. Females should not ingest them over a long time as they let them long for a male. *Supplementary Records by Famous Physicians.*

"Herb swaying even in the absence of wind." Unidentified
21-A102

Chen Cangqi: Worn on the body it stimulates love between husband and wife.

Li Shizhen: *Notopterygium, gastrodia,* umbrella leaf herb, and wood ragwort, these four items are all named "herb that sways by itself even when there is no wind," but they are different items.

Duan Chengshi in his *A Miscellany from Youyang* says: "From Yaozhou comes a 'dancing herb.' It has three leaves, similar to fetid *cassia.* One leaf is at the tip of the stem. The other two leaves are located in the middle of the stem facing each other. When a person gets close and sings a song or claps the hands the leaves move as if dancing."

My comment: This is the "herb to mislead a beautiful woman." It, too, is one of those that sway by themselves without wind.

Also, according to the *Classic of Mountains and Seas*, "on the mountains of Gu yao the daughter of an emperor died and transformed to an herb named *yao* 䔄. Its leaves form layers above each other. The flower is yellow. The fruits are similar to *cuscuta* seeds. When it is ingested by a female it makes her attractive."

Peach-shaped red *atractylodes*
Vol. IV, 15-25-A01

Chen Cangqi: Peach-shaped red *atractylodes* grows in gardens. It is as fine as Chinese celery. The flowers are purple; the seeds form protuberances. When the protuberances are struck with a mirror from the side, the seeds will be emitted. The seeds are gathered on the fifth day of the fifth month. Worn on her clothes they will seduce a male to make love with that woman.

Uncovered oil lamp
Vol. VIII, 38-56

On the 15th day of the first month steal an uncovered oil lamp from a rich family and place it under the bed. This will let the people having intercourse on it have a child. Li Shizhen.

Locust
Oxya chinensis Thunberg. Vol. VIII, 41-28

Wait for them to mate on the fifth day of the fifth month, and collect them. When husband and wife wear them on their garments, this will stimulate their mutual love. Chen Cangqi.

Thunderball fungus
Polyporus mylittae Cook at Mass. Vol. VII, 37-05

Control. Thunderbolt fungi kill the three kinds of worms/bugs. They eliminate poison qi and heat in the stomach. They benefit husbands; they do not benefit females. *Original Classic*.

Rubbed in water to make a paste, they eliminate the hundreds of diseases affecting children. They expel evil qi and malign wind responsible for sweating. They remove accumulations of bound heat in the skin and *gu*-poison, white worms/bugs and tapeworms that leave the body continuously without end. Ingested for a long time, they cause yin member (i.e., penis) dysfunction. *Supplementary Records by Famous Physicians.*

Songaria cynomorium herb. *Cynomorium songaricum* Rupr.
Vol. III, 12-13

Li Shizhen: Songaria *cynomorium* herb comes from Suzhou.

According to Tao Jiucheng's *Records Taken while Stopping from Field Work*, "songaria *cynomorium* herb grows on fields in the Tartar region. When the essence/sperm of wild horses or flood dragons drops down and enters the ground, after a long time songaria *cynomorium* herb develops and rises like bamboo shoots. It is rich/thick above and frugal/thin below. It has scales lying close to each other and interconnected sinew vessels. It very much resembles a male yang member (i.e., penis). It belongs to the same group as *cistanche deserticola*. Some say, when it is inserted into a lustful woman's vagina it will unite with her and she is given yin qi and will experience a violent, lengthy orgasm."

Arsenolite
Arsenic trioxide. Vol. II, 10-14

My elder brother Wen'an gong, stationed in Jinling, during hot weather in autumn lost his appetite. Tang Sanyi, a physician, advised him to ingest pills with arsenic trioxide. Then he drank and ate everyday, and satisfied by the effects of the medication he decided to ingest ever more. After ten months the poison began to work. Through nosebleed he lost more than one peck of blood. This happened again and again, and did not end. Eventually, he had lost all his essence liquid and died."

I, Li Shizhen, venture to say that Hong Wen'an's disease was not necessarily caused by the poison of the arsenic alone. The fact is, it was also caused by his forceful eating habits. He loved rich food and he exhausted himself with sexual intercourse. He indulged in his pleasures without restraint until eventually his essence/sperm was used up and he died. Now, he ingested arsenic trioxide because he had lost his appetite. Once he began to eat again, his disease was gone. This was the moment when he should have stopped taking this medication. Still, he continued to ingest it without end. For his presumptious lifestyle he relied on this medication. So how could his death be the fault of this medication?

Muscovite
Vol. II, 08-39

The Master Embracing Simplicity: Other items when buried will rot, when set afire they will be scorched. But muscovite in all five colors may be given into a fierce fire for quite some time and it will not be scorched, and when buried it will not rot. Hence those who ingest it will enjoy a long life. When they enter a water, they will not be affected by moisture, and when they enter a fire they will not burn. Treading on thorns they will not be harmed.

Li Shizhen: In former times the people said that corpses covered with muscovite will not rot. Once robbers opened the tomb of a noble woman named Feng. Her physical appearance was that of a living person. Hence they all raped her. When the tomb of Duke You of Jin was opened, 100 corpses lay there in all directions, with their clothes they looked as if they were still alive. The reason was that all of them had been covered with muscovite.

Litharge
Lead oxide. Vol. II, 08-14

Bone impediment-illness, with the bones protruding. Another name is "multiple kindred sores." When every now and then a fine bone appears, this is because a mother after having conceived, in her first month of pregnancy, has had intercourse with any of her six relations, affecting her essence qi. Hence this is called "multiple kindred sores." Prepare an equal mixture of litharge powder and *vernicia* oil and apply this to the affected region. *Recipes from the Realm of Longevity*.

Gekko
Gekko swinhonis Gunther. Vol. VIII, 43-07

Tao Hongjing: Gekkos love to be on fences and walls. One feeds them with cinnabar until they have assumed a weight of three *jin*, and then kills them. The dry powder is then applied to the body of women, and will fall off when they have sex. As long as they do not have sex, they will remain marked red. Hence gekkos are named "guardians of the palace." Now, lizards, too, are named "guardians of the palace," and this makes it difficult to distinguish between them. An example of such confusion is Dongfang Shuo's statement: "If it is not a guardian of the palace, then it is a lizard."

Su Gong: Gekkos are also named "scorpion tigers." Because they are always found on the walls of homes they are called "guardians of the palace," and also "palace protector." That they are fed with cinnabar to mark women is absurd rhetoric.

Dried ginger
Zingiber officinalis L. Vol. VI, 26-18

Yin and yang exchange disease. A woman, following a harm caused by cold episode, although she was cured, for the next 100 days she should not have intercourse with a man lest one of them or both fall ill with a tense contraction of hands and feet and an abdominal pain letting one wish to die. When the husband falls ill it is called "yin exchange." When the woman falls ill it is called "yang exchange." To cure them a sweating must be induced right away. After four days, it can no longer be healed. Grind four ounces of dried ginger into powder. Each time let the patient ingest half an ounce mixed with clear, boiled water. Cover the patient with clothing or a quilt. After a sweating the hands and the feet can be stretched out again, and that is the healing. *Categorized Essential Recipes on Harm caused by Cold.*

Allium sativum L. Hardneck garlic
Vol. VI, 26-09

Sun Simiao: Eating garlic in the fourth and eighth month harms the spirit, and causes panting with palpitation. It strengthens the taste sensation in the mouth. Eating a lot of fresh garlic and then engaging in sexual intercourse harms the liver qi and leads to a loss of complexion.

Slenderstyle *acanthopanax*
Acanthopanax gracilistylus W.W. Smith. Vol. VII, 36-23

In ancient times, Meng Chuozi and Dong Shigu said to each other that they preferred a handful of slenderstyle *acanthopanax* to a cart filled with gold and jade. That they preferred one pound of *sanguisorba* root to the precious pearl that glows in the dark.[28] Also, in ancient times, the mother of Duke Ding of Lu ingested slenderstyle *acanthopanax* wine. She escaped death and simply left her corpse and departed. Zhang Zisheng, Yang Ji-

---

28 A reference to a report in *Sou shen ji* ch. 20 of a severely injured snake that was saved by someone who put a medicinal bandage on. More than a year later the snake returned with a large pearl in its mouth that was sufficiently luminous to light up an entire chamber.

anshi, Wang Shucai and Yu Shiyan, they all ingested this wine and never stopped having sexual intercourse. Their long life lasted 300 years.

Pepper. *Piper nigrum*
Vol. VI, 32-06

Bedroom exhaustion and yin poison. Pound seven peppercorns, a two and a half *cun* long piece of an onion stalk with one-tenth of a mace of musk to a pulpy mass, mix it with melted beeswax, and form sticks. Insert them into the yin orifice (i.e., glans penis). After a short while the patient sweats and is cured. *Mr. Sun's Collected Efficacious Recipes.*

Depletion and weakness
Vol. I, 03-56-02.

For females with a presence of cold qi in the yin (i.e., genital) region, chew medicinal *evodia* fruit into a fine paste and insert it into the vagina. After an extended period of time it will burn like fire.

Schisandra chinensis Turcz. Baill
Vol V. 18-02

Failure of the yang affair (i.e., penis) to rise. Grind one pound of new schisandra chinensis into powder and with wine ingest the amount held by a square inch spoon. To be ingested three times a day. During this therapy pork, fish, garlic, and vinegar are to be avoided. When one dose is ingested for full, the patient will gain strength. After ingesting it for one hundred days or more, he can copulate with ten girls. If the ingestion of this medication is not stopped at any time during the four seasons, the function of this pharmaceutical drug will be apparent. *Recipes Worth a Thousand in Gold.*

Chinese *asparagus*
Asparagus cochinchinensis (Lour.) Merr. Vol. V, 18-22

Zhang Yuxi: *The Master Embracing Simplicity* says: "Those who enter the mountains to live there can simply steam or boil Chinese asparagus and eat it, and this is sufficient to stop eating grain. Strong persons may consume it for their pleasure. Or it is prepared into powder and ingested with wine. Or it is pounded and the resulting juice is prepared to a liquid that is ingested as a paste. After 100 days one's strength will have doubled, and this occurs even faster than following an ingestion of *atractylodes* rhizome or Solomon's seal root. Within 200 days it strengthens sinews and marrow, preserves a youthful complexion, and ingested prepared with heat refined pine resin and honey to pills, it is especially good. Du Ziwei ingested them and copulated with 80 concubines.

Garments worn during menstruation
Vol. IX, 52-16

Li Shizhen: When a woman enters her monthly period, she emits a malign fluid that has the stench of fish and is filthy. Hence a gentleman stays away from her. Because of her being unclean, she can harm his yang qi and generate disease. All those who prepare medications such as concocting a paste, who suffer from outbreaks of smallpox or who observe Buddhist discipline, and those who practice refinement of their nature to guard their life, they must avoid these women for this very reason.

Recurrent heat disease because of exhaustion through intercourse with women. A husband's heat disease had been cured and breaks out again following sexual intercourse. All of a sudden, his testicles are drawn into his intestines, and his intestines are so painful that he comes close to dying. Burn a garment of a woman that was turned red by her menstrual liquid and grind the residue to powder. The amount held by a square inch spoon is to be ingested with hot water. This will stabilize his condition. *Recipes of Bian Que.*

They resolve the poison of arrows and serve to cure relapse into diseases because of exhaustion from intercourse with women. Tao Hongjing.

Alum
Potash. Vol. II, 11-17

Yellow *dan*-illness of women. Irregular menstruation caused by abnormal sexual activity. Grind half an ounce each of white alum and yellow beeswax with three maces of tangerine peels to a powder. Transform it in beeswax to pills the size of *firmiana* seeds. Each time ingest 50 pills, to be sent down either with the "decoction to nourish blood" or with the "decoction to regulate menstruation."

Chinese small onion
Allium fistulosum L. Vol. VI, 26-03

Recurrence of harm caused by cold because of exhaustion through sexual intercourse, with abdominal pain and swollen testicles. Pound onion white into a pulpy mass and drink it mixed with one cup of bitter wine. *Recipes Worth a Thousand in Gold.*

Desert broomrape
Cistanche deserticola Y. C. Ma. Vol. II, 12-11

It supplements the center. It removes painful alternating sensations of cold and heat from within the penis. It nourishes the five long-term depots. It stiffens the yin (i.e., male member), it boosts the essence/sperm qi, and lets one have many children. It serves to cure concretion-illness and conglomeration-illness of women. ... It boosts the marrow, cheers up one's complexion, extends the years of life, massively supplements and strengthens the yang qi (i.e., male sexual strength), and more than doubles the daily performance of sexual intercourse. Zhen Quan.

Apricot leaf ladybell
Adenophora trachelioides Maxim. Vol. II, 12-05

Sun Simiao in his *Recipes Worth a Thousand in Gold* resorts to apricot leaf ladybell to cure the disease of stiff center, that is, when the penis extends in an erection, filled with essence/sperm, and ejaculates without intercourse.

Depletion and detriment
Vol. I, 03-34

Ginseng root. For five types of exhaustion, seven types of harm, in the case of qi depletion with much dreaming, add it to the medication to supplement the center and nourish the camp qi. For qi depletion, exhaustion and heat effusion, boil it in water together with sickle leaved hare's ear and ingest the liquid. For blood spitting after an exhausting sexual intercourse, boil ginseng alone in water and ingest the decoction.

Ashes of the tip of a writing brush
Vol. IX, 51-33-01

Ingested with water, they serve to cure blocked urination, frequent and difficult urination with dripping, swollen yin (i.e., genital region) and prolapsed anus, as well as being struck by the malign. *Materia Medica of the Tang.*

Two maces ingested with wine serve to cure penis dysfunction of males on the wedding night. *Discourse on the Properties of Pharmaceutical Substances.*

Polygonum hydropiper L. Water pepper fruit
Vol. IV, 16-47-

Relapse of harm caused by cold because of overexertion. When following sexual intercourse the testicles swell, or are drawn back with pain into the abdomen. Rub a handful of water pepper seeds in water and drink one ounce of the resulting juice. *Recipes to be Kept Close at Hand.*

Injured bladder
Vol. I, 04-39-08

Yellow, thin, tough silk (38-02). For women whose urinary bladder is injured during sexual intercourse or while giving birth, with unending dripping of urine, boil yellow, thin, tough silk until it has turned into a rotten matter in the juice obtained by pouring water on charcoal ashes, add beeswax, floss grass root, and puffball, boil this in water, and let the woman ingest the decoction every day. Another recipe recommends to grind it together with white *paeonia* tree bark and common *bletilla* into powder, boil it in water, and to let the woman ingest this every day.

Refined white human urine sediments
Vol. IX, 52-12

Ye Mengde in his *Records of Waters and Clouds* gave them highest praise as a refinement of yin and yang, while the *Records of Trivial Things* stated that "'autumn minerals' have a salty flavor and follow the blood, so that the water is unable to check the fire. If ingested over a long time autumn minerals let one develop a thirst ailment."

The fact is, this substance has undergone a refinement through calcination. Hence its qi are warmed. Those who ingest it are often licentious persons. They resort to this substance to engage in sex without limits. They deplete their yang qi by meaningless activity, and their true water is ever more dried up. How could it be that they do not develop thirst? Furthermore, when they engage in sex excessively, they add medication to increase their yang qi. Does not this support the evil fire?

Rhubarb root
Rheum palmatum L. Vol. IV, 17-01-01

Marriage pain of women, with a painful swelling of the vagina. Boil one ounce of rhubarb root in one ounce of wine to bubbling and let the woman ingest this all at once. *Recipes Worth a Thousand in Gold.*

Husked glutinous rice
Oryza sativa L. Vol. V, 22-10-01

White, turbid urination. The "white husked glutinous rice pills." They serve to cure persons whose nocturnal urine has a white, turbid sediment. Old persons and persons with a depletion often have this disease sign. It may result in their sudden death as it massively diminishes their essence/sperm fluid and is responsible for a dizzy and heavy head. Grind five pints of husked glutinous rice, stir-fried until it assumes a red-black color, and one ounce of *angelica dahurica* root into powder and with husked glutinous rice flour paste form pills the size of *firmiana* seeds. Each time ingest 50 pills, to be ingested with a climbing fig decoction. If that is not available, resort to the "decoction to supplement kidney qi" outlined in the *Recipes from the Pharmaceutical Bureau.* If the patient is a young man with a timid and weak constitution, who has had excessive sex, who has frequent urination, with his water ducts blocked and rough, and the urine assuming a consistency of a greasy paste, add Japanese sweet flag root and oyster shell powder, and that is very effective. *Tried and Proven Good Recipes.*

White overflow of females. Stir-fry equal amounts of coarse glutinous rice and Chinese pepper and grind them into powder. With vinegar and wheat flour paste form pills the size of *firmiana* seeds. Each time let the patient ingest 30 to 40 pills, to be send down prior to a meal with a vinegar decoction. Yang Qi, *Simple and Convenient Recipes.*

Japanese rough potato
Metaplexis japonica (Thunb.) Makino. Vol. V, 18-50

To supplement and boost the qi in the case of depletion and injury. It greatly boosts the qi in the case of exhaustion through sexual intercourse. Grind four ounces of *metaplexis japonica* and three ounces each of *lycium* root skin, *schisandra* seeds, *arborvitae* seed kernels, jujube kernels, and dried Chinese foxglove roots into powder. Each time ingest the amount held by a square inch spoon and send it down with wine. *Recipes Worth a Thousand in Gold.*

Tao Hongjing: *Metaplexis japonica* grows as a vine. When it is plucked, a white milk sap appears. People often plant it. It has thick, large leaves. It can be eaten raw, and it is steamed or cooked to be consumed. A saying goes: "When travelling 1,000 *li* away from home, do not eat *metaplexis japonica* and *lycium* leaves." That is to say, *metaplexis japonica* supplements and boosts essence/sperm qi and strengthens the yin path (i.e., male sexual potency) similar to *lycium* leaves.

Chinese *photinia* leaf
Photinia serrulata Lindl. Vol. VII, 36-27-01

Zhen Quan: Although the leaves of Chinese *photinia* can nourish the kidneys, they can also induce a yin (i.e., genital/sexual) dysfunction/impotence.

Li Shizhen: In ancient recipes they are an important pharmaceutical drug to cure blockage related to wind intrusion and kidney weakness. Today, people definitely do not know of their usage and very few people are familiar with them. The fact is, this is a result of Mr. Zhen Quan's report in his *Discourse on the Properties of Pharmaceutical Substances* of the potential of these leaves to cause yin (i.e., genital/sexual) dysfunction/impotence. They do not know that ingesting this pharmaceutical drug can strengthen the kidneys. People driven by lust resort to these leaves to indulge in sex without restraint until eventually this results in sexual dysfunction and impotence. When they blame the medication, this is truly regrettable.

Floss grass root
Imperata cylindrica (L.) Beauv. var. *major* (Nees) C. E. Hubb
Vol. III, 13-19

Five types of jaundice. They include yellow *dan*-illness, grain *dan*-illness, wine *dan*-illness, female *dan*-illness, and exhaustion *dan*-illness. Yellow sweat results from massive sweating and repeatedly entering water.[29] The body is slightly bloated and sweat leaves similar to the juice of *phellodendron* root. Prepare a gruel from a handful of fresh floss grass root, cut into small pieces, and one pound of pork, and ingest this. *Recipes to be Kept Close at Hand*.

---

29 *Ru shui* 入水, "to enter water," is also a reference to "having sexual intercourse."

Oil rape seeds
Brassica campestris L. Vol. VI, 26-11-02

Loss of essence/sperm while dreaming of sexual intercourse with demons. Sun Simiao.

Extract the oil and apply it to the patient's head to let the hair grow long and remain black. Chen Cangqi. It stimulates the passage of sluggish blood, breaks up cold qi accumulation, dissolves swelling, disperses nodular qi concretions, and serves to cure all types of illness in the central and abdominal region related to difficult delivery and following childbirth. Cinnabar red swelling with heat. Wounds caused by metal objects/weapons and bleeding piles. Li Shizhen.

Sumatra benzoin
Styrax benzoin Dryand. Vol. VII, 34-26

To treat women who dream of sexual intercourse with demons, burn it together with realgar and with the fumes steam the cinnabar field acupuncture needle insertion hole (CV 5, CV 7). The dreams end forever. Li Xun.

Burn it to drive away demons and invite spirits to come. Xiao Bing. It serves to cure being struck by the malign, nightmares, and exhaustion consumption through corpse qi transmission. Li Shizhen.

10. The significance of reproduction: Fertility and pregnancy, abortion and birth

Since the rise of Confucius's teachings to a dominant social ideology in China, a patrilinear orientation was pursued at least by the Han-Chinese upper social class. To achieve the required sex-selected reproduction generation after generation, attention was paid to female and child health quite early. Zhang Ji, author of the famous *Discourse on Harm Caused by Cold* of the 3rd c. CE, devoted almost 10% of the recipes collected in his *Essentials of the Golden Casket* to female health problems. In chapter 20 he discussed ailments related to pregnancy. In chapter 21 he focused on post-partum issues. Chapter 22 concentrated on "miscellaneous diseases" of women. One thousand years later, social and economic changes, as well as deliberate political initiatives during the Song era, lead to a new awareness of people's health. This also included women's reproductive well-being. A separate "specialty concerned with women" with its own literature emerged. Chen Ziming (1190 – 1270), one of the first influential authors of such texts, wrote a book "Good Recipes for a Complete Recovery of Women." He is often cited by Li Shizhen.

Charlotte Furth is right when she states: "Basic bodily functions, menstruation, conception, childbirth, lactation, stand across cultures as stable, materially grounded forms of human embodiment."[30] It is for this reason that when reading all the many recipes on the reproductive health of females encountered in the *Ben cao gang mu*, there is never a feeling of entering a foreign, or even mysterious cultural setting. All the essential reproductive organs, of males and females, outside and within were known for their position and function, probably since times immemorial. References to them are immediately understandable; they require no further explanation. Even the numerous magical interventions, mostly to ease birth, find their near-equivalents in the history of European medicine. Pouring wine through an iron muzzle-loading firearm and letting the mother-to-be drink it, or tying the bowstring from a crossbow around the woman's waist, these are pieces of advice meant to stimulate a release of the fetus as quickly as the firing of a bullet from a gun or a bolt from a crossbow. They were not enigmatic to a medieval European.

An intention to become pregnant requires not only a union of female and male essence. It requires that the woman be prepared to become preg-

---

30 Charlotte Furth, *A Flourishing Yin. Gender in China's Medical History, 960 – 1665.* University of California Press. Berkeley and Los Angeles, 1999, 14.

nant in the first place. Without any moralizing value judgement, the *Ben cao gang mu* offers advice on how to prevent conception and pregnancy either once or for good. Being prepared for conception may also be related to biological facts. The reproductive organs may be too cold and thus prevent pregnancy for years. The *Ben cao gang mu* offers recipes on how to generate the required warmth. A male partner's essence/sperm, too, may be too cold, or the amount given to the woman may be too scant. Recipes are available to change this.

Regardless of whether a pregnancy is desired or not, it is good for several reasons to know as soon as possible whether conception has occurred. Shen Gua (1031 – 1095), an often-quoted medical theorist, describes a pregnancy test and is quoted by Li Shizhen. If the pregnancy was undesirable for one reason or another, or even dangerous to health, the possibility of abortion remained. Both Confucianism and Buddhism are known to speak against abortion. Apparently, in the health care arena as defined by Li Shizhen, such objections need not be mentioned. Different ways to end a pregnancy were outlined in detail. However, experience with such remedies had also shown that they are not always harmless to pregnant women and can be fatal. This has to be taken into account.

A pregnancy test could also reveal the sex of the fetus. In the previous section, we have already learned of methods believed suitable for changing a female into a male fetus. A woman who wants to make very sure that she gives birth to a boy in the first place, is, for example, advised to hold in her hands while pregnant certain items associated with malehood. The size of the fetus is another issue discussed during pregnancy. Zhu Zhenheng (1281 – 1358), influential medical theorist, knew what he spoke of when he told the story of his sister. She was overweight and rarely moved, and because his family was not rich, she was to take supplemental medication to ease her delivery. This, he explained, was the opposite of expectant mothers from the affluent upper class. They, too, were obese, but the reason was good food. They, too, rarely moved, but the reason was that they were waited upon by servants. Their fetuses most likely were already oversized in the womb, with a difficult birth highly likely. Methods were also developed to "shrink a fetus to ease delivery."

Pregnancy can be accompanied by numerous health problems. Women may experience painful urination. They may be plagued by edematose swelling rising in the body from the toes. They may complain of lower back pain. A woman may lose blood or yellow fluid, a condition called "leaking fetus." The fetus may move and push against the woman's heart.

Excessive sexual intercourse may cause such movement and result in the expectant mother's critical condition. Stimuli are known to cause a child to develop congenital birth defects. It may have a dark face or a sixth finger. This is to be prevented.

When delivery is due, the position of the fetus should permit a smooth release. A transverse position is to be corrected. In unfortunate cases, when a child has died in the mother's abdomen and fails to be delivered, methods are recommended for aborting it. Eventually, the due date arrives. Numerous interventions were believed to ease birth, including manual therapies, ingestions of medication, and magic spells. Single Chinese characters were to be written, for example, on a lotus flower then eaten by the woman, or a castor bean pulp was to be applied to the soles of the mother's feet. Not every child seems to know when its due date has arrived; some are known to be born even 15 months after conception.

Many references dealing with fertility, pregnancy and delivery can be found scattered throughout the *Ben cao gang mu*. Taken together, they offer a more comprehensive overview of these facets of ancient Chinese culture than does any other early work.

Chinese ash tree bark
Fraxinus rhynchophylla Hance. Vol. VII, 35-19

Li Shizhen: Chinese ash tree bark is greenish in color; its qi are cold. The flavor is bitter and by its nature it is astringent. Hence, it is a pharmaceutical drug for the ceasing yin liver and minor yang gallbladder conduits. It is for this reason that when it serves to cure diseases of the eyes and fright epilepsy one takes advantage of its ability to balance/level the qi of the phase of wood. When it is used to cure discharge with free-flux illness, collapsing center, and discharge from below the belt, one takes advantage of its ability to gather and astringe. In addition, it can serve to cure a diminished essence/sperm amount released by males. It boosts the essence and lets him have children. For all these therapeutic ends one takes advantage of its potential to astringe and supplement.

Husked glutinous rice
Oryza sativa L. Vol. V, 22-10-01

Long-lasting outflow with a decrease in the amount of food eaten. Soak one ounce of *nuo mi* in water for one night. Drip off the water and dry the *nuo mi.* Slowly stir-fry it until done, grind it and pass it through a sieve. Add to the powder one ounce of Chinese yam. Every morning add to half a cup of this powder two spoons of sugar and a little Chinese pepper powder, mix it with hot water by forcefully stirring it and eat this. It has an extremely good flavor, and is very nourishing. Ingested over a long time it warms a man's essence/sperm and lets him have children. A secret recipe. Songhuang, *Tried and Proven Recipes.*

Wheat
Triticum aestivum L. Vol. V, 22-04

It eliminates visitor heat and ends vexing thirst with a dry pharynx. It stimulates urination, nourishes the liver qi, and ends blood leaking and blood spitting. It helps women to get pregnant easily. *Supplementary Records by Famous Physicians.*

Sichuan lovage
Ligusticum chuanxiong Hort. Vol. III, 14-02

Pregnancy test when the menstruation is blocked. A method to make a pregnancy test when there has been no menstruation for three months. Grind unprepared Sichuan lovage to powder, boil it with common mugwort, and ingest this decoction, as much as is held by a spoon, on an empty stomach. If this stimulates a slight movement in the abdomen, it is a fetus. If no movement results, there is no fetus. *Recipes from the Numinous Garden.*

The white section on onion stems
Allium fistulosum L. Vol. VI, 26-03-01

Movement of a fetus in the sixth month of a pregnancy, entering a critical condition that makes it difficult to save the child. Boil one generous handful of onion white in three pints of water down to one ounce, remove the dregs, and let the woman ingest the liquid all at once. *Mr. Yang's Book on Childbirth and Nursing.*

Movement of a fetus with a discharge of blood, with pain in the lower back knocking against the heart. Boil onion white to obtain a thick juice and let the woman ingest it. If the fetus has not yet died, it will be calmed. If it has already died, it will be released. If no effect shows, let her ingest the juice a second time. Another recipe: Add Sichuan *ligusticum* root. Another recipe: Boil the juice in a silver vessel together with husked rice to prepare a congee and a thick soup and let her eat this. *Recipes of Master Mei.*

Masaikai cape
Capparis masaikai Lévl. Vol. VI, 31-30

For difficult childbirth, when the time has come chew several seed kernels to a fine mass and send it down with well splendor water. The effect takes place after a short time. Then remove the shell of four seed kernels and let the woman hold two of them in each hand. This leads to a discharge of lochia. If you wish to end birthing, regularly chew two seed kernels and send the resulting pulp down with water. After a long time the uterus will be cold and she will not become pregnant. Wang Ji.

Wheat flour
Vol. V, 22-04-04

Contraception for women. Boil one ounce of white wheat flour in one ounce of wine to bubbling, remove the dregs, and ingest the liquid divided into three portions. To be ingested at night the day before menstruation sets in, the next day in the early morning and during the day.

Black soybeans
Glycine max (L.) Merr. Vol. V, 24-01

Lower back pain during pregnancy. Boil one ounce of soybeans in three pints of wine down to seven *ge* and let the woman drink this on an empty stomach. *Heart Mirror of Diet Physicians.* ... A child has died in the abdomen prior to the due date, with the mother feeling heart-pressure as if she was going to die. Boil three pints of soybeans in vinegar to obtain a thick juice and let her ingest it all at once. The dead child will be released immediately. *Collected and Proven Recipes for Childbirth and Nursing.*

Wild hop
Humulus scandens (Lour.) Merr. Vol. V, 18-54

Sweating of blood of a woman giving birth, with her clothes turned red. Recipe identical with the one above.

Red mung bean
Vigna umbellata (Thunb.) Ohwi et Ohashi. Vol. V, 24-04.

When a few months into pregnancy menstruation sets in, that is called "leaking fetus." If it is caused because of chamber (i.e., sexual) activity, it is called "harmed fetus." Let the woman ingest red mung bean powder with warm wine. Three times a day. End this therapy when an effect is achieved. Li Shizhen, quoted from *Recipes for Universal Benefit*.

Failure of the placenta to come down. Let the mother swallow red mung beans with water flowing toward the East. If the child borne is a boy, she ingests seven beans. If it is a girl, two times seven beans. *Recipes for Rescue in Emergencies.*

Job's tears
Coix lacryma L. Vol. V, 23-16

It serves to discharge the three types of worms/bugs. *Original Classic.*

Boiled in water and eaten prepared as a very fragrant gruel, it removes roundworms. Very effective.

Tao Hongjing. Boiled in water and ingested, it causes abortion.

Broomcorn millet
Panicum miliaceum L. Nonglutinous panicled millet. Vol. V, 23-01

Difficult delivery with transverse position. On the double yang day (ninth day of the ninth month) dry broomcorn millet root, also called "dragon with claws," in the yin (i.e., shade), burn it with its nature retained, and grind it into powder. Let the woman ingest with wine two maces and the child will come down.

Polished, non-glutinous rice
Vol. V, 22-11

Abdominal pain caused by fetal movement, with a sudden discharge of yellow juice. Boil five pints of polished, non-glutinous rice and six ounces of *astragalus* root in seven pints of water down to two pints and ingest this divided into four portions. *Sheng hui.*

Japanese brome
Bromus japonicus Thunb. Vol. V, 22-07

A fetus has died in the abdomen, and the placenta does not descend, striking upward against the heart. Boil one handful of Japanese brome in five pints of water down to two pints and let the woman ingest this warm. *Secret Records About Children and Mothers.*

Seeds of Chinese lantern plant
Physalis alkekengi L. var. *franchetii* (Mast.) Makino. Vol. IV, 16-16-02

The "pills with Chinese lantern plant fruit." They serve to cure hidden heat in the Triple Burner, the intestines and the stomach, as well as fetal heat and difficult delivery of women. Use the following items. Five ounces of Chinese lantern plant fruit. Three ounces of *amaranth* fruit. Three ounces of Chinese iris seeds. Two ounces each of large salt chunks and Siberian elm bark, fried. One ounce each of *bupleurum* root, *scutellaria* root, *trichosanthes* root, and spurge. Grind them into powder and form with heat prepared honey pills the size of *firmiana* seeds. Each time ingest 30 pills, to be sent down with *costus* root decoction. *General Records of Sagely Benefaction.*

Yellow day lily
Hemerocallis citrina Baroni. Vol. IV, 16-06

Master Dong Zhongshu states: "If you wish to let someone forget his worries, send him yellow day lilies as a present, because they are also named 'forget your worries'." The seedling is boiled to be eaten. It has qi and flavor similar to onions. There are nine types of herbs eaten by deer to resolve poison, and yellow day lilies are one of them. Therefore it is also called "deer's onion."

Zhou Chu in his *Records of Customs and Geographical Surroundings* states: "When a pregnant woman wears this flower at her belt, she will give birth to a boy." Hence it is named "suitable to attract a male."

Loving bamboo juice. *Phyllostachys nigra* (Lodd. ex Lindl.) Munro var. *henonis* (Mitf.) Stapf ex Rendle. Vol. VII, 37-13-14.

Fetal movement in women. When a pregnant woman, following a sexual intercourse activity by her husband, is in a critical condition. Let her drink one ounce of bamboo juice and she will be cured immediately. *Jewels of Childbirth.*

Indian lotus rootstock
Nelumbo nucifera Gaertn. Vol VI, 33-10

Harm caused by cold of women during pregnancy, with massive heat and vexing thirst, threatening to harm the qi of the fetus. Grind half an ounce of tender, curled lotus leaves, baked over a slow fire, and two and a half maces of fresh water mussel powder into a powder. Each time let the woman ingest three maces, to be ingested mixed with newly drawn water to which is added some honey. Also, apply this to her abdomen. The recipe is called "powder to cover the fetus." *Mr. Zheng's Recipes.*

Fetal movement during pregnancy, with yellow water already appearing. Grind one roasted lotus leaf stalk into powder, mix it with one wine cup of water in which glutinous rice has been washed and let the woman ingest this to calm the fetus. *Tried and Proven Recipes.*

Male cinnamon
Cinnamomum cassia Presl. Vol VII, 34-04-03

Cinnamon by its nature is acrid and disperses. It is able to penetrate the uterus and break up blood accumulation. Hence, the *Supplementary Records by Famous Physicians* says that it induces abortion.

Pang Anshi states that once it is stir-fried it no longer harms the fetus.

Rape turnip
Brassica rapa L. Vol. VI, 26-15

Rough urination during pregnancy. Ingest with water rape turnip seed powder, the amount held by a square inch spoon. To be ingested twice a day. *Secret Records About Children and Mothers.*

Root, vine and leaf of grape vine
Vitis vinifera L. Vol. VI, 33-03-02

Boil them in water to generate a thick juice and drink it in small portions to stop vomiting and retching, and nausea in the aftermath of cholera. When the child in a pregnant woman rises and rushes against the heart, let her drink the juice. The fetus descends again and remains quiet. Meng Shen.

Nutgrass
Cyperus rotundus L. Vol. III, 14-30.

To correct the position of a fetus when delivery is imminent. Let the woman ingest this in the ninth or tenth month and she will deliver without fright and fear. The "powder for the good fortune of a fetus." Grind four ounces of nutgrass, three ounces of *amomum villosum* kernels, fried, and one ounce of *glycyrrhiza* root, roasted, to powder. Each time let her ingest two maces, to be sent down with a rice beverage. *Mr. Zhu's collected and Proven Recipes.*

Peach seed kernels
Amygdalus persica L. Vol. VI, 29-06-03

Women with difficult childbirth, when the child does not come out for several days. Open a peach kernel. On one of the pieces write the character for "can"; on the other write the character for "come out." Let the woman ingest them and the child will be born. *Recipes with the Superfluous Deleted.*

Amaranth
Amaranthus tricolor L. Vol. VI, 27-10.

Meng Shen: On the fifth day of the fifth month collect *amaranthus tricolor*. Mix it with an equal amount of purslane and grind it into fine powder. Let a pregnant woman eat this regularly and she will have an easy delivery. Zhu Zhenheng: Red amaranth prefers to enter the blood section. For this reason, when it is ingested together with *amaranthus tricolor* it can send down a fetus. Or, when it is boiled in water it eases delivery.

Zingiber officinale L. Fresh ginger
Vol. VI, 26-17

Tao Hongjing: Ingested over a long time, it weakens one's mind and knowledge, and harms the qi of the heart. Ginger is the most often consumed acrid, peppery item today. Hence, the *Analects* of Confucius states: "In every meal, do not omit ginger." That is to say, it can be eaten continuously, but not in great amounts. For patients it may be appropriate.

Su Gong: The *Original Classic* says: "Ginger ingested for a long time enables communication with spirit brilliance and it controls phlegm qi disorder." That is, it may be eaten continuously. What Mr. Tao Hongjing says on this has no factual basis.

Sun Simiao: Those who eat much ginger in the eighth and ninth month often suffer from ailments of the eyes in spring. It is detrimental to longevity and diminishes the strength of the sinews. When pregnant women eat it, their child will have a surplus finger.

Rice vinegar
Vol. V, 25-23-01

A dead fetus does not come down, prior to the due date. Boil soybeans in vinegar and let the woman ingest three pints. The fetus will separate itself instantly. If it fails to come down, let the woman ingest the liquid a second time. *Secret Records About Children and Mothers.*

The placenta fails to come down. When the woman has a feeling of fullness in her abdomen, that will kill her. Add water to a little vinegar and spirt it out of your mouth on the woman's face. Divinely effective. *Sagely and Benevolent Recipes.*

Fermented soybean. Soybean relish
Vol.V, 25-01

Difficult birth. When an infant's headrest is broken and the child is enclosed by decayed blood. Remove the decayed blood with the "powder superior to gold" and the birth will proceed smoothly. Wrap one ounce of salted soybean relish in an old, greenish piece of cloth, heat it until it has turned red, grind it into a fine powder, add one mace of musk, and grind this into powder. Heat a counterpose until it has turned red, dip it into wine, and let the woman ingest one generous bowl of the wine mixed with the aforementioned powder. *Guo Jizhong's Recipes.*

Sprouted naked barley
Vol. V, 20-18-03

To abort a fetus during pregnancy. The Arcane Essential Recipes from the Outer Censorate recommends to cure a pregnant woman who wishes to abort a fetus as follows. Let her ingest one ounce of sprouted barley with one ounce of honey, and the fetus will be discharged.

Yeast/ferment made of husked rice
Vol. V, 25-15-01

A fetus moves and fails to rest, or it moves up and pushes against the heart, with a discharge of blood. Grind a fresh yeast cake into powder, mix it with water, squeeze it to obtain a juice, and let the woman ingest three pints. *Recipes to be Kept Close at Hand*.

White Egyptian kidney bean
Dolichos lablab L. Vol. V, 24-12-01

Poisonous medication to induce an abortion. When females ingest herbal pharmaceutical drugs to induce an abortion and suffer from abdominal pain. Remove the skin from fresh, white Egyption kidney beans and grind them into powder. Let the woman ingest, with a rice beverage, the amount held by a square inch spoon. To boil the beans in water to obtain a thick juice and drink this, is possible, too. Whenever the qi of the fetus are damaged by ingesting such pharmaceutical drugs with the fetus not aborted, the mother may be affected by lockjaw and stiff hands, spontaneous sweating and lowered head, similar to wind stroke. Nine patients die and only one survives. Physicians often fail to recognize the true cause of this condition and cure a wind stroke. This results in the patient's death, without any doubt.

Sesamum indicum L. Sesame
Vol. V, 22-01

A fetus has died in the abdomen. Give equal amounts of clear sesame seed oil and honey into hot water and let the woman ingest it all at once. *Recipes of Universal Benefit*.

Leaking fetus and difficult delivery. The reason is dryness and a rough passage of blood. Boil half an ounce of clear sesame seed oil and one ounce of good honey together several tens of times to bubbling and let the woman ingest this warm. The child will come down smoothly. When other medication has proved to be inadequate, this recipe effectively assists the blood. *What one should know about pregnancy and birth*.

"Double head lotus." Unidentified
Vol. V, 21-A143

Li Shizhen: Alternative name: The "herb that expedites delivery." Control: Women with difficult delivery. They should hold it in their left hand and will give birth.

Dutchman's pipe
Aristolochia debilis Sieb. et Zucc. Vol. V, 18-64.

Water swelling during pregnancy. It begins from the two feet and gradually reaches upward until it causes panting and heart-pressure, similar to water. Water comes out of the toes. This is called "child qi." It is related to a long-lasting presence of wind qi in the pregnant woman, or to a blood and wind intrusion in the throughway and controller vessels. In such a situation decoctions for water disorder must not be given indiscriminately. The "powder with dutchman's pipe" is appropriate. Grind equal amounts of dutchman's pipe, washed and slightly stir-fried, nutgrass, stir-fried, tangerine peels, *glycyrrhiza* root, and *lindera* root into powder. Each time let the patient ingest three maces. Boil one such dose in one large cup of water with three ginger slices, three quince slices, and three *perilla* leaves down to 70% and let the patient ingest this on an empty stomach. To be ingested three times a day. When the urine flows freely, the movement of qi in the vessels is unimpeded, and the swelling gradually decreases, do not ingest much more. This is a secret recipe of Chen Jingchu, a renowned physician in Huainan. It was obtained from Li Boshi's family. Chen Ziming, *Good recipes for Women*.

Human abnormalities
Vol. IX, 52-37

When a fetus has reached the tenth month, it will be born. That is the general principle. But there are those that are born after seven or eight months, or as late as after 12 or 13, even 14 or 15 months. These are sometimes said to be cases of "qi depletion." Wang Bing, *Secret Conversations on the Mysterious Pearl*.

Touch-me-not
Impatiens balsamina L. Vol. IV, 17-32

To hasten birth in cases of difficult delivery. Grind two maces of touch-me-not seeds into powder and let the woman ingest it with water. It must not come close to her teeth. For an external application, pound a number of castor beans corresponding to her age and apply the resulting pulp to the soles of her feet. *Simple Recipes from the Collection of Li Binhu*.

Assumption lily root
Hosta plantaginea (Lam.) Ascherson. Vol. V, 17-31-01

To end the reproductive faculties of a woman. Pound one and a half maces of assumption lily root and white touch-me-not seeds, two and a half maces of trumpet flower and two maces of cinnabar into powder and form with honey pills the size of *firmiana* seeds. Ingest them with half a cup of wine within 30 days after a birth. They must not touch the teeth. They could injure the teeth. *Selected Profound Recipes.*

Daphne flower
Daphne Genkwa Sieb. et Zucc. Vol. IV, 17-36

To speed up birth and remove a dead fetus. Cut the skin from a daphne flower root, wrap it in silk fabric, dip it in musk, and insert it three inches deep into the woman's yin opening (i.e., vagina). This serves to discharge the baby/fetus. *Miraculous Recipes to Conserve Life.*

Sweet basil
Ocimum basilicum L. Vol. III, 14-43-01

To interrupt the ability of women to give birth. Grind sweet basil to powder and ingest with wine two maces. Each time ingest up to one ounce and there will be no pregnancy for one year. The fact is, when blood smells fragrance it will disperse. *Collected Essentials from the Forest of Medicine.*

Undigested soybeans in ox dung
Vol. IX, 50-05-36

Women with difficult birth. One soybean found in ox dung is cut in two pieces. Write the character for "father" on one of them, and the character for "child" on the other. Then add them together again, have the mother swallow them with water, and she will deliver immediately. Zan Yin, *Jewels of Childbirth.*

Lotus flower
Nelumbo nucifera Gaertn. 33-10-07

To speed up the birthing process when delivery is difficult. Take one lotus flower leaf, write the character 人, "human," on it and let the woman swallow it. That makes the birth easier. *Recipes to be Kept Close at Hand.*

Xylosma congestum (Lour.) Merr. Shiny *xylosma* tree bark
Vol. VII, 36-41-01

Women with difficult childbirth. The "beverage with shiny *xylosma* wood to expedite birth." Regardless of whether a transverse position or a breech position is concerned, or whether the fetus has died in the abdomen, an application of this beverage has often been effective. It is a recipe of Zhang Buyu from Shang cai. Wash a one foot long piece of a big shiny *xylosma* twig clean. Break it into one inch long pieces and do the same with a big *glycyrrhiza* root. Put both items with three and a half pint of newly drawn water into a new earthenware jar and firmly seal it with three layers of paper. Heat it over a mild fire first and a strong fire later until one and a half pint of the liquid are left. Wait until the woman feels a painful heaviness in her lower back and abdomen and wishes to take place on straw to give birth. Then she should drink one cup of the warm liquid. This will immediately give her a feeling of physical relaxation below her heart. She should drink one more cup, eventually up to three or four cups, and when she has a sensation of heaviness in her lower body parts she will give birth without any further trouble. Still, she should not get down on the straw too early, as is the case if her delivery is accompanied by an incompetent old woman/midwife. Zan Yin, *Jewels of Childbirth.*

Iron muzzle-loading firearm
Vol. II, 08-28-03

To hasten birth, heat it until it is red, pour wine into the muzzle, and let it flow out again through the hole further down in the barrel. Have the woman drink the wine while it is still hot, and this prompts the birth of the child. An old muzzle-loader is especially good.

Winged spindle tree
Euonimus alatus (Thunb.) Sieb. Vol. VII, 36-19

Blood decay following birth. An infant's headrest hardening with intermittent pain, or an internal attack by wind and cold taking advantage of a woman's qi depletion following birth, with uncomfortable lochia and a hardened distension of the navel and abdominal region. The powder with Chinese *angelica* root. Prepare a mixture of one ounce each of Chinese *angelica* root, stir-fried, winged spindle tree twigs, with the core wood removed, and safflowers. Each time ingest three maces, boiled in one large cup of wine down to 70%, to be ingested warm prior to a meal. *Recipes from the Pharmaceutical Bureau.*

Bitter orange
Citrus aurantium L. Vol. VII, 36-05

The *Recipes of Du Ren* has a record of "the Princess of Huyang who suffered from difficult childbirth. A recipe master introduced a 'beverage for emaciating a fetus.' This recipe suggests to grind four ounces of bitter orange fruits and two ounces of *glycyrrhiza* root into a powder and each time ingest one mace, to be ingested dripped into clear, boiled water. If this is ingested once a day beginning the with the fifth month of a pregnancy until the month of the due date, it not only eases delivery it also prevents malign diseases in the fetus."

Zhang Jiegu in his *Crucial Points of the Laws of Life* changed this to "pills with bitter oranges and *atractylodes macrocephala* rhizome" to be ingested every day. They let a fetus remain emaciated and ease birth. They are called "pills to restrain the growth of a fetus."

Now, Kou Zongshi in his *Extended Meanings of Materia Medica* says: "When a fetus is robust, the child has strength and is born easily. If the mother is asked to ingest bitter orange medication, the mother, contrary to one's intentions, will have no strength and the child, too, has weak qi and is difficult to nourish. When it is said 'to shrink a fetus to ease delivery,' this is certainly not the case."

To consider this rationally, Mr. Kou Zongshi's statement seems to get straight to the point. If prior to delivery a woman experiences an obstruction and sluggishness of abounding qi, it is advisable to use such medication. For the so-called eighth, ninth month fetus it is required to use bitter orange fruits and *perilla* stalks to adjust the flow of qi. If there is no qi stagnation prior to birth, there will be no depletion after delivery. For persons endowed with weak qi, this medication is entirely inappropriate.

Zhu Zhenheng: Difficult births are often seen in persons with pent-up qi, heart-pressure having an easy and comfortable life, in households of the rich and noble that are supported and waited upon. The "beverage to emaciate a fetus" was designed for the Princess of Hu yang. My own sister suffered from difficult childbirth. She was fat and loved to sit. I reckoned that she was exactly the opposite of the princess. The qi of persons supported and waited upon must be replete. Hence, their qi are diminished to reach a balanced state allowing for an easy delivery. Here now, my sister was fat and her qi were depleted. And as she sat down for long times, her qi did not move. Hence, it was essential to support the qi of the mother. She was let to ingest a *perilla* beverage with a medication designed to increase her qi ten times or more and eventually experienced a quick delivery.

Frankincense
Boswellia carteri Birdw. Vol. VII, 34-22

The *Sagely and Benevolent Recipes* recommends to grind a bean-size piece of transparent frankincense into a powder, put it in one cup of newly drawn water, and add a little vinegar. Let the woman in labor hold with both hands a spirifer fossil, recite "looking forward to medication" three times, and drink the liquid. Then she walks several steps and the child comes down.

To accelerate childbirth if delivery is difficult. The *Simple and Convenient Recipes to Benefit the Masses* recommends to grind five maces of yellow, transparent frankincense into a powder. Mix it with a sow's blood and form pills the size of *firmiana* seeds. Each time let the woman ingest with wine five pills.

The *Tried and Proven Recipes* recommends to perform the following on the fifth day of the fifth month at noon. Let one person stand inside the house at a wall holding a mortar in his hands. On the outside of that wall a boy sends by means of a writing pen tube frankincense pellets one by one through a crack in the wall to the person inside to grind them in the mortar into fine pieces to be formed with water to pills the size of *Euryale* seeds. Each time let the woman ingest one pill, to be sent down with ash-free wine.

Bugleweed
Lycopus lucidus Turcz. Vol. III, 14-45

Wounds caused by metal objects/weapons. Swelling and sores with pus related to obstruction-illness. *Original Classic.*

Stagnant blood blocking the vagina following a wound caused by a knife during birth. *Supplementary Records by Famous Physicians.*

Abdominal pain following delivery. Blood and qi weakness and cold following several births, resulting in exhaustion and emaciation. Blood dripping and lower back pain of women.

Medicinal *evodia* fruit
Evodia rutaecarpa (Juss.) Benth. Vol. VI, 32-08.

Cold in the yin (i.e., private, genital region) of women, letting her have
no children for ten years. Grind one ounce each of medicinal *evodia* fruit
and prickly-ash from Sichuan into a powder and form with heat prepared
honey pills the size of bullets. Wrap them in silk floss and insert one of
them into her yin orifice (i.e., vagina). Replace them daily. This will open
her uterus and she can have children. *Records of the Core of Classics*.

Iron axe
Vol. II, 08-28-04

Li Shizhen: A method practiced by the ancients to change a female into a
male is as follows. "The third month of a pregnancy is called 'beginning of
the fetus'. Its blood does not yet flow through the vessels, and the physical
appearance undergoes a change. At this time it is suitable to ingest medication and to place an axe at the bottom of her bed, fastened in a way
that the blade is directed downward. The woman must not be informed
of this." There were those who doubted the effects of this method and
failed to believe in it. They tested it on chicken and, as a result, the chicks
in the nest were all males. The method of fetus transformation is based
on natural principles. Hence, to eat roosters is to obtain yang essence as
perfect as it is produced by heaven. To wear realgar on one's garments is
to obtain yang essence as perfect as it is produced by the earth. To hold a
bow and arrows, and to handle axes and weights, is to acquire hard items
evidently used by male humans. Corresponding qi invisibly affect each
other, resulting in the creation's secret alterations – and these are unavoidable consequences of the principles underlying all items. Hence, when
pregnant women see spirit images or strange items, they will often give
birth to ghosts and monsters. This is the proof. The line design of ivory
and rhinoceros horns follows that of elephants. The physical appearance
of *dioscorea* root and *celosia* flower changes in accordance with the physical
appearance of the humans raising them. To inform the spirit of the kitchen
stove with chicken eggs results in the hatching of nestlings. To brush cats
with a broom made of rushes lets them become pregnant. If items are re-
sponsive to such affects, how much more does this apply to humans!

Chen Cangqi: When one has tumorous flesh growths on his body, as soon
as he hears the sound of a nail struck into someone's coffin with an axe, he
should immediately stroke these flesh growths with his hands two times

seven times. As a result, some time later, they will dissolve and the surface will be flat again. Women giving birth must not apply this treatment.

Straw shoe
Vol. VIII, 38-21

To hasten childbirth. Wash a worn straw sandal found at the roadside clean and burn it to ashes. Let the woman ingest with wine two maces. If the sandal found was for a left foot, the child to be born will be male. If it was for a right foot, it will be a girl. If it had lain upside down, the child will be dead. It if had lain on its side, the child will suffer from fright. These are the principles of nature. *Mr. Xu's Recipes for Pregnancy and Birth.*

Bowstring and crossbow string
Vol. VIII, 38-43

Tao Hongjing: For difficult birth, wind a bowstring or crossbow string around the woman's waist. Also, burn the trigger of a crossbow, put it in wine, and let the woman drink it. All these therapies are based on the idea of the ability of bows and crossbows to release their arrows quickly.

Li Shizhen: To hasten birth with a bowstring and a crossbow string makes use of their ability to quickly send something off. To end bleeding with broken bowstrings makes use of their being ruptured.

The *Record of Rites* states: "When a boy is born, shoot with a bow made from mulberry wood arrows made from fleabane into the four cardinal directions to demonstrate the tasks of boys."

Chao Yuanfang in his discourse on how to educate an embryo states: "When a woman is in the third month pregnant and wishes to give birth to a boy she should hold a bow and arrows while riding a male horse."

Sun Simiao in his *Recipes Worth a Thousand in Gold* states: "When a woman just notices that she is pregnant, she should take a bowstring or a crossbow string, put it in a pouch, and wear it on her left arm. This will transform a girl fetus into a boy fetus."

The *Classic of the Chambers* states: "Whenever you realize that a woman is pregnant, take a bowstring or crossbow string and tie it around her waist. After one hundred days untie it again. This is a secretly transmitted recipe of the Jade Girl in the Purple Mansion."

Oil rape seeds
Brassica campestris L. Vol. VI, 26-11-02

Li Shizhen: The therapeutic potential of oil rape seeds and leaves is identical. Their flavor is acrid and their qi are warm. They can warm and they can disperse. They are especially useful to stimulate the movement of sluggish qi, and to break up qi nodes. Hence, ancient recipes use them in all types of medication to cure painful qi and blood disorder in the central and abdominal region following childbirth, all types of roaming wind cinnabar-red poison, and sores and piles associated with heat and swelling. Following menstruation they let the women add them to the "decoction with four items," claiming that this prevents further conception.

11. Case records:
Assessment and justification of therapeutic strategies

Li Shizhen's *Ben cao gang mu* is the first truly inclusive encyclopedia of natural history and pharmacotherapy in China. Nothing comparable existed in the medical literature earlier in China and elsewhere on the Eurasian continent. *Materia medica* literature had hitherto been dedicated to the description of individual substances. It was Li Shizhen who integrated numerous assessments of therapeutic interventions. Records of individual therapies have a long history in China, reaching back to divinatory writings on bones during the Shang era. The grand historian Sima Qian included in his *Historical Records* of 90 BCE in the biography of the physician Chunyu Yi 淳於意 (205 – 150 BCE) examples of his treatments. Beginning with the Yuan dynasty, an increasing number of physicians chose to publish characteristic (and successful) examples of therapies they had performed. Their intention most likely was to transmit their own understanding of proper medicine and health care.

At a time when no licensing boards existed to certify the competence of a healer, various methods of advertising one's skills were applied. Healers did not want merely to impress a still skeptical public. Often enough, the family and friends of a patient had enough medical knowledge to critically observe an unknown practitioner's approaches. During the Ming, as Christopher Cullen has shown,[31] records of therapeutic performances developed to a point where they formed a literary genre of its own, focussing on "medical cases," a term deliberately resonating with the term "legal cases." Medical practice, despite an increased influx of persons well educated in Confucian and other scholarship, still required all types of efforts if it was to be recognized as a pursuit worthy of a gentleman. Proof of two millennia of literacy, from the ancient classics to the present, was one of the avenues chosen to reach a higher status.

Li Shizhen was not interested in proving his own expertise when he integrated reports of therapies in his *materia medica* work. His motivation appears to have been different. A rich literature of case records already stood at Li Shizhen's disposal. He quoted not only ordinary case records left behind by physicians. What he wanted to say he also illustrated with anecdotes found in non-medical, historical accounts. He used all these reports

---

31 Christopher Cullen, "Yi'an (case statements): the origins of a genre of Chinese medical literature," in Elisabeth Hsü (ed.), *Innovation in Chinese Medicine*. Cambridge University Press, Cambridge, 2001, 297-323.

to achieve at least two ends, the first being to convincingly demonstrate the therapeutic potential of individual substances and specific formulas. Cases tied to real persons, their symptoms and eventually their cure, more vividly served his purpose than theoretical explications. At the same time, Li Shizhen regularly ended his case studies with a theoretical conclusion to help readers understand the therapeutic course described, and possibly act competently themselves.

Second is his emphasis on flexibility. Flexibility, the reader is told, is required when in the course of a treatment prior symptoms give way to new signs of an illness. The healer must react, and his competence enables him to turn to a wide spectrum of varied approaches, always re-adapted to changing conditions. Flexibility is also required, as Li Shizhen emphasizes again and again, when it becomes necessary sometimes to abandon seemingly irrefutable principles and adapt a substance's application to a specific challenge not met by a therapy guided by long held certainties. An example is his own successful treatment, recorded in chapter 35, of "an old woman over 60 years old" who had suffered from viscous outflow, i.e., some form of diarrhea, for an extended period of time. No established therapy had been able to end her suffering. Li Shizhen followed a recommendation by the Tang physician Wang Bing, who had traced viscous outflow to an excessive accumulation of cold. He resorted to *croton* seeds to counteract the cold responsible for that particular patient's illness.

Since antiquity, though, *croton* seeds had been described in Chinese *materia medica* literature not only as an extremely "hot" substance but also as a most violent purgative. Li Shizhen had also read the Yuan era author Wang Haogu, who had pointed out for the first time, that, given an appropriate pharmaceutical processing, *croton* seeds could also be applied to stop diarrhea. Hence, Li Shizhen counted on the extreme heat of *croton* seeds to attack the accumulated cold in the old woman. He treated her with pills prepared with *croton* seeds and coated with beeswax, and thus achieved a cure.

Li Shizhen offers only a few examples of his own reading of a patient's specific needs. He includes a record of an illness episode of his own at the age of 20, when he was successfully cured by his father. He adds it to a case giving him an opportunity to admonish his audience to advance beyond the written words of a text and to approach the underlying principles first, before following the advice given. Primarily, Li Shizhen provides details of earlier healers' creative approaches to difficult therapeutic situations.

The implicit goal underlying most such case records and anecdotes is to promote adaptability rather than show stubborn adherence to superficial principles. Hence, Li Shizhen praises previous healers for their ingeniously individualized therapies. Nor is he afraid to criticize trained doctors or even court physicians for their incompetence. Here, as in 13, a characteristic of Li Shizhen's attitude towards information management is obvious. The healers he cites and portrays are not necessarily scholarly physicians. The *Ben cao gang mu* offers a stage to a much wider range of experts.

Skullcap root
Scutellaria baicalensis Georgi. Vol. III, 13-03

To carefully read the texts requires first to approach their underlying principles and not to strictly cling to the written words.

Wang Haicang states: "Why should learned persons not be flexible? When I myself was 20 years old, because of an affection by the malicious I suffered from cough for a long time. Also, I violated the rules of an appropriate therapy and eventually suffered from bone steaming and heat effusion. My skin was like a blazing fire. Each time the phlegm I threw up filled more than a bowl. This was during the hot summer months. I felt vexation and thirst, and I could neither sleep nor eat. The movements in the six vessels were floating and vast. I ingested all medication such as *bupleurum* root, *ophiopogon* tuber and *schizonepeta* sap, but the disease became more serious month after month. Everybody thought I was going to die. Then my father thought of Li Dongyuan's therapy for lung heat resembling blazing fire, associated with restlessness, thirst, and a peak during daytime indicating heat in the qi section. He recommended as suitable a decoction with skullcap root as its sole ingredient; it was to drain the fire from the qi section of the lung conduits. According to the recipe, one ounce of flat skullcap root was boiled in two cups of water down to one cup, and I ingested this all at once. The next day, the body heat had completely disappeared. Phlegm and cough had been cured. When a medication is aimed at the heart of the matter, its effects will follow as promptly as a drum reacts to the drumstick. This is an example of the wondrous abilities of medicine.

Yellow soil, loess
Vol. II, 07-04

Also, the *The Records of Yijian* states: "Wu Shaoshi once fell ill and suffered from increasing emaciation for several months. Everyday, when beverages and food entered his throat, it was as if a myriad worms/bugs had assembled there to attack. He felt an itch and he felt pain, and everybody thought that this was an exhaustion consumption. Eventually, he met the famous physician Zhang Rui who diagnosed his disease. Zhang Rui asked him not to eat anything the next morning. He ordered a servant to walk a road for more than ten miles, to remove red soil from the road and to bring it back. The red soil was then mixed with two pints of warm wine. A hundred medication pellets were given into the liquid and the patient was asked to drink it. He felt an almost unbearable pain and went to the latrine where he defecated more than a thousand leeches, half of them wriggling, the other half dead. Wu Shaoshi felt extremely tired, but felt fine again after having received good care for three days. Asked for a possible cause of his illness, he said that 'during the summer months, when he was out on a military mission, he was thirsty and drank a cup of water from a mountain stream. He immediately sensed that some item had entered his throat and subsequently acquired this disease'. Zhang Rui said: 'When worms/bugs enter one's long-term depots, they inevitably will breed offspring there. When they are hungry, they will gather and suck their host's essence and blood. When they are filled, they scatter and settle in all the long-term depots and short-term repositories. If one only kills them but fails to completely remove them, a therapy will be of no use. This is why I asked you, Sir, to attract them with an empty abdomen. The worms/bugs had not eaten soil for a long time, and they also love wine. Hence they all gathered where you felt hungry, and with one dose of a liquid medication they were all wiped out'. The general was very pleased. He expressed his gratitude with a rich present and had the physician escorted home with all due honors."

Hardneck garlic
Allium sativum L. Vol. VI, 26-09

Shi Yuan in his records of the potential of garlic cauterization states: "My mother once suffered from an itching shoulder blade on her back, with a red halo of a half a *cun* diameter and white grains similar to millet. Two times seven cones were burned and the redness gradually vanished. Two nights later a red stream two *cun* long descended. All the family laid the blame on the cauterization. A physician from outside used an ointment to save her, but the halo increased in size every day. Twenty-two days later it had assumed a diameter of six to seven inches, and the pain was unbearable. Someone said that a nun had had this disease and was cured with cauterization. I rushed to her to ask her. The nun said: 'At the time the suffering was too severe. I was confused and did not recognize other people. I was told that Fan Fengyi kept watch over me and applied 800 or more moxa cauterizations until I came back to my senses. He had used up an entire sieve of mugwort leaves'. I quickly returned and with moxa cones the size of a gingko fruit applied more than ten cauterizations. My mother felt nothing. Then I applied cauterization on all four sides of the red area and they all were painful. With each cone burned down, the red area shrank in size. After more than 30 cones were burned, the red halo had vanished. The fact is, as the cauterization was delayed, the flesh at the point from where the halo had emerged had already been damaged. Hence, there was no pain. Only when the area with good flesh was cauterized, my mother felt a pain. That night, the fire radiated through her entire back. The sore formed an elevation and was hot. Still, she calmed down and slept that night. The next morning the elevation had assumed the size of a bowl turned upside down, about three to four inches tall. It had hundreds of small holes and was completely black in color. After having been given appropriate care, my mother was cured. The fact is, such a tall elevation is the release of the poison toward outside. As there are many small apertures, the poison cannot accumulate. The color was completely black because the skin and the flesh had rotted. If the fire of the mugwort leaves had not released the fire from within the rotten flesh, it would have advanced toward the five long-term depots and that would have resulted in a critical condition. When common physicians speak of applying cold to such a hot swelling to dissolve and disperse the poison, how could anybody believe it?"

Vol. I, 01-05-15

There was a woman with a warmth disease. It had already lasted for 12 days. An examination of the movement in her vessels revealed that it arrived six or seven times within one breathing period and was rough. It was slightly increased at the *cun* section, and it was slightly decreased at the foot-long wrist section. The woman developed alternative sensations of cold and heat; her cheeks were red and her mouth was dry. She did not understand clearly what others said, her ears were deaf. When asked, she responded that several days after the disease had commenced, she still had menstruation. This was a case of minor yang heat having entered the blood chamber. It results in death if the treatment fails to exactly confront the disease. She was advised to ingest the "decoction with sickle leaved hare's ear" for two days. Then she was asked to ingest for one day the "decoction with cinnamon twigs and dry ginger root," and the sensations of cold and heat stopped. But she said: "I feel tension and pain below the navel," and was given to ingest the "pills with leeches." A slight free-flow set in, the pain ended and the body turned cool. But she still had problems to understand others. Now she was given the "minor decoction with sickle leaved hare's ear," and the following day she stated: "In my chest, I sense heat and parchedness; my mouth and my nose are dry." Then she was given a small dose of the "decoction to regulate the stomach and maintain the qi." No free-flow resulted and she was given the "pills for a chest sunken in deeply." Before she had ingested half of the dose she had three bowel movements. The next day she experienced qi depletion and vexation and was restless. She had hallucinations and uttered mad words. The physician realized that her feces had hardened, but because of her state of extreme qi depletion, he did not dare to launch an attack. He let her ingest a "bamboo leaf decoction" to eliminate her vexation and heat, and defecation set in again as a result, including many lumps of hard feces. Her madness and vexation were resolved completely. Only her cough and her spitting of foam continued. This was a case of lung qi depletion. If it is not treated, it may end up as a lung dysfunction. A "minor decoction with sickle leaved hare's ear" was given her to ingest, with the ginseng root, fresh ginger, and Chinese dates omitted, and dry ginger root and *schisandra* seeds added instead. Within one day the cough subsided; within two days she was cured.

Summer ice
Vol. II, 05-10

Li Shizhen: Emperor Hui zong of the Song ate too much ice and suffered from a spleen disease. The state physicians failed to cure him. He then ordered Yang Jie to examine him, and Yang Jie resorted to the "pills to massively bring back to order the center." The Emperor said: "I have ingested this several times already." Yang Jie replied: "The Emperor suffers from this disease because he consumed ice. I, your official, will therefore boil this medication with ice water to cure the origin of the disease." The Emperor ingested the medication prepared with ice water and was cured.

That is, Yang Jie can be said to have been a scholar who flexibly adapted a standard treatment to the special circumstances of an illness.

Human urine
Vol. IX, 52-10

Sunstroke with dizziness and heart pressure. When during summer months someone on the road is struck by heat and dies, he is to be quickly moved to a yin i.e., cool, shady location. Then take a handful of hot soil from the road and form a pit on the patient's navel. Let some other person urinate into it to have warm qi penetrate the navel, and the patient will regain his consciousness. Then he should ingest drugs such as the clear liquid filtered from a mud pool and garlic water.

Lin Yi remarked: This method originates from Zhang Zhongjing. Its meaning is extraordinary, and remains inaccessible to common logic. Hence it was shunned by *materia medica* literature, but represents, in fact, a great technique of emergency rescue. The fact is, the navel is the base of life. If someone suffers from a heatstroke and has his qi harmed, the idea is to add warmth to his navel to get a hold of his original qi.

St. Paulswort
Siegesbeckia orientalis L. Vol. IV, 15-44

Tang Shenwei: The "St. Paulswort pill recipe memorandum" submitted to the Emperor by Cheng Na, stationed in Jianglingfu as Military Commissioner, reads: "I, your subject, have a younger brother, Yan, who at the age of 21 years was struck by wind. He stayed in bed for five years. A hundred physicians were unable to cure him. Then a Daoist named Zhong Zhen saw his suffering and said: 'He can take St. Paulswort pills, and he will definitely be cured. Much of this herb grows on fertile land. It is more than three feet tall. Leaves grow facing each other at the nodes. It must be gathered in summer beginning with the fifth month. Each time cut it five inches above the ground. Wash it clean with warm water to remove muddy soil and select the leaves and the tips of the twigs. Always steam them nine times and dry them in the sun nine times. They must not become too dry, though. Stop when there is sufficient moisture left. Then heat it, pound it, and form the powder with heat prepared honey to pills the size of *firmiana* seeds. Send down on an empty stomach with warm wine or a rice beverage 20 to 30 pills. Let the patient ingest up to 2,000 pills. When the suffering increases, do not worry. This is a sign of the strength of the medication.

When 4,000 pills are ingested, a restoration of health will be achieved. By the time 5,000 pills are ingested, the patient will be very strong.' I, your subject, prepared the medication as prescribed and let my younger brother Yan ingest it. The result was as the Daoist had predicted. After ingesting this medication one must eat three to five spoons of cooked rice to press it down. The herb collected on the fifth day of the fifth month is excellent." On request of the Emperor, the memorandum was submitted to the Medical Office for detailed recording.

Ephedra sinica Stopf
Vol. IV, 15-49.

Li Shizhen: Chinese *ephedra* is a pharmaceutical drug especially for the lung conduits. Hence, it is often used to cure lung diseases. When Zhang Zhongjing cured harm caused by cold without sweating, he used Chinese ephedra. For harm caused by cold with sweating, he used *cassia* twigs. In the course of history, when famous physicians explained their therapeutic approach they followed him, clinging to his texts without further consideration. There has never been an investigation of the seminal essentials underlying Zhang Zhongjing's treatments. I, Li Shizhen have always thought about an explanation. When eventually I arrived at it, it differed from the explanations offered by persons of former times, as follows.

Body liquids form the sweat, and sweat is blood. In terms of camp qi it is blood; in terms of guardian qi it is sweat. Now, cold harms the camp qi. When the camp qi are locked down in the interior, they are unable to communicate with the guardian qi in the exterior. When the guardian qi are blocked and shut in, the body liquids fail to pass. Hence there is no sweating. Heat effusion and an aversion to cold result. Now, when wind harms the guardian qi, the guardian qi flow off toward the outside and are unable to offer protection to the camp qi inside. When the camp qi are depleted and weak, the body liquids are unstable. This then results in sweating, an effusion of heat and an aversion to wind.

As it is, the evil qi of wind and cold always enter the body via skin and hair. Skin and hair form a union with the lung. The lung controls the guardian qi, enclosing the entire body like a net. This is the image of heaven. Although the illness signs listed above belong to major yang, it is a lung repletion resulting from its having received evil qi.

The illness signs may include a red face with anger and depression, cough with phlegm, panting, and a feeling of fullness in the chest. When all such signs appear, is this not a lung disease? The fact is, when skin and hair are closed on the outside, evil heat attacks internally and the lung qi are pent up. Therefore, one resorts to Chinese ephedra and *glycyrrhica* root joined by *cassia* twigs to lead away the evil qi in the camp qi section, guiding them to the exterior section of the muscles. This is assisted by apricot seeds to drain the lung and free the flow of its qi. If following sweating no great heat effuses, with the patient panting, one adds gypsum. Zhu Gong in his *The Book for Saving People's Lives* recommends to "add gypsum and *ane-marrhena* root after Summer Solstice (June 21)." Both are drugs draining lung fire.

That is, even though the "decoction with Chinese *ephedra*" is an important preparation stimulating sweating in the major yang region, it is truly a pharmaceutical drug serving to effuse and disperse pent-up fire in the lung conduits. When the intersticial structures are not closed, the body liquids flow off toward the outside and the lung qi will be depleted as a result. "In the case of such a depletion, one supplements qi in the long-term depot lung's mother i.e., the long-term depot spleen." Hence *cassia* twigs and *glycyrrhiza* root are used to disperse the evil qi of wind and safeguard the exterior body section in the outer region and to fell the liver associated with the phase wood in the interior to protect the spleen associated with the phase soil, the mother phase of metal, associated with the lung. This is assisted by *paeonia* root medication, serving to drain wood i.e., liver qi and to stabilize the spleen.

That is, one drains in the East to supplement in the West. Ginger and Chinese dates serve as guiding substances to stimulate the passage of the body liquids of the spleen and to harmonize the communication of camp and guardian qi. If following such a therapy patients suffer from slight panting, add *magnolia* bark and apricot seeds to free the passage of lung qi. If after the sweating the movement in the vessels is in the depth, add ginseng root to boost the lung qi. Zhu Gong adds *scutellaria* root to create the "decoction for a daybreak of yang qi," to drain lung heat. All these are medications for the spleen and the lung.

That is, although *cassia* twigs are a light preparation to resolve muscle qi in the major yang section, they are really a pharmaceutical drug to order spleen qi in order to safeguard the lung. This is a secret aim that has never been disclosed since a thousand years before. Hence I have published it here. Also, for a minor yin disease with heat effusion and a deep movement in the vessels, the "decoction with Chinese ephedra, *aconitum* accessory tuber, and *asarum heteropoides* root" and the "decoction with Chinese *ephedra, aconitum* accessory tuber, and *glycyrrhiza* root" are available. A minor yin and major yang constitute outside and inside. This corresponds to what Zhao Sizhen has said to require a combination of *aconitum* accessory tuber with Chinese *ephedra*, that is an effusion within supplementation.

An embroidered-uniform guard once in a summer month drank wine until daybreak and then suffered from a watery outflow that lasted for several days. Water and grain consumed left the body right away. He ingested all types of medication to rearrange the flow of liquid and solid food, to dissolve and lead off evil qi, and to raise the qi responsible for unending discharge, but contrary to expectations, the disease only increased in severity. I, Li Shizhen diagnosed his condition. The movement in the vessels was in the depth and slowed. His large intestine had descended to generate a tumorous flesh growth, repeatedly developing bleeding piles. This had resulted from an excessive mixture of meat, raw and cold items, tea and water, repressing and holding back yang qi below. The wood i.e., the liver qi flourished, while the soil i.e., the spleen qi was weakened. This was a case termed in the *Basic Questions* "outflow of undigested food caused by wind." The appropriate therapeutic approach requires "to raise, to lift." Hence I prescribed the "minor decoction to prolong life." One single ingestion resulted in a cure.

False hellebore
Veratrum nigrum L. Vol. IV, 17-15-01

According to Zhang Zihe in his *How Scholars Should Serve Their Parents*, "there was a woman who suffered from epilepsy related to wind intrusion. When she was six or seven years old, she was affected by fright and wind intrusion. After this, the disease recurred every year or every second year. From five to seven years later, it recurred five to seven times. From her 30th to her 40th year of age it recurred every day, sometimes in the course of one day more than ten times. Eventually she became lethargic, then succumbed to idiocy and forgetfulness. She just sought to die, and reach an end. That year there was a great famine and she collected hundreds of herbs to eat. In the wild she saw an herb similar in shape to onions. She collected it, took it back, steamed it until done, and ate it to her repletion. In the early morning hours of the next day she felt uneasy in her stomach/heart and spat out saliva similar to glue. This did not end for several consecutive days, altogether one or two pecks. She perspired as if she was washed, eventually she fell into a coma and three days later felt light and healthy. Her disease was gone and she could eat. All the movements in her vessels were harmonious. Then she took the onions she had consumed to consult with someone and was told that these are the seedlings of 'naïve onion,' which is the false hellebore recorded in the *Materia medica*. The *Illustrated Classic of Materia Medica* says that it can cure wind intrusion disease. This case of that woman is an example of using this herb as a method encountered by chance to stimulate vomiting."

During our present dynasty, Ms. Liu, a concubine of Prince He of Jing, at the age of 70 suffered from wind stroke and no longer recognized persons or anything else, with severe lockjaw. All physicians were helpless. Eventually my father Yuechi weng, an attendant to the Imperial Physicians, examined her. It proved impossible to have her take the medication he had described. The attempts continued from *wu* hours (11 – 13) to *zi* hours (23 – 1), but to no avail. Then they struck out one of her teeth and force-fed her with a thick decoction of boiled false hellebore. Within short a sound of belching qi was heard, she spat out phlegm and regained consciousness. She was given harmonizing medication and eventually enjoyed health again. A saying is: "If a medication fails to cause nausea, illnesses of qi recession are not healed." This is true.

Bugbane
Cimicifuga foetida L. Vol. III, 13-11-01

Li Shizhen: Bugbane root leads the clear qi of the yang brilliance conduits to move upward. *Bupleurum* root leads clear qi of the minor yang conduits to move upward. These are most important spleen and stomach guiding pharmaceutical drugs in the case of a weak natural constitution with the original qi depleted and internal harm caused by a generation of cold resulting from exhaustion and hunger or overeating. The "decoction with bugbane root and grass cloth rhizome" is a medication to disperse wind and cold from the yang brilliance conduits. I, Li Shizhen use this recipe to cure pent-up yang qi and all types of diseases associated with a sinking down of original qi, with epidemic red eyes, and this has always been effective.

Anybody with a clear vision on the nature of disease, how could he cling to established recipes? There was a person addicted to drinking wine. During the cold months he wept because of the loss of his mother and was entered by cold. As a consequence, he suffered from a disease of cold center. He could eat only when his food included ginger and garlic. When summer came, he drank a lot of water and he felt grievous and depressed. Because he suffered from painful distension at some location in his right lower back that drew on his right flanks, and above reached his chest and mouth, he felt he always wanted to sleep. When his disease was active, he felt an urge to defecate with a feeling of heaviness in his behind, and often went to the latrine. He frequently urinated for a long time. Sometimes he suffered from sour regurgitation, or threw up water, or he experienced outflow, or his yang (i.e,. sexual) member did not function, or there was yang qi recession with counterflow, and occasionally all this ended when he was given wine, or the disease signs subsided a little when he was exposed to heat. But once he was exposed to cold or consumed cold food, or when he overexerted himself, had sex, got angry or was hungry, the disease signs returned. When the disease signs were all swept away, it was as if he had no disease. When they were extremely active, they broke out several times a day. He ingested all types of medication to warm the spleen, to conquer moisture, to nourish and supplement, and to melt and lead off evil qi. They caused a little standstill before the disease effused again.

I, Li Shizhen thought about this. This disease was caused by irregular eating and exhaustion that had internally harmed the original qi. The clear yang qi had descended and were held back so that they were unable to ascend again. As a consequence I resorted to the "decoction with bugbane root and *pueraria* root" together with the "four rulers decoction," added *bupleurum* root, black *atractylodes* rhizome, and *astragalus* root, and let the patient ingest this decoction. After he had ingested it, he drank one or two cups of wine to assist the medication. Once it had entered his abdomen, he felt the clear yang qi rise, and he experienced a pleasant sensation in his chest and diaphragm region. His hands and feet became warm. His head and his eyes cleared up and his spirit quickly recovered. It was as if all his disease signs had been swept away. Whenever the disease effused again, it ended after only one ingestion.

This was a divine effect, beyond any comparison. If bugbane root or *pueraria* root had been diminished, or if he had not drunk the wine, the results would have been slow. In general, after the age of 50, one's qi increasingly melt away, and there is little growth. Most qi descend, only a few ascend. The orders of autumn and winter (that is, of collecting and storing) are many; the orders of spring and summer (that is, of coming to life and blossoming) are few. If someone has a weak constitution and shows the aforementioned disease signs, this medication, based on a flexible pattern of adding and omitting individual ingredients, will cure him.

The *Basic Questions* states: "Where yin essence is presented from below, the people enjoy longevity. Where yang essence is bestowed from above, the people experience early death." In the course of the past millennium, there have been only two persons, Zhang Jiegu and Li Dongyuan, who have perceived the profound nature of this therapy and who were able to disclose it to others.

Garden shallot bulbs
Allium macrostemon Bunge. Vol. VI, 26-06-01

Wang Zhen states: "The qi of fresh/raw Chinese chives are acrid; when they are heat prepared, they are sweet and delicious. When they are planted, they are not eaten by moths, when they are eaten they benefit man. It is for this reason that persons who study the DAO value them; and old people should eat them." Still, the Daoists regard Chinese chives as one of the five strong-odored/polluting items. How can it be that all the venerable experts say that they are not polluting?

Croton tree
Croton tiglium L. Vol. VII, 35-47

Li Shizhen: *Croton* seeds used as a drastic measure can suppress disorder and eliminate disease. Used in minor doses they yield wondrous results of pacifying and harmonizing the center. This can be compared to figures like Xiao He, Cao Shen, Jiang (i.e., Zhou Bo), and Guan Ying. They were courageous and relentless warriors. But serving as ministers they also were able to maintain great peace. When Wang Haicang says that *croton* seeds can penetrate the intestines and are able to stop outflow, this is a revelation of an eternal secret.

An old woman of more than 60 years had suffered from outflow for five years. When she ate meat, oily things, or fresh and cold items, this was an offense and an outflow occurred. She ingested all types of medication, those aimed at regulating her spleen qi, others with an ascending and lifting faculty, and still others to stop outflow and to astringe the intestines. Once they entered her abdomen, the outflow became even worse. They consulted me to examine her. Her movement in the vessels was in the depth and smooth, signalling that her spleen and stomach had been damaged for a long time, resulting in accumulation, congealing and stagnation because of cold. As Director of the Imperial Stud Wang Bing had said: "When severe cold congeals internally, this results in a long-lasting free flow and outflow." Cure and relapse may follow each other for years.

The method to be applied is to cause a discharge by means of heat. As a result the cold leaves and the free flow ends. Hence, I administered beeswax coated *croton* seed pills as medication, and let her ingest 50 pills. For two days she had no defecation and there was no free flow. The outflow was healed thereafter. From this time on, *croton* seeds were used to cure all types of diseases of both outflow and free-flow illness and accumulation and stagnation. Almost a hundred persons no longer suffered from outflow and their disease was cured.

If the pharmaceutical items are combined in perfect accordance with the case at hand, the medication and the disease are opposed to each other. If pharmaceutical drugs are used that should not be used, then it goes against the warning that even a small dose can reduce the yin qi.

Pharbitis nil (L.) Choisy
Vol. V, 18-13

A woman of the imperial clan, almost 60 years old, had suffered from constipation all her life. She had one bowel movement every ten days, and this was even more painful than giving birth to a child. When she ingested medication to nourish her blood and moisten dryness, this only closed her diaphragm and remained without effect. When she ingested medication to open passages, such as mirabilite and rhubarb root, they, too, remained without noticeable effect. This had continued for more than 30 years when I, Li Shizhen examined her.

She was fat, ate rich, oily food, and was often grieved. Every day she spat out more than a bowl full of sour phlegm, and then felt a little better. In addition, she often had a fire disease. This was a case of pent-up, sluggish qi in the Triple Burner. The qi ascended but failed to descend. All the body fluids transformed to phlegm rheum; they were unable to move down to nourish the intestinal short-term repositories. This was not just a dryness of blood. Preparations aimed at moistening retained the sluggish qi. Mirabilite and rhubarb root entered the blood section but were unable to clear the passage of qi. They were confronted by a phlegm barrier and, therefore, remained without effect.

Then I resorted to pills with *pharbitis nil* powder and *gleditsia* pods/seeds paste and let her ingest them. They freed the passage of defecation and urination relief. From this time on, when she noticed bound qi in her intestines, she would ingest these pills once and the passage of stools and urine was normalized. Also, she could eat safely and regained her essence. The fact is, *pharbitis nil* rapidly enters the qi section and penetrates the Triple Burner. Once the movement of qi is normalized, the phlegm is eliminated and phlegm rheums are dissolved.

My nephew Liu Qiao was addicted to wine and sex. He suffered from an extremely painful distension in his lower body parts, and the passage of both defecation and urination relief was blocked. He could neither sit nor lie down. He groaned and cried for seven days and nights. Physicians resorted to medication aimed at freeing the passage of defecation and urination, but this remained without effect. Then he sent someone to call me. I imagined that this was a case of evil qi of moisture and heat in his essence/sperm duct causing an obstruction of passage ways with distension. The disease was located between the two yin (i.e., anus and scrotum) regions. Hence, in front urination was blocked, and behind defecation was blocked. This disease was not located in the large intestine or in the bladder. Based on this, I resorted to pharmaceutical drugs such as Persian lilac fruit, fennel, and pangolin scales plus a doubled dose of *pharbitis nil*. This was boiled in water and given to him to ingest. With one ingestion his problems subsided. After three ingestions he was cured. *Pharbitis nil* is able to enter the right kidney (i.e., the Gate of Life), and the essence/sperm duct.

Allium sativum L. Hardneck garlic
Vol. VI, 26-09

Chen Cangqi: In former times, someone suffered from string-illness and aggregation-illness. Then he dreamed of a person who taught him to eat three bulbs of garlic day after day. In the beginning he felt dizziness and closed his eyes, and he vomited with qi counterflow. In his lower body parts it felt like fire. Later, someone told him to take several pieces of garlic, retain the skin but cut off both ends, and swallow this. This is called "internal cauterization." Eventually, it showed a strong effect.

Su Song: The classic states: "Garlic disperses obstruction-illness swelling."

According to Li Jiang's *Recipes Collected by Hand from the Ministry of War*, "nobody knows how to differentiate sores related to poison and swelling with poison causing patients to yell and making it impossible to lie down and sleep. Take two bulbs of single clove garlic and pound them into a pulpy mass. Add sesame oil and apply a thick layer to the affected region. When it dries, replace it with a moist layer. This recipe has often been used and it has saved the lives of people. There was not a single instance where it was not divinely effective.

Vice-Director Lu Tan developed a sore on his shoulder. The pain involved his heart and he suffered from heart-pressure. He resorted to this recipe and was cured.

Vice-Director Li suffered from an obstruction-illness in his brain that remained without cure for a long time. Lu Tan gave him this recipe, and he, too, was cured."

Dandelion
Taraxacum mongolicum Hand-Mazz. Vol. VI, 27-18-01

Su Song: A recipe to cure malign sores caused by piercing copied from Sun Simiao's *Recipes Worth a Thousand in Gold*. The "preface" states: "I, Sun Simiao in the night of the 15th day of the seventh month in the fifth year of the reign period "Uprightness Held in High Regard" (631) was in the courtyard when the back of the middle finger of my left hand was touched by a tree. By the next morning I suffered from an unbearable pain. For the next ten days, the pain increased every day, and the sore developed an every higher and bigger swelling. It was colored like a boiled mung bean. I had often heard of some senior discussing this recipe, and eventually I used it to cure myself. Healing took place in no time at all. The pain had vanished and the sore was cured. Within ten days my finger was restored to its previous condition."

White plum
Armeniaca mume Sieb. Vol. VI, 29-04-03

The *Medical Anecdotes* records the following case: "Duke Zeng of Lu suffered from free-flux illness with blood for more than 100 days. The state-employed physicians were unable to heal him. Chen Yingzhi ground the meat of one plum stored in salt water into a pulpy mass, mixed it with tea of the 12th month, added vinegar and let the duke ingest it. He took a sip and was cured. Grand Counselor Liang Zhuangsu gong also suffered from free-flux illness with blood. Chen Yingzhi prepared a powder of equal amounts of smoked plums and *picrorhiza* rhizome, mixed it with tea, and let the patient ingest it. This, too, proved to be effective.

The fact is, when blood is exposed to sour flavor it is held back. When it is exposed to cold its flow ends. When it is exposed to bitter flavor it is astringed. That white plums serve to erode malign sores and tumorous flesh growth may be a function of sour flavor's ability to contract and that is a wondrous facet of the principles underlying things. To say so is based on the *Original Classic*.

Peach tree leaves
Amygdalus persica L. 29-06-07

Chen Linqiu in his *Recipes from the Small Essays* has a record of Yuan Henan's "method of steaming with peach tree leaves." It states that if a permanent sweating is required, and if no sweat leaves the body, the patient dies. The steaming follows the same method as the one applied for wind stroke. Burn fire on the ground. When it is hot, remove the fire and spray a little water on the hot ground. Spread a two or three inches thick layer of peach tree flowers there, place a mat on the leaves, and let the patient lie down on it with a warm cover to induce a massive sweating. While the patient is covered apply a powder to absorb the sweat and achieve complete dryness. This results in a cure. The leaves of arborvitae trees, wheat bran or silkworm feces may all be used for this method.

Zhang Miao says: "Once someone was extremely tired and sweated. He lay down on a grass mat and caught a cold. He suffered from sensations of cold and was tired. For four days a therapy to induce sweating was performed, but he would not sweat. Then this method was applied and a cure was achieved."

Li Shizhen: According to Xu Shuwei's *Recipes Based on Facts*, "in the case of harm caused by cold, physicians must inspect the patient's outer and inner condition, and a treatment should follow a definite order. In former times, Fan Yun who served as an official under Emperor Wu di of the Liang dynasty had a heat illness caused by a seasonal epidemic. Xu Wenbo was called in to examine him. At this time, Wu di had ordered to bestow on Fan Yun the nine most precious gifts in recognition of his service and there was very little time left. Fan Yun feared that he would not be ready for the ceremony and requested a quick cure. Xu Wenbo said: 'This is very easy. I only fear that after two more years you will not get up again.' Fan Yun said: 'Those who obtain the WAY in the morning, may as well die in the evening. How much more does this apply if there are another two years?' Then Xu Wenbo heated the ground with a fire. He spread peach tree and arborvitae tree leaves on the hot ground and asked Fan Yun to lie down there. Within short, Fan Yun sweated and then he was powdered. The next day he was cured. Two years later Fan Yun died.

To induce sweating prior to the right time may shorten longevity. How much more is this true if the outer and inner condition of a patient and the right moment for an intervention are neglected?! Now, there is this wondrous method of inducing sweating by means of a peach tree leaf decoction. And yet, there are such warnings. Is not that reason enough to be careful?"

Dried Chinese dates
Zizyphus jujuba Mill. Vol. VI, 29-09-02

According to Xu Shuwei's *Recipes Based on Facts*, "once a woman suffered from dryness in the long-term depots, with grief and unending weeping. Prayers were said in all possible ways. I recalled that to cure this condition, ancient recipes recommend to use a big/dried date decoction. Hence, it was prepared and given her to ingest. She took the entire dose and was cured. So wonderful are the knowledge that ancient people had about diseases and the recipes they developed for treating them."

Also, Chen Ziming in his *Good Recipes for Women* states: "When Chen Huqing's wife was pregnant in the fourth to fifth month, all day long she felt miserable and was full of sorrow. She often cried as if there was something that gave her a reason to behave like this. Physicians and sorcerers joined to cure her, but all their efforts remained without a good result. Guan Bozhou said: 'Such a condition has been discussed by former people. A therapy must rely on a big/dried date decoction to achieve a cure.' Chen Huqing obtained such a recipe and had the medication prepared. She took it once and was healed." The recipe is listed here further down.

Cherry
Cerasus pseudocerasus (Lindl.) G. Don. Vol. VI, 30-25

Zhu Zhenheng: Cherries are associated with the phase fire; by their nature they are very hot and stimulate the effusion of moisture. People who formerly suffered from heat disease, with panting and coughing, when they are affected by the heat of cherries they will have this disease again in a moment, and some may die.

Li Shizhen: According to Zhang Zihe's *How Scholars Should Serve Their Parents*, "in Wushui a rich family had two children who loved to eat purple cherries. Day after day they consumed one or two pints. After half a month the elder one developed lung dysfunction, the younger one developed lung obstruction-illness. One died after the other. What a pity! The hundreds of fruits grow to nourish the people, they are not intended to harm people! In rich and noble families they unrestrainedly follow their lust, and why do they die? Because of heaven? Because of their fate? Shao Yaofu in a poem states: 'To overly please the mouth with any item may end in illness.' This is well said."

Japanese raisin tree seed/fruits
Hovenia dulcis Th. Vol. VI, 31-31-01

Zhu Zhenheng: A male person, aged 30 years, drank wine and as a result developed heat. In addition, he was affected by depletion and weariness following an exhaustion with sexual intercourse. He ingested medication to supplement qi and blood, and added *pueraria* root to resolve the wine poison. He sweated a little and contrary to his expectations felt as sluggish and hot as before. This was a case of qi and blood depletion, and the patient was unable to withstand the dispersing effects of *pueraria* root. In such a situation it is essential to resolve the poison with Japanese raisin tree fruits. Therefore, they were added to a decoction of further pharmaceutical drugs. He ingested it and was cured.

Li Shizhen: Of Japanese raisin tree fruit/seeds, the *Materia Medica* says only that it can ruin wine, and Mr. Zhu Danxi frequently uses Japanese raisin tree fruit/seeds fruits to cure diseases caused by wine. The therapeutic effects are identical to ruining wine. According to Su Dongpo, "Jie Yingchen of Meishan suffered from melting with thirst. Every day he drank several *dou* of water, he ate several times more than usual, and he urinated frequently. He ingested medication for melting with thirst for a year, but his illness increased day after day, until he was convinced he had to die. I asked him to invite Zhang Gong, a physician from Shu, to attend and examine him. Zhang Gong said with a laughter: 'You might soon have died because of this mistaken treatment.' He took musk, moistened it with wine and prepared a little more than ten pills, and asked the patient to swallow them with a Japanese raisin tree fruit decoction. That resulted in his cure.

Asked for the reason behind this approach, Jie Gong responded: 'Melting with thirst and melting center are always related to spleen weakness and kidney destruction. That is, the phase soil is unable to check the phase water and an illness results. In the present case, Yingchen had extreme heat in his spleen vessels, while his kidney qi had not weakened. Because of an excessive consumption of fruits and wine the heat had accumulated in his spleen and, for this reason, he ate a lot and drank water. When he drank that much water, his urination had to increase. This was neither a 'melting' nor a 'thirst.' Musk is able to check wine, fruits, flowers, and wood. Japanese raising tree fruits, too, overcome the effects of wine. If such trees are outside of a house, the wine brewed inside that house will never be excellent. It is for this reason that these two items are used to prepare a medication to eliminate the poison of the wine and of fruits."

Zanthoxylum bungeanum Maxim
Carpel of red prickly-ash from Shu. Vol. VI, 32-02-01

Li Shizhen: Prickly ash is an item of pure yang; it is a pharmaceutical drug for the qi section on the hand and foot major yin conduits and the right kidney (i.e., the Gate of Life). Its flavor is acrid and numbing; its qi are warm and provide heat. It is endowed with the yang qi of the South and has received the yin qi of the West. Hence, it can enter the lung and dispel cold, and serves to cure coughing. It enters the spleen and removes moisture, and serves to cure blockage related to wind intrusion and the presence of cold and moisture, as well as water swelling and outflow with free-flux illness. It enters the right kidney and supplements its fire, and serves to cure yang (i.e., male sexual) weakness and frequent uncontrolled urination, weak feet, and long-lasting free-flux illness – all such conditions.

There was a woman, more than 70 years of age. She had suffered from outflow for five years, and not one of the hundreds of medications applied showed an effect. I let her take 50 of the "pills letting you feel a response." For two days she had no major relief (i.e., defecation). Then I gave her pills to ingest made from a medication to balance the stomach to which I added red prickly-ash carpels, fennel and date meat, and she was healed. Everytime when she got angry, she ate too much and the illness broke out again. Then she ingested the medication I had recommended to her and the illness ended. This is an effective medication to dispel moisture and dissolve food, to warm the spleen and supplement kidney qi.

According to the *Records of the Annual Seasons in Jing and Chu*, "in the morning of New Year's Day drink the 'wine with prickly ash and *phellodendron* bark to ward off epidemics'. Prickly ash is the essence of the Alioth star; eating it lets your body become strong, and prevents aging. *Phellodendron* bark is the essence of the hundred woods/trees. It is a pharmaceutical drug of hermits/immortals because it can subdue evil demons."

Wu Meng, a true man, in his *Instructions for Ingesting Pepper* states: "Prickly ash grows endowed with the qi of the Five Phases. Its leaves are greenish. Its skin is red. Its flowers are yellow. Its membrane is white. The seeds are black. Its qi are extremely fragrant; by their nature they move into the lower body parts and are able to guide the heat of fire to reach the lower body parts rather than to rise and steam the upper body parts. Among all the fragrant herbs there is not one that could reach its quality." For its recipes, see below.

I, Li Shizhen, humbly say: Although the pills with prickly-ash carpels are said to supplement kidney qi, if it remains unclear whether the case in question is a condition of water or fire, a mistaken treatment of that person is inevitable. Basically, this recipe is suitable only for treatments of depletion cold with pent-up moisture qi affecting spleen, stomach, and the Gate of Life. If it is a case of pure heat affecting lung and stomach, one should definitely not resort to it.

Hence, Mr. Zhu Danxi states: "Prickly ash is associated with the phase fire and it is able to reach the lower body parts. Ingested over a long time, fire develops out of the water (i.e., the kidneys). Therefore none of those who ingest prickly ash regularly will avoid poisoning."

Sugar cane
Saccharum sinensis Roxb. Vol. VI, 33-06-01

The *Unofficial Histories* states: "Lu Jiang was struck by a malaria ailment and suffered from weariness consumption. Suddenly he dreamed of a woman in a white garment who told him: 'Eat sugar cane; it can cure you.'

The next day he bought several sticks of sugar cane and ate them. The next day he was cured." Is this not another example of sugar cane's effects of supporting the spleen qi and harmonizing the center?

Unscraped bark of larger, older cinnamon trees
Vol. VII, 34-04

Someone suffered from painful, swollen red eyes, with a spleen qi depletion making it impossible to drink and eat. The movement in the liver vessels was in abundance, that in the spleen vessels was weak. An application of a cooling medication to cure the liver resulted in an increased depletion of spleen qi. When warming medication was applied to cure the spleen, the liver qi were even more in abundance. The only appropriate therapy was to add "fleshy cinnamon" to a warming and balancing medication; it killed excess liver qi and boosted insufficient spleen qi. That is, one curative approach had two effects."

Tradition has it that "when wood is contacted by cinnamon, it withers." That is correct. All this is in perfect agreement with the idea underlying the statement in the *Supplementary Records by Famous Physicians* that "cinnamon frees the passage of liver and lung qi, and that unscraped bark of older cinnamon trees serves to cure aching flanks and wind intrusion in the flanks." As people do not know this, it is pointed out here. Li Shizhen.

12. Neglected heritage: Tool-supported therapy

The government of the newly founded People's Republic of China in 1949 was faced with a rather uncommon task of information management. Perhaps the most diverse and literally best documented health care tradition world-wide was to be scrutinized. How much should be retained; how much should be obliterated as part of the program to build a new China?

The easy defeat of the Qing Imperial troops, inflicted by British aggressors during the First Opium War 1839/1840, was only the beginning of a series of humiliations inflicted on China by Western European powers quickly joined by Tsarist Russia, democratic USA, and feudal Japan. It took a few decades for the Chinese government to realize that this onslaught could not be compared to the many invasions of neighboring powers from past times.

Imperial armies had been unable to repel invaders often enough during the previous two millennia. Foreign powers, most recently the Manchus and before them the Mongols, had ruled China for centuries. And yet, this time it was different. The Mongols and the Manchus, to mention only the two most recent successful invaders, had entered China well aware of the superiority of Chinese civilization. Once they had conquered the country, they retained enough facets of their own so as to remain distinct and recognized as non-Han Chinese. But they ruled China by integrating themselves into the established political order, continuing its many idiosyncratic traditions and developing them further through outstanding contributions. They could not become Han-Chinese, but they became Chinese.

The foreign powers who, it seemed, were playing games with China in the 19th and early 20th century never intended to become Chinese. They meant to make China a market for their products, a cheap source of more or less badly needed human and natural resources. Japan, above all, a neighboring East Asian people constructively influenced by Chinese culture for more than 1,000 years, left perhaps the deepest wound in the Chinese psyche. Its brutal behavior was no less than an attempt to colonize China. This caused a trauma that to this day has not been overcome. Why, the question arose early enough, was the chain of islands in the ocean to the east able to inflict such damage on China? The answer was soon given. Japan had switched from a China oriented technology, science, and medicine to a Western-type technology, science, and medicine. The political reaction of China was a rational one. In the course of only a few decades, radical reformers got the upper hand. The two millennia old political structure and social system were abandoned and forceful programs were initiated, dedicated to regaining the status of a respected "country in the center," as its name *zhong guo* demands.

A revolution in health care delivery was recognized as an urgent task. No reformer spoke a word of defense for the vast heritage of therapeutic strategies and their underlying doctrines. Once the political turmoil associated with the anti-Japanese war and the civil war between nationalists and communists had ended, the new government immediately took steps to examine the heritage for what could be transmitted to a Chinese society devoted to modern science and technology. A *xiangshan* committee, named after the venue in the Aromatic Mountains northwest of Beijing where it convened, was commissioned with this task in the 1950s and 1960s. Its members prepared a memorandum that was meant to prevent, first, an unchecked continuation of the many therapeutic approaches deemed harmful and absurd, and, second, to avoid a complete elimination of Chinese medicine as had been demanded for decades by Western trained physicians. The result was a very narrowly defined system of therapies, mostly based on pharmaceutical means and acupuncture, but also including suggestions for manual therapy, diet, life-style, and other soft approaches associated with remnants of historical theoretical foundations and now adapted to modern logic. This turned out to be a minute digest, disregarding a wealth of information from the historical therapeutic arsenal, of which the *Ben cao gang mu* is still a witness.

So-called Traditional Chinese Medicine (TCM) in western industrialized countries is even further separated from the historical reality than is TCM in China. Introduced not by persons who had gained sufficient knowledge of Chinese *Fachsprache*, Chinese medical history, and historical Chinese medical practice, this meant that a vast diversity of idiosyncratic intepretations, often based on misunderstandings and erroneous translations of key concepts, spread throughout the Western world and appealed to a receptive audience. The reinterpretation of the Chinese concept of qi as "energy" proved to have rapid success at a time when all the world was gripped by the first major energy crisis. The following anthology offers further information on any number of features that found no entry into TCM, often, it must be said, for good reason.

White bark of mulberry tree roots
Morus alba L. Vol. VII, 36-01-01.

Su Song: White mulberry bark is used to make threads for sewing up protruding intestines in wounds caused by metal objects/weapons. In addition, apply hot chicken blood. During the Tang era, An Jincang attempted to commit suicide and cut his abdomen. This method was used and he was cured.

Realgar
Arsenic disulphide. Vol. II, 09-07

Smallpox and pin-illness of children. Grind one mace of realgar and three maces of *arnebia* herb to a powder and mix it with liquid rouge. Then first pierce the affected region open with a silver hairpin and after this apply the medication there. Extremely wondrous. *Patterns and Treatment of Smallpox Papules.*

Vol. I, 04-08-03

For swollen, black lips with unbearable pain and itch, remove the blood with a porcelain blade, rub fat with an ancient coin, and apply this to the affected region.

Golden thread
Coptis chinensis Franch. Vol. III, 13-01

Sudden redness of the eyes and pain. File scraps from *huang lian* from Xuan, soak them in the clear contents of a chicken egg, bury them underground for one night, and filter the liquid the next morning. Dip a chicken feather into the liquid and drip it into the affected eye.

Decayed *imperata cylindrica* on a roof
Imperata cylindrica (L.) Beauv. var. *major* (Nees) C. E. Hubb
Vol. III, 13-19-04

Blocked defecation, with an ingestion of medication being unable to free its passage. Grind three maces of dark blue salt and seven nodes of rotten *imperata cylindrica* herbs from the eaves of a roof to powder. Each time blow through a bamboo tube one mace seven inches deep into the patient's anus and the passage will be freed. This recipe is called "powder promoting gold." *General Records of Sagely Benefaction.*

Cervus elaphus L
Deer blood. Vol. IX, 51-15-13

One or two male deer are raised and fed by having them drink, each day, one ounce of an aqueous ginseng root decoction. Also, mix the dregs of this decoction with locally produced fodder, rice, and beans, and have the deer eat this from time to time. Do not give it any additional water and herbs. After 100 days, a deer's sinew (i.e., penis) can be used as follows. The "method to feast." On the previous night decrease the food. The next morning, tie the deer with a piece of cloth onto a bench, with its head hanging down and its tail raised. Then have a strong person hold its front legs. If the deer has horns, they are to be held to fix the head. If it has no horns, a wooden frame is applied to keep its head from moving. Then take a needle with three edges and pierce the hole located in front of the inner canthi of the eyes, named "celestial pond hole." Next a silver tube of three *cun* length is punctured there toward the bridge of the nose, and the patient in a stable seating position is to suck the blood. Then he is to drink several cups of medicinal wine, and again suck and again drink until he is intoxicated. If blood flows out of the animal's nose it, too, can be collected and is drunk together with wine. After he has ended the drinking, the patient must avoid an exposure to wind, and he is to make gymnastic movements of raising and lowering his body. This then is one feast. Now apply a medication to make the muscles grow to the hole pierced into the deer, and further nourish it. This can be done once a month, and one deer can be used for six to seven years. Regardless of whether men or women, old or young persons ingest such deer blood, they will not fall ill their entire life and enjoy longevity. This is just one of the 24 items of elixir recipes consumed by hermits. The medicinal wine mentioned above is prepared with the "powder with the eight jewels" boiled in wine together with aloes wood and *aucklandia* root.

Shuttle head
Vol. VII, 38-45

For loss of voice and inability to speak and when someone stutters, pierce with a shuttle head the center of his palm to cause pain and he will speak. Of males pierce the left hand; of females pierce the right hand. Chen Cangqi.

Siberian motherwort stem
Leonurus japonicus Houtt. Vol. IV, 15-17-02

Acute or chronic pin-illness sores. The *Sagely and Benevolent Recipes* recommends to pound Siberian motherwort to a pulp and use it to seal the affected region. Also, wring it to obtain five *ge* of juice and ingest it. This will dissolve the pin. The *Great Compendium of Medical Recipies* recommends to collect Siberian motherwort with flowers in the fourth month and burn it with its nature retained. First cut a cross with a small, sharp knife to lay free the root of the pin-illness and cause a bleeding. Then cut around the root, sever it, and squeeze it until no more blood appears. Twist the burned *yi mu cao* drug with the fingers and insert it into the wound. Stop when red blood appears. On one day and one night insert the twisted drug three to five times.

In severe cases the root is softened and will come out the second day. In mild cases it comes out within one day. When the root of the sore swells and rises, this is a sign that the root comes out. Now pick it with a needle. Once it is removed apply the drug to the open wound. This will generate muscles and an easy cure is achieved. During the treatment wind and cold, sex, wine and meat, and all poisonous items are forbidden.

Black tin ashes made of lead and sulphur
Vol. II, 08-10-01

Li Shizhen: The nature of lead enables it to enter the flesh. Hence, when girls pierce their ears with lead pearls, eventually they will bore holes. When a barren girl has her vagina closed, a barb made of lead is used to pull on it day after day. Eventually, after a long time, it will open. All these are methods unknown to the people in ancient times.

Handle of a copper spoon
Vol. II, 08-19-03

For red and festering wind eyes and red eyes caused by wind and heat with a shade membrane, heat the handle of a copper spoon until it is hot and press it on the affected region. Repeated application will result in a wondrous effect. Li Shizhen.

Dust from a beam
Vol. II, 07-54

Sudden death of a person who has hanged himself. Form dust from a beam to pills the size of beans and insert one each into four bamboo tubes. Then have four persons simultaneously blow these pills through the bamboo tubes with utmost strength into that person's two ears and two nostrils. This will bring him back to life. *Arcane Essential Recipes from the Outer Censorate.*

Soil mushroom. Unidentified
Vol. VI, 28-28

Pin-illness swelling. When black bulls drop their dung on stones, mushrooms grow on them after a while. Bake them over a slow fire, dry them, and grind them with an equal amount of St. Paulswort into a powder. Remove the two ends of a bamboo tube, attach it with one end tightly to the pin-illness swelling, and fill it with one mace of a mixture of the powder with water. Within a short time, the liquid rises with bubbles, and then the root of the pin-illness is pulled out. If it fails to come out, repeat this application two or three times. *The Orthodox Transmission of Medical Studies.*

Calabash
Lagenaria siceraria (Molina) Standl. var. *microcarpa* (Naud.) Hara. Vol. VI, 28-04

Tumorous flesh growth and a film of blood covering the eyes. In autumn get a small calabash ladle or a small medicinal calabash vessel, dry it in the yin (i.e., shade), cut it apart at the narrowest circumference, and bore in it a small hole the size of an eye. Then open with your hand the afflicted eye by pulling the skin above and below it away from the eye and place the hole of the calabash firmly on the eye. In the beginning this is extremely painful, but gradually the tumorous flesh and the blood film are discharged. There is no harm to the pupil. Liu Songshi, *Tried and Proven Recipes.*

Leek
Allium tuberosum Rottl. ex Spreng. Vol. VI, 26-01

To fumigate teeth affected by worms/bugs. Calcine a roof tile until it has turned red, place several leek seeds on it, and drip some clear oil on it. Wait until fumes rise and inhale them with a tube to reach the location of the pain. After quite some time rinse the teeth with warm water. If you spit out small worms/bugs, that shows the effect of this therapy. If the pain does not entirely stop, then steam the teeth a second time. *Easy Recipes for Rescue in Emergencies.*

Croton tree seeds
Croton tiglium L. 35-47

A wind-intrusion disease with the presence of moisture and phlegm. Let that person sit in a closed chamber. On his left is a bowl with boiling water. On his right is a bowl with a charcoal fire. In front of him place a table with one book on it. First grind oil-free, newly collected *croton* seeds into a pulp. Press it with paper to remove any remaining oil and form three pies. If the disease is in the patient's left side, let him place his right hand on the book and place the medication on his right palm. Then place a bowl on the medication and pour hot water into it. When the water cools down, replace it. After quite some time the patient begins to sweat and a divine effect is seen immediately. If the disease is in the patient's right side, place the medication, etc. on his left palm. Another recipe states to place the medication in accordance with the location of the disease on the left or right side. *Tried and Proven Recipes from the Hall of Preserving Long Life.*

Vernicia tree seed oil
Vernicia fordii (Hemsl.) Airy-Shaw. Vol. VI, 35-13-01

In the case of vomiting phlegm related to wind intrusion with throat blockage and all other such illnesses, mix the oil with water and wipe it into the throat to induce vomiting. Or, grind the seeds into a powder and blow it into the throat to induce vomiting. Also, heat the tip of a copper chopstick in a lamp fire lighted by *vernicia* tree oil and cauterize a festering eye related to wind intrusion and heat. This is also wondrous. Li Shizhen

Chinese ash tree bark
Fraxinus rhynchophylla Hance. Vol. VII, 35-19-01

Red eyes with a sore. Soak one ounce of Chinese ash tree bark in one ounce of clear water in a white porcelain bowl, in spring and summer for at least as long as it takes to have a meal, and watch it until a jade-bluish color emerges. Then wind silk floss around the tip of a chopstick, dip it into the liquid, and let it drip into the affected eyes of the patient while he lies face up. A little pain is of no concern. After letting the liquid trickle into the eyes for quite some time, remove the heat juice that is released. If at least ten such applications are conducted each day, a cure is achieved after no more than two days. *Arcane Essential Recipes from the Outer Censorate.*

Boswellia carteri Birdw. Frankincense
Vol. VII, 34-22

The *Mr. Zhu's Collected and Proven Recipes* recommends to insert a bean-size amount of frankincense into the hole in the affected tooth. Then heat a chopstick until it develops smoke, touch the affected tooth to let the frankincense melt and the pain stops immediately.

Persian lilac tree fruits
Melia azedarach L. Vol. VII, 35-15

Longworms (i.e., roundworms) in the abdomen. Soak Persian lilac tree fruits in unmixed, bitter wine for one night. Wrap them in silk floss and insert this into the "grain pathway"/the anus about three inches deep. Exchange it twice a day. *Wai tai bi yao.*

Sudden heat and swelling of the ears. Pound five *ge* of Persian lilac tree fruits into a pulpy mass, wrap it in silk floss, and insert this into the affected ears. To be repeatedly replaced. *Sagely and Benevolent Recipes.*

Assumption lily root
Hosta plantaginea (Lam.) Ascherson. Vol. IV, 17-31-01

To discharge a fish bone stuck in the throat. Pound assumption lily root and hawthorne root to obtain a natural juice and force-feed it by means of a bamboo tube into the patient's throat. The bone will be discharged. Do not touch the teeth. Quxian, *Vitality in Heaven and Earth.*

Daphne flower
Daphne Genkwa Sieb. et Zucc. Vol. IV, 17-36

Piles with teat-like kernels. Wash one handful of daphne genkwa roots clean and pound them in a wooden mortar to a pulpy mass. Add a little water and squeeze it to obtain a juice. Boil this in a stone vessel over a slow fire to generate a paste. Pull a silk thread several times through the paste and use it to tie off the piles. This will cause some pain. Wait until the piles have dried and fall off. Then dip a paper stick into the paste and insert it into the opening to remove the root of the piles. This serves to eliminate the root forever.

Another recipe. Simply pound the roots, soak the silk thread in the resulting juice for one night, and then apply it. This does not require water. *Tried and Proven Recipes.*

Iron fragments
Vol. II, 08-22

When iron fragments are fried until they are hot and are then dropped into wine and the wine is drunk, this serves to heal robber wind spasms. Also, wrapped in a piece of fabric and pressed hot on the armpits, iron fragments effectively heal barbarian stench. Su Gong.

They level the liver qi and remove timidity. They serve to cure a tendency to be angry and outbreaks of madness. Li Shizhen.

Vol. I, 04-07

Grind common mugwort together with Chinese wild ginger, black *atractylodes* rhizome, and Sichuan lovage into powder and place it, separated by a piece of cloth, on the gate on the top of the skull. Press it down with a hot flat iron.

Vol. I, 04-05-03

For kernels of earwax in the ears that are painful and cannot be moved, drip burnt wine into the affected ear. After one hour the kernels can be removed with pincers.

Trichosanthes kirilowii Maxim
Vol. V, 18-18-02

Extremely painful unilateral elevation-illness. Wrap the scrotum warm with silk fabric. Soak five maces of *trichosanthes kirilowii* root in one bowl of pure wine from *mao* 卯 hours (5 – 7) to *wu* 午 hours (11 – 13). Briefly boil it and leave it in the open for one night. The next morning let the patient sit on a low bench and hold his knees with his hands. *Ben cao meng quan.*

13. Sources of therapeutic expertise: Beggar and sovereign, chance encounters and dreams

Reports of illnesses, mostly those of rulers or members of the ruling class, date back in China to the earliest written evidence. Cures were sought from numinous forces known to exist alongside mankind and to have power over human life. It was only late in the Zhou era or early in the Han era that a character depicting a *wu* medium, displaying a quiver containing an arrow and a hand holding a weapon, was modified to signify a new approach to health care. The element "*wu* medium" was replaced by the character for "mature wine." Medicine, the new character was to point out, relies on medicinal wines, that is, on pharmacotherapy. Still, the quiver with the arrow remained in the character, and so did the hand holding a weapon. When Chinese characters were simplified in the early years of the People's Republic, the character was shortened, but the quiver with the arrow was retained. This combination of symbols has remained characteristic of health care and disease therapy in China ever since.

Physicians found professionalization difficult. As is the case in all cultures and at all times, any type of attention and sympathy, no matter what its theoretical foundation may be, will successfully "heal" enough patients to acquire an image of being "effective." Hence, when a new type of healers emerged, encouraged by a new world view to compete with sorcerers and priests who had satisfied their clientele for times immemorial, they themselves may have believed in the superiority of their *materia medica*. However, there was little general evidence to prove this to the public.

Also, the types of healers who gathered under the new character for "medicine" were themselves marked by a competition between two approaches to health care and disease treatment.

The authors of the *Yellow Thearch's Inner Classic* promised health to those who lived in agreement with the laws of nature, outlined by the yin yang and Five Phases doctrines. Minor health problems could be corrected by diet change and needle stimuli. Pharmaceutical drugs went unnoticed. At the same time, though, a knowledge of the curative potential of natural substances, mostly herbs, was gaining momentum.

Practitioners of pharmacotherapy based their recommendations on experience, but continued a belief in the power of spirits and neglected the doctrines of natural laws. They appear to have been much more successful than their competitors. A literature of recipe collections and descriptions of the curative powers of individual herbal, mineral, and animal substances developed. It grew more quickly than the medical literature based on complex and demanding theoretical reasoning.

Sima Qian, the author of the *Historical Records* of 90 BCE, is the first historian known to have paid attention to healers. He included two biographies, those of Chunyu Yi and Bian Que, although it is not quite clear whether he meant to honor "physicians" or to question their calling. Sima Qian recounted 25 cases treated by Chunyu Yi, ten of which ended in the patient's death. Bian Que left the court of a marquis when the latter failed to listen to him so as to prevent the first signs of an illness from taking a deadly course. When the marquis saw the physician depart, he remarked: "Physicians look out for profit. Therefore, they try to be of use to those who are not sick." Later Bian Que's prognosis fulfilled itself, and the marquis died. Still, his assessment survived as a shadow following physicians for many centuries to come.

Health care and disease therapy remained in the hands of numerous diverse experts and practitioners. Confucianism in many ways, and often successfully, acted to prevent specialization in any occupation that might have jeopardized a social structure in which social and political decision making rested with the omniscient scholar official and gentleman. Sun Simiao (581 – 682?) was the first who sat down and wrote an essay "On the absolute sincerity of physicians."

The main focus of physicians' professionalizing efforts, both in Europe and China, has been to replace an enduring suspicion with trust. Sun Simiao asserted that his therapies were based on the doctrines of systematic correspondences outlined in the *Yellow Thearch's Inner Classic*. He tried to convince his readers his was a value system devoted to compassion and humanity, "to aid every life and every man." Sun Simiao was well aware that the widespread habit of physicians belittling their colleagues' competence harmed the entire group's professional interests. He spoke strongly against such slandering. At the conclusion of his essay, he maintains that the wrongful behavior of healers will certainly be punished in the afterworld. In the course of the following centuries, Confucian authors countered such claims and warned families not to entrust their loved ones to those who pretended to practice humanity, but in reality were only exploiting anxieties to make money.

At the time Li Shizhen was working on his *Ben cao gang mu*, individuals educated in classical Confucian scholarship turned increasingly to medicine when they failed to obtain one of the coveted positions in the bureaucracy. This trend had begun during the preceding Yuan dynasty and had led to strategies devised by a new group of "scholar physicians" to distance themselves from what they called "common physicians." A background in Confucian scholarship was used as an argument in seeking recognition as practitioners. That is, scholar physicians fought on two fronts. They sought to stand up to conservative Confucianists who opposed all professional practice of medicine and advised family members to acquire enough competence to treat their own loved ones. As they denounced such lay treatments as dangerous dilettantism, the scholar physicians also emphasized profound differences distinguishing them from practitioners without higher learning.

And yet, the reach of all these physicians remained limited, despite the ever-increasing output of an ever more sophisticated literature. The largest group of healers caring for the Chinese people were itinerant doctors of dubious competence. They were well aware of the distrust they were met with wherever they appeared. They had developed a psychologically highly effective rhetoric to encourage patients to come forward and ask for a cure. Buddhist and Daoist priests on the road and in temples and monasteries were always ready to apply their prayers, spells, and magical techniques in seeking the aid of spirits and gods, or they might also use exorcism to eliminate demons that had entered a patient's body. Li Shizhen paid tribute to this diversity. He saw beggars and convicts, physicians and pharmacists, noblemen and sovereigns as legitimate sources of therapeutic expertise whenever their advice proved to be effective. He also saw no problem in setting down advice conveyed in dreams or even inscribed by the hands of spirits on a wall.

Lesser galangal root
Alpinia officinarum Hance. Vol. III, 14-16-01

Painful teeth with swelling related to wind intrusion. Grind a two inches long piece of lesser galagal root and one complete scorpion, baked, to powder and rub the teeth with it. Spit out the resulting saliva and rinse the mouth with a salt decoction. This has been transmitted by a beggar in Leqing. When Bao Jiming was affected by this disease, he resorted to it and it was effective. Wang Qiu, *101 Select Recipes*.

Golden thread root
Coptis chinensis Franch. Vol. III, 13-01-01

The "pills with sheep/goat liver" of Liu Yuxi's *Transmitted Core Recipes*. They serve to cure insufficient qi in the liver conduits, with wind and heat rising to attack above. The eyes have only dim vision and shy light, resulting in screens and green blindness. Pound one ounce of golden thread root powder with one sheep/goat liver, the membrane removed, to a pappy substance and form pills the size of *firmiana* seeds. Each time, following a meal, swallow 14 pills with warm fermented water of foxtail millet. A cure will be achieved after five consecutive doses.

Formerly, Cui Chengyuan pardoned a prisoner convicted to death. Later, the prisoner died of a disease. One morning, Cui suffered from an internal eye screen that lasted for more than a year. Once at midnight when he sat all by himself he heard steps as if someone was rushing on the stairs. He asked who this was and the answer was: "I am the formerly pardoned prisoner. Today I wish to pay my debt of gratitude." Then he informed him of this recipe and disappeared. Cui ingested it. After only a few months he had regained his eyesight. Hence, he shared it with the world.

Chinese small onion
Allium fistulosum L. Vol. VI. 26-03

Also, Tang Yao in his *Tried and Proven Recipes* recommends to mix onion juice with a small amount of honey and ingest this. This, too, is excellent. He states that "in his neighborhood an old woman used this recipe and it was very effective. An old servant tried it and again it proved to be effective."

The two items i.e., onion leaves and honey eaten together are harmful. How can it be that they are able to cure this illness? Presumably, the spleen and the stomach differ from person to person, and if it is not an extremely critical condition, they must not be tested lightly.

Dutchman's pipe
Aristolochia debilis Sieb. et Zucc. Vol. V, 18-64

Water swelling during pregnancy. It begins from the two feet and gradually reaches upward until it causes panting and heart-pressure, similar to water. Water comes out of the toes. This is called "child qi." It is related to a long-lasting presence of wind qi in the pregnant woman, or to a blood and wind intrusion in the throughway and controller vessels. In such a situation decoctions for water disorder must not be given indiscriminately. The "powder with dutchman's pipe" is appropriate.

Grind equal amounts of Dutchman's pipe, washed and slightly stir-fried; nutgrass, stir-fried; tangerine peels; *glycyrrhiza* root; and *lindera* root into powder. Each time let the patient ingest three maces. Boil one such dose in one large cup of water with three ginger slices, three quince slices, and three *perilla* leaves down to 70% and let the patient ingest this on an empty stomach. To be ingested three times a day. When the urine flows freely, the movement of qi in the vessels is unimpeded, and the swelling gradually decreases, do not ingest much more. This is a secret recipe of Chen Jingchu, a renowned physician in Huainan. It was obtained from Li Boshi's family. Chen Ziming, *Good recipes for Women.*

"Dry moss."
Ulva prolifera (Muell.) J. AG. Vol. V, 21-02

Li Shizhen: Mr. Hong Mai in his *The Records of Yijian* states: "In a monastery in Henan, all the monks suffered from a goiter illness. Then a monk from Luoyang shared a hut with them and each time they ate together they consumed preserved moss food. After several months the tumorous growth at the monks' nape had dissolved. Then they knew that items from the sea can eliminate such an illness.

Maltose. Malt sugar
Vol. V, 25-19

Li Shizhen: The *Records Collecting the Extraordinary* states: "Xing Caojin was a mighty general in Heshuo. Once a flying arrow hit one of his eyes. He pulled out the arrow but the arrowhead remained stuck in his eye. They tried to remove it with a pair of pincers, but to no avail. The general suffered from excruciating pain and he awaited his death. Then, suddenly, in his dreams a Hu monk advised him to drip rice juice into the wounded eye as that would certainly cure him. The general enquired with his entourage what that was meant to say but nobody understood it. Another day, a monk came to beg for food. He resembled the one in his dream, so the general kotowed in front of him. The monk said: 'You only need to drip malt sugar from the Cold Food day into the wounded eye.' The general applied it as prescribed and felt a cooling and refreshing effect. His suffering was mitigated immediately. During the night the wound itched, and with a forceful pair of pincers the arrowhead could be removed. Within ten days the general was cured."

Aconitum tuber as small as "seeds leaking from a basket."
Aconitum carmichaeli Debx. Vol. IV, 17-20

Also, as the *Categorized Compilation* states: "Someone developed sores on his two feet. They released a malodorous stench making it difficult to approach that person. One night he rested in the Ancestral Temple of the Five Ladies, and dreamed of a spirit offering him the following recipe. 'Grind one fresh *aconitum* tuber as small as seeds leaking from a basket into powder, add a little calomel, mix it with well water, and spit it on the affected region.' He started a cure following this advice and eventually was healed." The fact is, this item is not suitable for an ingestion. It is only used externally on sores.

Introductory Notes
Vol. I, 01-05-15

In the more than 100 chapters of the *Recipes of Fan Wang* and in Ge Hong's *Recipes to be Kept Close at Hand*, a small number of classic drugs applied as single substances, and also approaches tested by farmers, are recorded, and also arts from closed spheres with unusual knowledge. For example, that lotus root skin disperses blood is knowledge introduced by cooks. That *pharbitis nil* seeds serve to drive out water is knowledge originating from old peasants nearby. The garlic and leeks from noodle shops are pharmaceutical drugs to discharge snakes. Sickle leaved hare's ear from the roadside is a secret drug to cure wounds caused by metal objects/weapons. That is so because of the items to be found between heaven and earth, there is not one that has no use between heaven and earth. When people come into contact with them, they understand their usage without these items introducing themselves.

Walnut
Juglans regia L. Vol. VI, 30-28-02

Hong Mai states: "Once I had a phlegm ailment and because of it I came late to an audience. The sovereign had a recipe revealed to me recommending the following. To chew the meat of three walnuts with three ginger slices at bedtime and to ingest the resulting pulp by drinking two or three sips of boiled water. And to chew the walnuts and the ginger several times again as before, and then lie down calmly. This should result in a cure. When I, Hong Mai, returned to the Jade Hall, I ingested this medication as recommended, and the next morning the phlegm was dissolved and the coughing had ended."

Also, in Liyang, the young child of Hong Ji suffered from phlegm panting, and for five days and nights it failed to accept nursing milk or any other food. The physician informed the family of the child's critical condition. Hong Ji's wife that night dreamed of Guan yin who gave her a recipe recommending to let the child ingest a 'decoction with ginseng root and walnut kernels.' Hong Ji quickly obtained a more than one inches long ginseng root from Xin luo and the meat of one walnut. They were boiled and as much as is held by a corbicula shell was forcefed to the child. That ended the panting. The next morning a decoction was prepared with walnuts whose shells had been removed, but the panting began again. Then walnuts with their shell/skin still present were used, and two nights later the child was healed.

This recipe is not recorded in the literature. The fact is, it is effective because ginseng root cures panting, and walnuts with their skin astringe the lung.

Dung beetle heart
Catharsius molossus L. Vol. VIII, 41-18-02.

Pin sores. Su Song: According to the *Liuzhou's Recipes for Rescue from the Three Kinds of Death*, compiled by Liu Yuxi, the author had acquired a pin sore in the eleventh year of the reign period "Original Harmony" (816). After 14 days, the disease became ever more serious, and even the application of good medications remained without effect. Eventually, Mr. Jia Fangbo from Chang le advised him to resort to the hearts of dung beetles. Within one night all his suffering had ended. The next year, in the first month, he ate mutton, and the disease massively broke out again. Again he used dung beetle hearts and they were divinely effective.

The method to apply them is as follows. Remove the hearts of dung beetles from below their abdomen. Their meat is somewhat white. Paste them onto the sores for a little longer than half a day, and then replace them with new ones. Once the bleeding has ended, and the root of the pin has come out, a cure is achieved. Dung beetles fear mutton. Hence, once he had eaten mutton, the disease broke out again. This method of treating this disease originates from Ge Hong's *Recipes to be Kept Close at Hand*.

Chinese small onion
Allium fistulosum L. Vol. VI. 26-03

Su Song: For a cure with simmered onion leaves of injuries caused by a blow or fall see Liu Yuxi's *Transmitted Core Recipes*. He states that "he had obtained it from the Executive Assistant Cui. Simmer newly broken onion leaves, heat them over a fire, remove the skin with its mucus and apply it to the location of the injury. Simmer many onion leaves and continuously replace leaves that have cooled with hot leaves. Cui states: 'Once when I and Li Baozhen served as judges in Ze and Lu we played a ball game with others. As Director Li was hitting a ball with his ball stick, a general with his stick crossed Li's stick. As a result Director Li's thumb was hurt and his fingernail was cut in two. He hastily required to have the thumb wrapped with some medication for wounds caused by metal objects/weapons, and he insisted on drinking wine. His face assumed a greenish color and he suffered from unending pain. A military official told him of this recipe and Director Li applied it. After three replacements his face turned red again, and after a short while the pain stopped. He wrapped his finger more than ten times with the heated onion leaves and their mucus, and eventually everyone who had attended the party talked laughing'."

Li Shizhen: According to the *Zhang shi jing yan fang*, "for bleeding wounds caused by metal objects/weapons and fracture harm, simmer onion white stalks with the leaves until they are hot, or bake them in a pan and stir-fry them until they are hot, pound them into a pulpy mass and apply it to the affected region. When it cools, replace it. Dai Yaochen, commander in Shicheng, tested a horse and hurt his thumb. It bled profusely. I used this recipe. After two replacements the pain stopped. The next day when he washed his face he did not discover any scars. Judge Song and District Governor Bao, they both got hold of this recipe. Whenever someone is killed or harmed with the flow of his qi not yet interrupted, quickly apply this recipe. It has saved the lives of many people."

Also, whenever someone feels a heaviness in his head and eyes, with heart-pressure and pain, I, Li Shizhen, insert onion leaves two or three inches deep into the patient's nose and ears. Once the passage of qi is freed, the patient will feel good again.

Indian coral tree
Erythrina variegata L. Vol. VII, 35-14

During the Southern Tang dynasty, Wang Shaoyan, Prefect in Yunzhou, in his *Sequel to the Recipes Transmitted with Verification* stated: "A year or so ago I was in Gu shu and suffered from an unbearable pain in the lower back and knees. Physicians treated me with all types of medication for wind poison affecting the kidney long-term depot, but did not achieve a cure. Then I read Liu Yuxi's *Transmitted Core Recipes* where this recipe was recommended as effective. I prepared and ingested one preparation and the pain decreased by one half. The recipe recommends to prepare a mixture of two ounces of Indian coral tree bark, one ounce each of *achyranthes* leaves, *ligusticum* root, *notopterygium* root, *lycium* root bark and *acanthopanax* root bark, half an ounce of *glycyrrhiza* root, two ounces of Job's tears, and ten ounces of fresh Chinese foxglove rhizome. Wash them clean, bake them over a slow fire until they are dry, and cut them into small pieces. Wrap them in silk fabric and soak this in two pecks of ash-free wine. In winter for two times seven days; in summer for seven days. Drink one cup on an empty stomach, once every day in the morning, at noon, and in the evening. Patients should be kept in a state of drunkenness at all times. Nothing should be added to or removed from this recipe. During its application poisonous food is forbidden."

Li Shizhen: The bark of Indian coral trees can pass through the conduits and network vessels to reach the location of a disease. It also enters the blood section. It removes wind and kills worms/bugs.

Asafetida
Ferula assa foetida L. Vol. VII, 34-32

According to Wang Qiu's *101 Select Recipes*, "Tan Kui in Kuizhou suffered from malaria for half a year. An old friend, Dou Cangsou, gave him a recipe recommending to grind one ounce each of true asafetida and good cinnabar into an even mixture, and with rice paste form pills the size of Chinese honey locust tree seeds. Each time the patient should ingest, on an empty stomach, one pill dissolved in a ginseng decoction. This results in a cure.

Today, when people cure malaria, they always resort to *dichroa* root and arsenic, and they often cause injuries. This recipe is balanced and easy to prepare, but people are unaware of it."

Weeping willow
Salix babylonica L. Vol. VII, 35-29

Piles sores resembling cucumbers, with the swelling aching as if burned. Boil willow twigs in water to obtain a thick decoction and use it to wash the affected region. Apply three to five mugwort leaf cauterizations. Gentleman of the Interior Wang Ji once had this disease. An official at a post on his journey treated him with this recipe and applied cauterization. Wang Ji felt hot qi entering his intestines and then had a massive and extremely painful discharge of blood and dirt. After a while the piles had dissolved. Wang Ji mounted his horse and left the post. *Recipes Based on Facts.*

Mimosa
Albizzia julibrissin Durazz. Vol. VII, 35-20

According to Pang Anshi's *Discourse on All Diseases from Harm Caused by Cold*, "in the fifth year of the reign period "Protection of the Origin" (1090), from spring to autumn, people in the two prefectures Qi and Huang suffered from sudden throat closure. Out of ten, eight or nine died. The disease progressed rapidly; patients died within half a day or within one day. Pan Anchang, judge in Huangzhou, obtained a recipe for a 'black dragon ointment.' He saved the lives of dozens of persons." This recipe serves to cure nine types of throat blockage: Acute throat closure, throat-constricting wind, bound throat, festering throat, run-away bug, worm-gnawing, doubled tongue, wooden tongue, and flying silk threads having entered the throat.

Chinese honey locust tree
Gleditsia sinensis Lam. Vol. VIII, 35-21-02

The *Biographies of Divine Immortals* states: "Cavalry Officer Cui Yan one morning got a malign illness of massive wind. Both eyes were darkened and blinded. His eyebrows fell off, his nasal bridge collapsed. His condition seemed hopeless. Then he met a strange person who gave him a recipe. It suggested to burn three pounds of soapbean tree thorns to ashes, steam them for as long as two hours, dry them in the sun and grind them into a powder. The amount held by a spoon should be drunk after a meal mixed with a thick rhubarb root decoction. Ten days later his eyebrows had grown again. His muscles were moist and his eyesight was clear. Later he went into the mountains to devote himself to the DAO. It is unknown how he ended."

Apricot kernels
Armeniaca vulgaris Lam. Vol. VI, 29-02-02

The *Leisure-hours Conversations of Rustics* states: "When the Han lin schol-ar Xin Rensun was in a Daoist monastery on Mount Qingchengshan, in a dream an august maiden said to him: 'You can ingest apricot kernels, they add to your intelligence. You will be old and remain strong. The strength of your heart does not weaken.' He asked for the recipe and it is as follows. Every morning after you have washed your face and rinsed the mouth put seven apricot kernels into the mouth. After quite a long time when the skin has come off spit it out to remove it. Finely chew the remaining parts of the kernels and swallow them with the saliva. Eat them every day. Within one year the blood will have been exchanged, and this relieves your body of its weight. This is a recipe of Heavenly Master Shen."

Centipede spec
Spirobolus bungei Brandt.Vol. VIII, 42-10

Sun the Perfected One in his *Recipes Worth a Thousand in Gold* states: "I myself once, in the sixth month, acquired such a sore, and for five, six days treatments remained without effect. Then there was someone who drew the image of an earwig on the ground. He cut with a knife a small piece of soil from its abdomen, mixed it with saliva and applied it to the affected region. After he had applied this twice, I was cured. This lets one know that the myriad things are interrelated; the final cause remains unknown."

Nelumbo nucifera Gaertn
Indian lotus rootstock. Vol. VI, 33-10

Tao Hongjing: The root has entered the homes of spirit hermits/immor-tals. During the Song era, the Provisioner responsible for preparing meals for the court once prepared a meal from thick cattle blood. When the cook cut the skin of a lotus rootstock it accidentally fell into the blood, and as a result the blood failed to coagulate. Hence, physicians successfully use lotus rootstocks to break up blood accumulations.

Fritillaria unibracteata Hsiao et K.C. Hsia
Sichuan *fritillaria*. Vol. III, 13-15-01

Inability of a nursing mother to let milk sap. The "powder with the two ingredients named 'mother' (*mu*)." Grind equal amounts of Sichuan *frit-illaria* bulbs (*bei mu*), *anemarrhena* root (*zhi mu*), and oyster powder to fine powder. Each time let the woman ingest two maces mixed with a pig trotter decoction. This is a recipe transmitted by the ancestors. Wang Haicang, *Materia Medica for Decoctions*.

Mung bean
Vigna radiata (L.) R. Wilczak. Vol. V, 24-06-01

Injury harm caused by a blow or fall. Stir-fry mung bean powder in a new pot until it has assumed a purple color, mix it with newly drawn well water, apply this to the affected region, and fasten it with Chinese cedar tree bark. Divinely effective. This is a recipe transmitted to Mr. Chen from Ding in a dream. *Recipes of the Tranquil Hut*.

Chinese bitter cucumber
Momordica cochinchinensis (Lour.) Spreng. Vol. V, 18-08-01

Leg qi with painful swelling. Cut Chinese bitter cucumber seeds into two pieces and fry them with wheat bran. Then cut them into small pieces and fry them again until all their oil has left. For each ounce of Chinese cucumber seeds add half an ounce of thick *cassia* bark and grind this into powder. Two maces are ingested with hot wine to reach an intoxication. When the patient sweats, healing is achieved. This is a recipe mysteriously obtained in a dream. *Eternal Key Recipes*.

Li Binhu's *Simple Recipes from his Collection* recommends to mix five female and five male Chinese cucumber kernels, still moist, with a nursing mother's milk and prepare seven pills. Cover them with an upside-down bowl at a damp place to prevent them from drying. Each time open one pill by dissolving it with saliva and attach it to piles. This ends the pain. One pill dissolves the piles in the course of one night. In Jiangxi, in the "Temple of the Iron Buddha," monk Cai suffered from this disease. The pain was unbearable. Someone gave him this recipe and he was healed. He then used it to cure numerous persons, and it always turned out to be effective.

Buckwheat
Fagopyrum esculentum Moench. Vol. V, 22-08

According to Yang Qi's *Simple and Convenient Recipes*, "in the case of a rather mild abdominal pain with an outflow, but in small amounts, and several bowel movements during day and night, prepare a cooked dish of *qiao mai* flour and nothing else and eat this three or four times in a row.

That will lead to healing. When I was in a robust age I suffered from this for two months. I was emaciated and extremely nervous. An application of various medications to dissolve food and transform qi remained without effect. A monk suggested this to me and I was healed. I used it on other occasions, and it always proved to be effective."

Red knotweed flowers
Polygonum orientale L. Vol. IV, 16-50-02

Painful stomach duct related to blood and qi disorder. Boil one generous handful of red knotweed flowers in two cups of water down to one cup and ingest this. This is a recipe of the company commander Mao Juzhuang; it has repeatedly proved to be effective. Dong Bing, *Collected and Proven Recipes Recorded while Avoiding the Floods.*

Rhubarb root
Rheum palmatum L. Vol. V, 17-01-01

Harm caused by scalds and burns. Grind fresh rhubarb root from Zhuanglang to powder, mix it with honey, and apply this to the affected region. This will not only end the pain, it also minimizes the scars. This is a recipe handed over by a divine person from Jinshan monastery. Hong Mai, *The Records of Yijian.*

Pinellia ternata (Thunb.) Breit
Vol. V, 17-26-01

Heat qi and phlegm in the upper section on the Triple Burner. Prepare with one ounce of processd *pinellia ternata*, two maces of sliced *scutellaria* root powder, and ginger juice a wheat flour paste to form pills the size of mung beans. Each time ingest 70 pills, to be ingested with a bland ginger decoction after a meal. This is a recipe designed by Prince Zhou Xian wang in person. *Precious Recipes to Be Kept up the Sleeve.*

Sudden death with unconsciousness. Blow *pinellia ternata* powder into the patient's nose and he/she will return to life. This is a recipe of the Lady of Nanyue, the Original Sovereign Wei of the Purple Numinosity.

Vertigo with a tendency of qi movements being cut off. Mix *pinellia ternata* powder with cold water and form pills the size of soybeans. Insert them into the woman's nose and she will be cured. This is a method of Bian Que. *Recipes to be Kept Close at Hand.*

Frankincense
Boswellia carteri Birdw. Vol. VII, 34-22

To avert warmth epidemics. From every 24th day of the 12th month at the fifth nightwatch to the fifth nightwatch of New Year's Day soak frankincense in the first water drawn from a well. From young people to adults, everybody ingests one piece of frankincense with three sips of the water. This prevents a misfortune for the whole year. Kong Pingzhou: "This is a recipe of the Venerable Sage Confucius. It has been in use by the Kong family for more than 70 generations."

Trichosanthes kirilowii Maxim
Vol. V, 18-18

Long-lasting free-flux illness in all five colors. Calcine one big, ripe *trichosanthes kirilowii* fruit by retaining its nature and then allow the fire poison to leave again. Grind the calcined fruit into powder and ingest it all at once. To be ingested with warm wine. A servant of Hu Daqing suffered from free-flux illness for half a year. A Daoist from Hangzhou gave him this recipe and he was cured. *Recipes Based on Facts.*

Bushy knotweed root
Polygonum cuspidatum Sieb. et Zucc. Vol. IV, 16-57-01

Xu Xueshi in his *Recipes Based on Facts* recommends to "cure all types of urinary dripping illness of males and women as follows. Wash bushy knotweed roots clean and cut one-tenth of a pint into fine pieces. Boil them in five-tenths of a pint of water down to one small cup full. Discard the dregs, add small amounts of frankincense and musk, and ingest this.

The wife of Geng Mengde, Commandant in Yinjian, suffered from sand and stone urinary dripping for 13 years. Each time she urinated, she was plagued by an unbearable pain, and when she urinated into a chamber pot, the sound of the sand and stones was heard. None of the hundreds of recipes was effective. It was by chance that she obtained this recipe and ingested it. After one night she was cured. I have witnessed this with my own eyes."

Sclerotium of *poria cocos* (Schw.) Wolf. *Poria*
Vol. VII, 37-01

Heart qi depletion with uncontrolled outflow of sperm during dreams, or white, turbid urine. Send down two maces of white *poria* powder mixed with a rice decoction. To be ingested twice a day. A recipe of Su Dongpo. *Straightforward Guide to Recipes.*

Croton tree
Croton tiglium L. Vol. VII, 35-47

Yin poison and harm caused by cold. Qi nodes in the central region that are very painful when pressed. Blocked major (i.e., defecation) and minor (i.e., urination) relief, releasing only slightly warmed qi. Quickly take ten *croton* seeds and grind them. Add one mace of wheat flour, and knead this to form a cake. Place it on the navel and perform five cauterizations with small moxa cones. Once their qi reach the abdomen, defecation/urination is freed. This is a recipe of Grand Preceptor Chen Beishan. Renzhai, *Straightforward Guide to Recipes.*

Lacquer Tree
Toxicodendrum vernicifluum (Stokes) F. A. Barkl. Vol. VII, 35-08

Su Song: A record in the Biography of Hua Tuo is as follows: "In his youth Fan A of Peng cheng followed Hua Tuo as his teacher. Hua Tuo taught him how to apply the recipe for the 'powder with fragrant Solomon's seal and lacquer tree leaves,' stating that when it is ingested it removes the three worms/bugs, frees the passage through the five long-term depots, relieves the body of its weight, boosts the qi, and prevents the head from turning white. Fan A followed his advice and lived for more than 500 years."

Lacquer tree leaves can be found everywhere. Fragrant Solomon's seal grows in Fengpai, Pengcheng, and Chaoge. It is also called "ground nodes" and yellow *ganoderma*. It orders the qi in the five long-term depots and boosts the essence qi. The origin of this recipe is that someone got lost in the mountains and saw an hermit/immortal ingest it. He informed Hua Tuo of this recipe. Hua identified it as an excellent medication and he in turn related it to Fan A. Fan A kept it secret. People close to Fan A saw that he enjoyed longevity with the full vigor of his qi retained and they asked him about his secret. Because he was drunk he accidentally told them about the recipe. The people ingested it with much success. Later on, people no longer knew of fragrant Solomon's seal leaves. Some said that these were the leaves of ordinary Solomon's seal.

Li Shizhen: Ge Hong in his *The Master Embracing Simplicity* states: "Lacquer tree leaves and fragrant Solomon's seal leaves are common herbal items. Fan A ingested them and reached a long life of 200 years, with his ears and eyes still sharp and clear. They appear to be capable of replacing needle and pharmaceutical drugs to cure disease."

This is a fact of recent times, reported and commented on in trustworthy historical texts. Ge Hong comes close to the underlying principle. Before it was said that Fan A lived 500 years. That is wrong.

Purple willow
Salix sinopurpurea C. Wang et Ch. Y. Yang. Vol. VII, 35-31

Wei Zhi in his *The Heart Mirror of Universal Love* states: The bathing serves to let warm qi pass through and cause a comfortable steaming to stimulate a penetration by qi and blood, with an effect that is by no means superficial. If medication is ingested to support the qi and the blood, it will rise with the steam and the effects will be even faster. Once I saw an old woman in a village who applied this therapy with success. I asked her and she gave me the recipe. I applied it a hundred times and it hit the target a hundred times. Be careful not to modify it. It truly has a wondrously adjusting effect. The fact is, when the yellow bell is rung and the hibernating worms/bugs begin to move, when the East wind blows and the hard ice melts, the treatment with this recipe results in a comparable spring." None of the many books has a record of this therapeutic method. Hence, it is noted here in such detail.

Black myrobalan plum tree
Terminalia chebula Retz. Vol. VII, 35-26

The Tang author Liu Yuxi in his *Transmitted Core Recipes* states: "Once I suffered from red and white discharge. I ingested all types of medication but was not healed for a long time. Eventually the items discharged turned into white pus. General Ling Hu gave me this recipe: Remove the skin of three black myrobalan plums, two roasted in a pan, one fresh, grind it into a powder, and ingest it with fermented water of foxtail millet heated to bubbling. If a case in question is simply a watery free-flux illness add as much *glycyrrhiza* root powder as is held by one spoon. If there is some pus and blood, add three spoons. If [the outflow] occurs with much blood, add three spoons, too."

Storax
Liquidambar orientalis Mill. Vol. VII, 34-27

As Shen Gua in his *Brush talks* states: "Defender-in-Chief Wang Wen-zheng gong suffered from diminished qi and was often ill. Song Emperor Zhen zong personally gave him a bottle with a medicinal wine, asking him to drink it on an empty abdomen, as it was supposed to harmonize qi and blood and to repel outside evil qi. Wang Wenzheng gong drank it and felt very much at ease and healthy. The next day he approached the Emperor to express his gratitude. His Highness said: 'This is storax wine. Add one ounce of storax pills to one peck of wine and boil this. It is very much able to regulate and harmonize the five long-term depots and to eliminate all illnesses from the abdomen. Whenever you are exposed to cold when you have got up early in the morning, it is advisable to drink one cup.' Since then all the people prepared this wine and the recipe was widely distributed."

The recipe was originally recorded in Tang Emperor Xuan zong's *Recipes for Extensive Assistance of the Reign Period "Opening a New Era"* under the name "pills with *atractylodes macrocephala* rhizome." Later people included it in the *Recipes Worth a Thousand in Gold* and *Arcane Essential Recipes from the Outer Censorate.* It very effectively heals illness.

Aloes
Aloe vera L. Vol. VII, 34-33

The Tang era Liu Yuxi's *Transmitted Core Recipes* states: "I myself in young years suffered from a skin illness. Initially it appeared in the region of my neck. Then it extended upwards to the left ear. Eventually, a moist sore developed full of liquid. I resorted to various pharmaceutical drugs, such as blister beetles, dog bile, and peach root. All they could contribute were some stings. The sores swelled further. Then I was in Chuzhou and met a drug seller who taught me to grind one ounce of aloes and half an ounce of roasted *glycyrrhiza* root into a powder. First I was required to wash the affected region with warm fermented water of foxtail millet. Then it was wiped clean and the powder was applied. The sores dried right away and within short I was cured. That was truly a divine and extraordinary success."

Fragrant rosewood
Dalbergia odorifera T. Chen. Vol. VII, 34-14

Li Shizhen: Fragrant Rosewood was not listed in the *Materia Medica* books of the Song era. Tang Shenwei was the first to add it, but he did not describe its therapeutic potential and uses. Today, practitioners often use knot thickening for fractures and wounds caused by metal objects/weapons. It is said that they can replace myrrh and dragon's blood.

As the *Records of Famous Physicians* states: "Naval officer Zhou captured a bandit and was hurt by his knife. The wound was bleeding endlessly. His sinews appeared to be severed; his bone appeared to be fractured. The 'powder with dolomite' was applied but without effect. A soldier named Li Gao closed the wound with the 'purple gold powder.' That ended the bleeding and stopped the pain. The next day a scab had formed like iron, and Zhou was cured. Also, no scars were left. Zhou kowtowed to the soldier to have him reveal the recipe. The powder was obtained by scratching purple vine aromatic/fragrant rosewood with a porcelain tile. This is the very best quality of fragrant rosewood; it has rescued tens of thousands of people."

Luo Tianyi has included this recipe in his *Precious Mirror to Protect Life*, too, stating that it is very effective.

Apricot kernels
Armeniaca vulgaris Lam. Vol. VI, 29-02-02

Su Song: The ancient recipes resorted to the following method to prepare apricot kernels. Steam them from morning to noon. Slightly stir-fry them on a slow fire for seven days and store them. Every morning eat them on an empty abdomen. Ingested for a very long time, they extend the years of your life with the original complexion maintained. This is said to be a method introduced by the imperial concubine Xia.

Taro leaves and stem
Colocasia esculenta (L.) Schott. Vol. VI, 27-32-02

Explication. Tang Shenwei: Shen Gua in his *Brush talks* states: "Retired scholar Liu Yang lived in seclusion on Mount Wangwushan when he observed how a spider was stung by a bee/wasp. It fell to the ground and its abdomen was about to break open. It slowly moved to the herbs and with its teeth severed the stalk of a taro plant. Then it approached the location of the stalk it had severed with its teeth and rubbed the sore generated by the bee's/wasp's sting against it. After quite some time the swelling of dissolved and the abdomen returned to its orginal size. That is the origin of the application of taro in later times to cure harm caused by bee/wasp stings."

Chinese radish
Raphanus sativus L. Vol. VI, 26-16

The *Medical Anecdotes* also states: "Someone loved to eat bean curd and eventually was poisoned. Physicians treated him, but without effect. Then suddenly he encountered someone who sold bean curd and who told him that his wife once had accidentally dropped a radish decoction into the cauldron used to boil the bean curd whereupon the bean curd failed to congeal. That man understood. He drank a radish decoction and was healed. The principles underlying the interaction of items are that wondrous."

Hardneck garlic
Allium sativum L. Vol. VI, 26-09

Ye Shilin in his *Records from the Summer Resort* states: "During a summer month a servant galloped on a horse when suddenly he fell to the ground and was about to die. His neighbor, Wang Xiang, taught those concerned with him to grind one handful each of garlic and hot soil from the road into a pulpy mass, mix it with a cup of newly drawn water, break the patient's teeth, and force-feed him the juice. Shortly afterwards he regained his senses.

Tradition has it that this recipe suddenly appeared inscribed on the city gate of Xuzhou, and everybody assumed that it was placed there by spirit immortals to save people."

Indian Lotus rootstock nodes
Nelumbo nucifera Gaertn. Vol. VI, 33-10-04

Zhao Jin in his *Literary Notes Written During Recuperation* states: "Song Emperor Xiao zong suffered from free-flux illness and all medical therapies remained unsuccessful. Then Emperor Gao zong (his father) happened to see a small apothecary's shop, called on the owner, and asked him about a suitable therapy. That man asked about the origin of that disease and was told that it was caused by eating lake crabs. Then he examined the patient's movements in the vessels and said: 'This is a free-flux illness related to the presence of cold.' He then ground newly collected lotus rootstock nodes into a pulp and let the patient send it down mixed with hot wine. Having ingested this several times, the patient was cured. Gao zong was very pleased and bestowed the pharmacist with a golden pestle and mortar to pound his medication in future. People thereafter called the pharmacist a 'strict defense specialist with a golden pestle and mortar.' This may be said to have been an encounter hardly occurring during a lifetime."

In general, lotus rootstock can dissolve stagnating blood, resolve heat, and open the stomach, and that is also why it resolves crab poison.

Wine brewing residue/sediment
Vol. V, 25-27-01

Li Shizhen: Wine brewing residue/sediment has the nature of yeast/ferment and sprouted grain. It can speed-up the movement of blood through the conduits and ends pain. Hence, it has the potential of curing harm and injury.

According to Xu Shuwei's *Recipes Based on Facts*, "it serves to cure fracture and harm affecting sinews and bones, with unbearable pain. Prepare a mixture of one pound of fresh Chinese foxglove rhizome, one pound of wine brewing residue/sediment stored together with melons and ginger, and four ounces of fresh ginger. Stir-fry this mixture until it is hot, and apply it, covered with a piece of cloth, to the injured location. When it has cooled down, replace it.

Once someone had a fracture harm. A physician ordered to catch a living tortoise and was going to kill it to use it in his treatment. During the night he dreamed of a tortoise giving him this recipe. He applied it and the patient was cured.

Hawthorne fruit
Crataegus pinnatifada Bunge var. major N.F. Br. Vol. VI, 30-09-01

According to the *Records of the Mutual Influences of Various Categories of Things*, "when you boil old chicken or hard meat, add several hawthorne fruits and they will turn tender easily." From this statement one can deduce the potential of hawthorne to dissolve food accumulations. A child in my, Li Shizhen's neighborhood because of a food accumulation turned yellow with a swelling. Its abdomen was bloated like a drum. It so happened that when it rested under a hawthorne tree it ate its fruits to repletion. When it returned home it massively vomited phlegm and water and its disease was cured.

Quince. *Chaenomeles speciosa* (Sweet) Nakai. Vol. VI, 30-05-01

Leg qi with a swelling and tension. Cut a quince fruit into pieces, put them in a pouch and let the patient tramp on it. Gu Anzhong from Guang de suffered from leg qi. His sinews were tense and his leg was swollen. Once on a boat he placed his foot on a bag and noticed that the pain gradually subsided. So, he asked the boatman: "What is in that bag?" He replied: "Quince from Xuanzhou." After his return home he prepared a bag with quince and used it to treat his disease. He stamped it with his foot and was cured. *Ming yi lu.*

Soybean leaves
Glycine max (L.) Merr. Vol. V, 24-01-03

Li Shizhen: According to *The Master Embracing Simplicity Nei pian*, "in the village of Counselor-in-Chief Zhang Wenwei there was a cave with weasels. Once their four kids were swallowed by a snake. The feelings of their parents were hurt and they thought of a plan. They built a dam of soil outside the cave to block its entrance. They envisaged that when eventually the head of the snake appeared, it would not be able to easily turn around. That way they could bite the lower back of the snake to sever it and they cut open its abdomen from where they took the four kids. They still had qi. The parents placed them outside the cave, chewed soybean leaves, and applied them to the kids. They all survived." When people later resorted to bean leaves to cure snakebite, it was based on this event.

Chinese clematis
Clematis chinensis Osbeck. Vol. V, 18-39-01

Su Song: Formerly, a person in Shangzhou suffered from a paralysis of hands and feet. For tens of years he was unable to walk on the ground. Good physicians had exhausted their skills but could not heal him. His relatives positioned him at the roadside to find help. Then a monk from Xinluo saw him and told him: "With this illness, there is one pharmaceutical drug that can return life to you. But I do not know whether it is available here." Hence, they urged him to go into the mountains and search for it. Eventually he got hold of it, and that was Chinese clematis. They let the patient ingest it and after several days he was able to walk. Later, Deng Siqi, a man living in the mountains, learnt of this and spread the message.

Piper wallichii (Miq.) Hand.-Mazz. var. *hupehense* (C. DC.) Hand.-Mazz. Vol. V, 18-66

Ma Zhi: According to the History of Southern Dynasties, Xie Shuqian, a man from Yanmen, one night prayed for his sick mother. He heard a voice from the void stating: "Get piper wallichii to treat her and she will be healed." He consulted physicians and the *ben cao* literature, but found nothing about this pharmaceutical drug. In the Yidu mountains he saw an old man who felled a tree. He stated: "This is piper wallichii; it heals wind intrusion." With tears Xie Shuqian politely asked him to give it to him. The old man also showed him how to soak it in wine. When Xie Shuqian had acquired the herb and the method to process it, the old man was no longer present. Xie Shuqian's mother ingested it and was healed.

Castor oil plant seeds
Ricinus communis L. Vol. II, 17-13-01

Distended tongue filling the mouth. Remove the shells of 40 castor oil plant seed kernels, grind them, and apply the oil to a piece of paper. Roll the paper into a stick, burn it, and expose the tongue to the fumes. If the distension fails to recede, fumigate it again. Continue until a cure is achieved. There was someone whose tongue was distended to a degree that it came out of his mouth. A fellow villager applied this method and he was cured. *Tried and Proven Good Recipes.*

Chinese quinine
Dichroa febrifuga Lour. Vol. IV, 17-14

Tan Yeweng in his *Tested and Proven Recipes* recommends to boil two maces each of Chinese quinine, *areca* nuts, and *glycyrrhiza* root together with one hundred grains of black soybeans in water and ingest it. This is a recipe transmitted by the Minister of Justice Peng.

Cocklebur
Xanthium sibiricum Patrin ex Widder. Vol. IV, 15-42

Zhu Duanzhang in his *Collected and Proven Recipes* states: "When I was appointed Tent Secretary in Huaixi, I suffered from massive toothache. A person selling knives and forceps let a pinch of an herbal drug soak in hot water for a short while. Then he dipped his finger into the hot water and rubbed the aching location. This ended the pain. Hence I asked him for the recipe and when I used it to cure people it was often effective."

Hedge bindweed
Calystegia sepium (L.) R. Br. Vol. V, 18-14

Li Shizhen. All plants that are vines and creepers resemble human sinews. Hence, they often serve to cure sinew diseases. The roots of hedge bindweed are as fine as sinews, and they are edible. Hence, the *Supplementary Records by Famous Physicians* says that "ingested for a long time they prevent hunger." When I, Li Shizhen returned from the Capital, I witnessed charioteers with every one of their vehicles loaded with them. When asked they stated that "after returning home in the evening they prepare a decoction that can supplement qi in the case of conditions of injury and other harm." This serves as evidence for the claim that it boosts the qi and reconnects sinews.

Climbing fig leaf
Ficus pumila L. Vol. V, 18-57-01.

Tang Shenwei: The *Illustrated Classic of Materia Medica* says: "Climbing fig leaves serve to cure sores on the back." Recently, in Yixingxian I met an old man who had been a successful candidate in the imperial examinations on the provincial level. He was more than 70 years old and suffered from an effusion on the back. There was no physician or medication available in his village. He quickly collected climbing fig leaves, ground them to a pappy mass and squeezed it to obtain a juice. He mixed it with honey and drank several *sheng*. Then he applied the dregs to the affected region. Later he applied further medication and was cured.

Dragon blood palm
Daemonorops margaritae (Hance) Becc. Vol. V, 18-69

Li Shizhen: Dragon blood palm is good at killing worms/bugs and stimulating urination.

Hong Mai in his *The Records of Yijian* states: "Zhao Zishan suffered from a tapeworm disease. A physician suggested to him to give up wine drinking, but he was addicted to it. One day he stayed in the Tian wang temple in Shao wu. At midnight he returned drunk and felt very thirsty. On the veranda he saw a jar with water that glittered in the moonlight. He drank all of it and it tasted as sweet as maltose. The next morning worms had left him and covered his mat. He felt better in his central and abdominal region and his old illness was cured. Everybody marveled at this and they inspected the water he had drunk. It was the water in which the temple servants had soaked the dragon blood palm roots that were used to weave straw sandals."

"The herb that will sober you up when you are drunk." Unidentified.
Vol. V, 21-A157

Li Shizhen: the *Forgotten Matters of the Kai yuan and Reign Periods "Heavenly Treasures"* states: Emperor Xuan zong planted it on the edge of Lake Xingqing. It grows as clusters. The leaves are purple, with a dark red center. Drunk guests picked the herb and smelled it. They were sober immediately. Hence the name.

St. Paulswort
Siegesbeckia orientalis L. Vol. IV, 15-44

A "Memorandum on St. Paulswort pills submitted" by Zhang Yong, governor of Yizhou, states: "I have eaten stones and drunk water and got delicacies filling the stomach. I have eaten pines and held cypresses in my mouth to realize their potential to rescue me from disease. That is, those who heal hunger will not shy away from the unusual, and those who cure disease, why should they be irritated by procedures that are different?! If a drug is acquired that helps in times of seasonal epidemics, then it should be propagated even if it is of a vulgar shape. One must not look at it narrow-mindedly, but propagate it to everybody. I, your subject, during the restoration of the Rising Dragon Monastery excavated a stele on which was written a procedure to nourish one's qi, accompanied by two recipes. Based on these recipes, I sent people out to make enquiries and gather information.

The herb mentioned on the stele is quite unique. It has golden edges and a silver thread, a plain stalk and purple roots. The leaves grow opposite at the nodes. In Shu, they call it "fire pillow." Stem and leaves are quite similar to those of cocklebur. There is no need to waste efforts to climb on high mountains and to pass through dangerous terrain, and each time obtain only a small amount of this herb. It is quickly collected without any difficulty, and large quantities are collected most easily. When it is ingested regularly and for a long time, its divine potential will be obvious. Who could imagine that in such an extremely cheap item such extraordinary effects are contained?!

When I, your subject, had ingested it 100 times, my eyes were cleared. When I had ingested it 1,000 times, my hair and beard had turned black. My sinews felt light and my strength had returned. So many effects and therapeutic successes.

In my, your subject's, prefecture a Chief Lackey Luo Shouyi was struck by wind and fell from his horse. He lost his voice and could no longer speak. I, your subject, gave him this herb to ingest it ten times and his disease was cured.

Also, the monk Zhi Yan, at the age of 70 years, suddenly suffered from a hemilateral wind stroke. His mouth and eyes were slanted and again and again he spat saliva. I, your subject, gave him, too, this herb to ingest it ten times and his health, too, was fully restored. Now I have put together 100 preparations and send the official Shi Yuan to submit it to Your Majesty."

Mulberry tree leaf
Morus alba L. Vol. VII, 36-01-04

Painful, rough, red eyes. Grind mulberry leaves into a powder, and burn it in a paper roll to let the smoke steam the nose until an effect is achieved. A recipe from overseas. *Recipes of Universal Benefit.*

14. Dealing with poison[32]

Nature, as was early recognized in China, is not a loving mother of mankind who does only good things for her loved ones. Nature, the ancient philosopher Lao zi's *Classic of the Way and of Virtue* acknowledged, "creates all things and stimulates their growth, brings them forth, forms them, and poisons them. Nature nourishes them, and it causes them to disappear once more." The term for "poison," *du*, had a long history preceding this statement. A pictographic character "snake in the grass" appears to have been chosen as an image revealing its meaning to everybody. However, even very early, the *Classic of Changes*, compiled in the second half of the first millennium BCE, used the term as a metaphor, that is, in the sense of "using poison to achieve a certain end." The 6th hexagram, "troops," devoted to a discussion of government and behavior during a war, states that "an unyielding center stands up to challenges from the outside; dangerous situations are mastered in an adaptable manner. If the king employs such means to lead his people through the war, as if he were using a poisonous medication to cure them from a disease, they will follow him."

The term *du*, "poison," entered Chinese medicine from the very beginning with these two meanings. Poison is a property inherent in a material substance. Poison may harm or even kill you, but it may also be used to help you in poisoning, or eliminating, your adversaries. These may be evil agents that have entered your body and cause disease there; they can also be creatures outside of your body that you wish to eliminate. The metaphorical use of "poison" as a means to cure a disease, or even to govern a people – which occasionally may necessitate acting as relentlessly as a poison – is also evident in *materia medica* literature from its very beginning.

The Divine Husbandman's Materia Medica, probably of the 1st or 2nd c. CE, categorized all 365 pharmaceutically used natural substances into three "ranks," a designation resonating with the "ranks" in the bureaucracy. The top rank, reflecting Daoist social ideology, was assigned to substances named "rulers." They were assumed to be responsible for an enduring harmony in the human body. They required no poison to achieve their ends. The third and lowest rank was reserved for the deputies, or messengers, who functioned as enforcers, possessing poison which was to be used where necessary. The middle rank was composed of substances both with

---

32 Additional Reading: Yan Liu, *Healing with Poisons. Potent Medicines in Medieval China.* University of Washington Press. Seattle, 2021.

and without poison; they acted as required, either to maintain harmony, or to apply strict measures.

By the time of the *Ben cao gang mu*, the ancient classificatory system had long since lost its dominant role. Insofar as the authors of *materia medica* texts acknowledged the inevitability of disease, they continued a rationale underlying pharmaceutical therapy from the beginning. The *Yellow Thearch's Inner Classic* had repeatedly emphasized "adhering to the law" as the only behavior guaranteeing health, with the unknown author concluding "where, if you follow the law, could a disease come from?" Li Shizhen, however, discarded the ancient categorization according to three ranks, as had done authors long before him. A historical awareness was important to Li Shizhen, but he acknowledged change and apparently saw no reason to return to the beginnings.

Virtually all the authors of the previous two millennia quoted in the *Ben cao gang mu* identified "poison" as an enemy. To eradicate this enemy it must be "killed." Another term used conveys an image of "freeing" oneself or a substance from an undesirable intruder or property. As in the military, a former enemy can be turned in order to work for you. Poison is always good as an ally to attack adversaries, whether inside your body or somewhere outside. When you plan to use such an ally, you should be fully aware that such a coalition may still lead to your own downfall. Hence, means are available to prevent "poisonous beings from causing harm." In pharmacotherapy, natural substances known to be poisonous were assessed as to their degree of toxicity, and they were processed to reduce unwanted toxicity. Admonishments not to use poisonous substances carelessly and to apply proper processing are widespread throughout the *Ben cao gang mu*.

The *Ben cao gang mu* lists a long range of possible carriers and transmitters of poison. In general, these may be food or beverages; food poisoning was a threat perceived throughout the centuries. Wine poisoning was an often observed and described phenomenon. Heat and fire, essential for human life, were transformed into poison when they invaded an organism. A mother could give birth to a child affected by too much of her heat during pregnancy, resulting in a disease known as "fetal heat." Minerals such as stalactites and those containing arsenic served as pharmaceutical drugs, and – if not applied appropriately – acted as more or less potent poisons. Snakes, dragons, mad dogs, wild animals, fox urine, fish, horse sweat, blister beetles, and lytta, or "rivulet bugs," they all represent threats lurking in nature as well as in one's private household. When such poisons were used to harm, attack or kill other persons, then the knowledge of such a natural resource was being used in applications contrary to pharmacotherapy. Examples are poisoned arrowheads, and the commissioning of a highly vicious bug-spirit, the so-called *gu*, to acquire material wealth owned by other humans. Entire families suspected of an alliance with *gu* were extinguished. The punishment for such a crime was among the severest on the Statute Books of Imperial China.

Realgar
Arsenic disulphide. Vol. II, 09-07

Alternating cold and heat sensations. Mouse fistula and malign sores. Impediment-illness, piles, and dead muscles. It kills essence items and malign demons, evil qi and the poison of the hundreds of worms/bugs. It helps to overcome wounds caused by the five types of weapons. Refined with heat and consumed it takes the weight of the body and lets one become a spirit immortal. *Original Classic.*

It serves to heal *jie*-illness with worms/bugs and sores with hidden worms/bugs, painful eyes, tumorous flesh growths in the nose, and severed sinews as well as broken bones. The hundreds of joints severely struck by wind, accumulations and aggregation-illness qi, being struck by the malign with abdominal pain, demon attachment illness. It kills the poison of all types of poisonous snakes and it resolves the poison of *veratrum* root. It makes the face appear happy and lustrous. When it is ingested for food, it flies into the brain and helps to overcome demons and spirits. It extends the years of life and boosts longevity. It protects the center and prevents hunger. Matched with copper it can become gold. *Supplementary Records by Famous Physicians.*

Zhen Quan: Realgar is able to kill the hundreds of poisons, to ward off the hundreds of evils, and to kill the poison of *gu*. When a person wears it on his garments, demon spirits will not dare to approach him. When he enters a forest, tigers and wolves will go into hiding. When he wades through river water, poisonous beings will not dare to harm him.

The Master Embracing Simplicity: When a person wears realgar on his garments and enters a forest, he must not be afraid of snakes. When a person is struck by a snake, he is to apply a small amount of realgar to the location of the bite, and he will be cured immediately. In the regions of Wu and Chu, summerheat and moisture cause a steaming atmosphere, and there are many poisonous worms/bugs, archers, and sand lice. To protect oneself all that is necessary is to pound equal amounts of realgar and large garlic cloves to a pulp, form one pill, and wear it on the garments. If he was struck already, to apply this pulp to the affected region will be good, too.

Also, the *Miscellaneous Records from the Time of Emperor Ming* states: "An Imperial Gatekeeper had returned from an official mission to Jiao and Guang and the Imperial physician Zhou Gu said: 'This person has in his abdomen a flood dragon (43-03)'. The Emperor was scared and asked the Imperial Gatekeeper whether he felt ill or not. He responded: 'Your subordinate rode a horse in the Da yu ling mountain range. I felt distressed by the heat and was thirsty. Hence I drank water from a mountain rivulet. A little later I had a feeling of a hard obstacle-illness in my abdomen, as if there were a stone'. Zhou Gu then had him ingest a decoction of nitrokalite and realgar, and he immediately vomited some creature. It was several *cun* long, and as big as a thumb. A close inspection showed that it was fully covered by scales."

All these cases are evidence of the potential of realgar to kill the poison of *gu*.

Su Song: Realgar is a valuable substance to cure sores and ulcers.

The *Rites of Zhou* states: "Ulcer physicians heal ulcers by attacking them with the five poisons."

Zheng Kangcheng in his comment states: "The recipes of today's physicians include a medication with five poisons. To prepare it give chalcanthite, cinnabar, realgar, arsenolite, and magnetite into a yellow earthenware pot, and heat them for three days and three nights. The smoke rises and attaches itself as a kind of soot to the lid of the pot. Scrape it off with a chicken feather and apply it to cure sores, malign flesh, and broken bones."

Yang Yi in his personal notes recorded the following. "In his youth, Yang Yu developed an ulcer on his cheek, involving his teeth, cheekbones, and gums. On the outside a swelling appeared like a bowl turned upside down. Inside it festered with pus and excreted blood. The pain was hard to bear. Hundreds of cures for several years brought no cure. Eventually, someone let him treat this according to Zheng Kangcheng's method of heating five poisons to prepare a medication. After a short while, the decayed bone and the adjacent teeth were excreted, and this brought the cure. This is trustworthy evidence of the speedy successes reached by attacking diseases with ancient recipes."

Li Shizhen: A "medication with five poisons" is referred to in Fan Wang's *Records of Fan Dongyang* with a changed name and indication as the "powder with the flying realgar." It serves to cure chronic impediment-illness and malign sores, as well as erosions of malign flesh. The method to prepare it is as follows. Take a pottery basin and place orpiment into its center, then cinnabar South of it, magnetite North of it, malachite East of it, quartz West of it and arsenolite on top of it, followed by gypsum to be placed on top again of the *yu shi*. Stalactite is placed underneath the orpiment. All this is covered with realgar and lies on a layer of muscovite. Each of the ingredients is entered as a powder, weighing two ounces. The basin is to be covered with a second basin, and the rims are tightly sealed with a mud with sheep hair. Now build a triangular furnace, place the two basins on top of it, and burn in it long kept reed stems for one day. Then remove the "flying realgar" from the inside of the upper basin, and it may be used for therapeutic purposes.

Now, realgar is an important medication to cure sores and to kill poison; it enters the qi section on the liver conduit. Hence it is resorted to with remarkable therapeutic successes for all types of diseases such as liver wind and liver qi, fright epilepsy with phlegm and saliva blockages, headache and dizziness with vertigo, summerheat malaria and outflow with free-flux illness, as well as accumulations. Also, it is able to transform blood into water. But the recipe masters propagate the effects of ingesting it after a heat refinement as miraculous, and as a result there are many cases of people being poisoned by it.

According to Hong Mai in his *The Records of Yijian*, "Yu Yunwen, Duke of Yong, was affected by a summerheat free-flux illness, and he was not cured for several months. Then all of a sudden in a dream he went somewhere where he saw a person who looked like an hermit/immortal. That person invited him to sit down with him. On a wall a pharmaceutical recipe was written, stating: 'Summerheat poison is in the spleen. Moisture qi affect the legs. If they are not discharged, this will result in free-flux illness. If there is no free-flux illness, it will result in malaria. The only way to cure this is to mix realgar and steamed cakes to a medication. If a physician conducts a different therapy, he commits a big mistake'. The Duke followed the advice of the recipe. He processed realgar with aqueous sublimation nine times and filled it into a bamboo tube. This he steamed seven times, and then he ground it to a powder and mixed it with steamed cakes to prepare pills the size of *firmiana* seeds. For each application he sent down seven pills with a *glycyrrhiza* root decoction, with three ingestions a day. Eventually he was cured."

The *Extensive Records of the Reign Period "Great Peace"* has a record of Liu Wuming from Chengdu ingesting realgar and achieving longevity. Such sayings of recipe masters are not trustworthy.

Being struck by poison in a beverage or food. Grind equal amounts of realgar and natural indigo to a powder. Each time let the patient ingest two maces, to be sent down with newly drawn water. *Deng Bifeng's Recipes.*

Worm/bug poison. *Gu* poison. Grind equal amounts of realgar and unprocessed alum to a powder, dissolve it in honey, and form pills the size of *firmiana* seeds. Each time ingest seven pills, to be sent down with boiled water, and recite the name of the God of Medicine Buddha seven times. *Good Recipes of Su Dongpo.*

Being struck by the poison of a medicated arrow. Apply realgar powder to the affected region. When a bubbling juice is released, the patient will be cured. *Arcane Essential Recipes from the Outer Censorate.*

To resolve the poison of *veratrum* root. Ingest with water one mace of realgar powder. Arcane Essential Recipes from the Outer Censorate.

Pin-illness sores with a malign poison. The *Recipes Worth a Thousand in Gold* recommends: Pierce the affected region on all four sides and in its center and apply realgar powder there. Proved to be divinely effective.

Orpiment
Arsenic trisulphide. Vol. II, 09-08

Qi and Flavor. Acrid, balanced, poisonous.

Supplementary Records by Famous Physicians: Very cold. It must not be resorted to for decoctions.

The True Lord of Saturn: *Ligusticum* root, Chinese foxglove rhizome, *kochia* fruit, *leonurus* seed, *rhododendron* flower, *sanguisorba* root, *acanthopanax* root bark, *orostachys* herb, and winter melon juice – all these substances are capable of checking and subduing the strength/poison of orpiment. Also, when orpiment is exposed to lead and lead carbonate, it will turn black. … Lung exhaustion with cough. Fill one ounce of orpiment into a pot made of baked clay and do not close it. Place it on the ground and cover it with a two inches thick layer of ashes. Fix the top of it with one pound of charcoal, light it, and calcinate the pot until one-third of the charcoal is used up. Then withdraw the fire and let the heat poison leave. Grind the contents of the pot to a powder, mix it with toadcake, and form pills the size of millet grains. Each time send down on an empty stomach three pills with a decoction of apricot seeds. *Recipes of the Big Dipper Gate*.

Gypsum, calcium sulphate
Vol. II, 09-09

Thirst resulting from stalactite mineral poison. Hold one piece of gypsum in the mouth until a healing is achieved. *General Records of Sagely Benefaction*.

Talc. Soapstone. Smooth stone/mineral
Vol. II, 09-13

Zhang Bo in his *Records of Wu* and in his *Geographical Records of the Reign Period "Great Well-being"* states: "In Lake Ma hu and on Mount Ma ling in Bu shanxian, Yu linzhou, there are snakes that are extremely poisonous and kill humans. Their poison can be resolved with soapstone. The color of this stone/mineral is red-black; its flavor is bitter. When scraps of 'cold stone' are applied to such a snake bite wound, and at the same time are rubbed on the patient's teeth, he will be brought back to life immediately. It is also named 'stone/mineral to be rubbed on the teeth'." Nowadays, the people often use soapstone to prepare a powder to cure seething rashes. Some say that this is talc, but their sweet and bitter flavors are not identical.

Wind poison associated with heat sores, with a yellow watery liquid released from all over the body. Apply talc powder from Gui fu to the affected region and a cure will be achieved the next day. But first wash the affected region clean with a decoction of equal amounts of bushy knotweed herb, peas, and *glycyrrhiza* root, and only then apply the talc powder. *Recipes of Universal Benefit*.

Strange diseases associated with heat poison. The eyes are red and the nose is bloated. Patients pant massively and macules appear all over their body. Their hair on the body and on the head is as stiff as iron. This is because the patient was struck by heat poison resulting in bound qi in the Lower Burner. Grind one ounce each of talc and alum to a powder and let the patient ingest this in one dose. Also, let him drink in one draft a decoction of three bowls of water boiled down to one half. Xia Ziyi, *Recipes of Unusual Illnesses*.

Stalactite
Calcium carbonate. Vol. II, 09-21

Sun Simiao: Stalactites must come from the right place, they must be clear white and of shiny glossiness, and with a net-like line design, like bird feathers or cicada wings. If they are white, they can be used for therapeutic purposes. Those that do not come from the right place must be handled carefully and cannot be ingested. They are more deadly for humans than the poison of the (legendary) *zhen* 鴆 bird.

Ma Zhi: A commentary in another volume states: To all stalactites developing in deep caves and dark holes the following applies. These are locations where dragons and snakes lie hidden and they may be affected by poison qi of dragons and snakes or by an unbalanced presence of yin and yang qi at the opening of a cave, or by a wind draught passing through. They may be rough like wild goose teeth, or they are yellow or red, and the milk stone lacks glossiness, or after being refined over fire their color may be unequal. If after a first boiling the water is not exchanged, fire poison is generated and when ingested lets one have dripping urine. Take stalactites from Shaozhou, regardless of whether they are thick or thin. They simply need to have a shiny, clear and glossy color to be suitable for a refinement with heat. Only those of the two colors yellow and red must not be used. Place them into a gold or silver vessel and fill it with water. Heat the vessel to boil the water until bubbles form resembling fish eyes. When the water is reduced, add new water. In the case of only small amounts of stalactites, continue the boiling for three days and three nights. In the case of large amounts, continue it for seven days and seven nights until the water has dried up. When the color of the stalactites has changed to yellow-white they are done. If you are not sure whether they are done continue the boiling for a total length of ten days, and this will yield the best results. Remove the stalactites from the vessel and discard any remaining water. Then boil them again in clear water for half a day. Once the color of the water remains clear and does not change, end the boiling. The stalactites are no longer poisonous now. Then give them into a porcelain or earthenware bowl, add a little water and pound them with a jade pestle. Whenever they appear dry and rough, add some water until it looks like water in which rice was washed. Continue the grinding for four to five days, wipe the powder until it is shiny and greasy, just like white fish described in literature, and then wash it with water. If the powder does not flow away with the water, it is done. If it flows away with the water it is to be ground again. Eventually the dregs are dried in the sun. Each time ingest one and a half *qian*, to be sent down mixed with warm wine on an empty abdomen. At the same time the stalactites are to be used as pills and powder. The yellow turbid water left after boiling stalactites must not be ingested. Ingesting it injures one's throat, harms the lung, and causes headache. In some cases it causes unending discharge with free-flux illness. Those who have violated this prohibition need to eat pork to resolve the poison of that water. Sun zhenren, *Recipes Worth a Thousand in Gold*.

Petroleum
Vol. II, 09-27

Kou Zongshi: Genuine petroleum is difficult to store. It often erodes and seeps through containers. It is only very rarely added to medication. Experts in refining substances with heat add ground, raw arsenic to petroleum and then grind it again to obtain a paste. They give it into a crucible, close it with a tile, and place it on a fire. When the oil has completely gone, they take the arsenic out, grind it again, add petroleum again, and refine it with heat again. This serves to eliminate the poison of the arsenic.

Flint
Vol. II, 09-28-A01

Qi and Flavor. Sweet, acrid, warm, poisonous. Li Shizhen: When humans are struck by the poison of coal qi, they experience clouding with dim vision and come close to dying. They only need to drink cold water to resolve this.

Dugu Tao: Flint serves to remove impurities of tin, and checks the effects of the three substances realgar, orpiment, and sulphur that have in their names the character "yellow," sal ammoniac, and nitrokalite.

Lime
Calcium oxide. Vol. II, 09-29

It stimulates the growth of muscles and flesh. It resolves the sour flavor of wine, and serves to cure wine poisoning. Da Ming.

It causes abortion. Han Baosheng.

Humans bitten by earthworms, with a poisoning similar to that of massive wind and a loss of eyebrows and beard hair. Soak the affected region in lime water. Good. *Tried and Proven Recipes*.

Pumice
Porous lava. Vol. II, 09-31

Boiled in water and the juice drunk serves to stop thirst, to cure dripping urine, and to kill the poison of wild animals. Da Ming.

It ends thirst. Tao Hong jing.

It removes eye shades. Kou Zongshi.

It cools metal i.e., the kidneys and causes fire to descend. It dissolves accumulation lumps and transforms old phlegm. Zhu Zhenheng.

Green skin malachite
Vol. II, 10-12-A01

Supplementary Records by Famous Physicians: Flavor acrid, salty, balanced, nonpoisonous. It controls worm/bug poison and malign sores caused by all types of poison of snakes, vegetables, and meat. It must not be ingested for a long time lest it cause emaciation. It grows in the mountain valleys of Yizhou.

Tao Hongjing: It is not used in common recipes and it is not recommended in the classics of hermits/immortals. The people simply do not know it.

Chalcanthite. Water soluble copper sulphate
Vol. II, 10-13

Li Shizhen: The qi of chalcanthite are cold; its flavor is sour and acrid. Qi and flavor enter the minor yang gallbladder conduits. By its nature chalcanthite is astringent and moves upward, and it is able to free the passage of phlegm and saliva caused by wind and heat. It disperses minister fire of wood/the liver excited by wind, and it is also able to kill worms/bugs. Hence in the treatment of sores with poison affecting the throat, the mouth, and the teeth, it is used with extraordinary success.

Zhou Mi in his *Rustic Conversations from East of Qi* states: "When I, Zhou Mi, passed through Nanpu, an old physician gave me a 'recipe to cure moribund patients affected by throat closure.' It advises to forcefeed to the patient genuine duck beak chalcanthite powder mixed with vinegar. This lets the patient vomit several pints of glue-like phlegm, and he will be cured. In Lin ting the wife of an old soldier suffered from this ailment. She had not consumed water or rice grains for three days already. When I applied to her the medication as required she was cured. I have used it many times, and never without a good result. It is a divine recipe."

Mad dog bite with poison. Apply chalcanthite powder to the affected region. A cure will be achieved immediately. *Recipes for Aid in Emergencies.*

All types of poison. Use chalcanthite powder and a paste of polished glutinous rice to prepare pills the size of euryale seeds, coated with cinnabar. During storage continuously repeat the coating with cinnabar to protect them against decay. At the time of their application dissolve one pill in cold water and let the patient ingest this. A cure will be achieved immediately. *Recipes Worth More than Gold.*

Having become a victim of the technique to "poke life" and *gu*-poisonings with painful chest and mouth. Soak two maces of chalcanthite in tea and ingest it. This will cause the poison to be released by vomiting. *Recipes from Lingnan to Protect Life.*

Red bayberry poison sores. Apply chalcanthite powder mixed with vinegar to them. When the pain is severe, add frankincense and myrrh. This will cause malign water to be released. After one or two applications the sores will have dried up.

Independently growing arsenolite. Colored asenolite
Vol. II, 10-15

Li Shizhen: Arsenolite appears in numerous kinds: white arsenolite, grey arsenolite, purple arsenolite, red skin arsenolite, peach blossom arsenolite, golden star arsenolite, silver star arsenolite, and independently growing arsenolite – they all are one identical item. By their nature all of them are hot and poisonous, and they all alike can poison mice/rats and check mercury. Only grey and white arsenolite are added to medication. All types of arsenolite grow in mountains and on these mountains herbs and trees do not grow, and frost and snow do not accumulate. When arsenolite grows in a water, this water will not freeze. Sometimes there are warm springs that are obviously endowed with the hot qi of arsenolite.

The *Jade Volume from the Years Geng to Xin* states: "Arsenolite is a yang stone/mineral. It grows in mountain valleys and waters. When it is washed clean it is similar to alum. That with horizontal line structures in the center is fine. It subdues fire and checks cinnabar and mercury. Its shape is somewhat similar to that of the 'stone/mineral that splits into rectangular pieces'. Still, when it is tossed into water and the water does not freeze, it is genuine arsenolite. Arsenolite originating in gold/metal caves is called 'arsenolite that holds the snow'."

Arsenic. Arsenic trioxide
Vol. II, 10-17

Chen Cheng: Nowadays, the people often use it to cure malaria. However, malaria basically is a harm caused by summerheat, and this item, as long as it is unprocessed, is capable of resolving heat poison. Today's common physicians do not investigate such underlying principles. Hence, when this substance is prepared with heat to a frost and then ingested, patients inevitably will be affected by massive vomiting and discharge. There are some who happily recover after such a therapy, but those who will be harmed are many more. One must be careful! In the beginning, when the arsenic frost is prepared with heat sublimation, the persons engaged in this process will take a position more than ten fathoms away in the direction where the wind comes from. In the direction where the wind blows, all herbs and trees will die. Also, they mix it with rice to poison rats/mice. When a cat or a dog eats the dead rats/mice, they will die, too.

Kou Zongshi: Nowadays, it is extracted in Xin from pits dug in the ground. These pits are often sealed and closed. There is a murky green water in the pits. It must be completely removed before digging further to extract the arsenic.

Li Shizhen: Acrid, sour, very hot, very poisonous.

Da Ming: Ingested together, it fears mung beans, cold water, and vinegar. It is added to medication and boiled in vinegar to kill its poison before it is used for therapeutic purposes.

The True Lord of Saturn: When the strength of arsenic is checked by heating it in water with herbs, a juice is generated with golden streaks forming on its surface. It will transform copper and dries mercury. Halite, *chenopodium* herb, nitrokalite, garlic, water pepper, *dichroa* root, *leonurus* seed, *kochia* fruit, poplar resin, *acorus* root, Indian sorrel, small *centipeda* herb, *spinacia* herb, *lactuca* herb– all these are able to subdue the poison of arsenic.

Kou Zongshi: Arsenic frost is used by malaria specialists. Sometimes they overdose it and this causes vomiting and free flow at the same time. In such cases it is imperative to let the patient drink the juice obtained by boiling mung beans together with cold water.

Liu Chun: Elixirs for malaria often use the very poisonous medication arsenic frost. The *Materia Medica* says it controls all types of malaria and wind phlegm in the chest and diaphragm region. Also, it can serve as an emetic. The fact is, since its nature is extremely violent, it is quite capable of drying phlegm. But even though it can dry phlegm, it massively harms the stomach qi. Those patients with a spleen and stomach depletion must abstain from it.

Li Shizhen: This is a medication of massive heat and of massive poison. And the poison of arsenic frost is especially violent. When rats/mice and sparrows eat only a small amount of it, they will die immediately. When cats and dogs eat these rats/mice and sparrows, they, too, will perish. Humans consuming up to one mace will die, too. Even the strength of the poison of yellow jessamine and aconite does not exceed the strength of this poison. Still, in their *materia medica* works, Song authors did not say much about this poison; how could this be? This substance was considered by the ancients a variety of arsenolite. When it is ingested with wine or brandy, it will erode the intestines and the stomach and kill a person within a short time. Even mung beans and cold water will hardly be able to resolve such poison.

Nowadays, those merchants who store wine in bottles often resort to the fumes of arsenic to fumigate the bottles. This way the wine will not spoil. This is yet another example of profit greed without an attitude of humaneness! Those who drink this wine and without realizing it are affected by the poison of the arsenic, they blame it solely on the wine.

This item is not to be drunk as a decoction; it is only added to elixir pills. Whenever it is used for phlegm malaria and snoring as well as panting, it is genuinely effective in curing the disease right away. But it must be swallowed with cold water, and neither a cup of beverages nor a spoon of food are to be consumed at the same time. Patients are to quietly lie down for one day or one night, and they must not be stimulated to vomit. Even small amounts of beverages and food will lead to outbursts and result in vomiting. Its very dry and hot nature is based on the same qi as that of brandy and nitrokalite. Hence it serves to eliminate illnesses associated with moisture and phlegm and to open pent-up qi associated with anger. Nowadays, specialists producing fireworks add small amounts of arsenic and the sound of the explosions will be even louder. All of this is evidence of the extremely violent nature of arsenic.

Green pebbles of foreign origin. Unidentifiable
Vol. II, 10-20

Su Song: The Hu people highly value it. Together with gold ornaments they wear it as finger rings. Whenever they are about to eat or have eaten, they take it into the mouth and suck it several times to avoid being poisoned. When nowadays someone obtains a piece as big as a fingertip, its worth is that of a hundred pieces of gold.

Stone arrowtip
Vol. II, 10-20-A01

Li Shizhen: Stone arrowtips originate in Sushen. The people there use the wood of dead trees to make arrows, and they use greenish stones to make arrowheads. They apply poison to these arrowheads and anyone struck by them dies. These stones grow in the mountains. "The arrowtips supplied by Jingzhou and Liangzhou," as mentioned in the Yu gong section of the *Book of History*, are made from this stone. Also, in the South, in Tengzhou, they use greenish stones to make knives and swords, as if these were copper and iron. The women use them to make rings. When the people of the country of Liuli cultivate their fields, they use these stones to make ploughshares of a length of more than one *chi*. All these are of that same group.

Crude salt
Vol. II, 10-01-01

To dissolve the poison of yellow flies. In the valleys of Mount Wumengshan are many yellow flies that live in the scales of poisonous snakes. When they gnaw on humans, at first nothing is felt. Slow by slow an itch develops, eventually resulting in sores. Do not scratch the itching regions. Only rinse them with cold water and apply small amounts of salt to them. This will prevent the formation of sores. *An Overall Survey of the Earth.*

To dissolve the poison of wolfsbane root. Let the patient drink a salt liquid. *Recipes Worth a Thousand in Gold.*

Poison qi resulting from medicated arrows. Apply salt to the wound and cauterize it with 30 moxa cones. Good. *Collected and Proven Recipes*.

Salt from the Rong. Crystal salt. Sodium chloride
Vol. II, 11-02

It clears the eyes and serves to cure painful eyes. It boosts the qi, strengthens muscles and bones, and removes *gu* poison. *Original Classic*.

It serves to cure heart and abdominal pain, urination with blood and vomiting with blood, as well as bleeding teeth and tongue. *Supplementary Records by Famous Physicians*.

It assists the water long-term depot, boosts essence/sperm qi, removes concretion-illness nodes from the five long-term depots, accumulations and collections, as well as painful sores, *jie*-illness, and *xuan*-illness. Da Ming.

It resolves the poison of *lytta* bugs and blister beetles/mylabris. Li Shizhen.

Chinese yam
Dioscorea opposita Thunb. Vol. VI, 27-34-01

Meng Shen: It benefits husbands in that it assists their yin (i.e., sexual) strength. Boil it until done and mix it with honey. Or boil it to ingest it as a decoction. Or grind it into powder/flour. All these preparations yield excellent results. When it is dried and then added to medication, this is particularly wondrous. Only when it is mixed with wheat flour to prepare rice cakes, it excites the movement of qi because it is unable to check the poison of wheat flour.

Root of Chinese artichoke
Stachys sieboldii Miq. Vol. VI, 27-39-01

Soaked in wine it eliminates wind and breaks up blood accumulation. Boiled in water it serves to cure rivulet bug poison. Chen Cangqi.

Baked over a slow fire until it has dried, it serves to control running influx (caused by) wind (intrusion), disperses wind and ends pain. The nodes, too, can be pounded into powder and this is ingested with wine. Su Song.

It harmonizes the five long-term depots, sends down qi, and clears the spirit. *Proper and Essential Things for the Emperor's Beverages and Food*.

Winter bamboo shoots
Phyllostachys nigra (Lodd. ex Lindl.)
Munro var. *henonis* (Mitf.) Stapf ex Rendle. Vol. VI, 27-40-05

Li Shizhen: Zan Ning's *Treatise on Bamboo Shoots* states: "Bamboo shoots may be sweet and delicious, and they may smooth and free the large intestine, but they are not good for the spleen, and they are commonly said to be a 'comb scratching the intestines.' Their poison is resolved only with fresh ginger and sesame oil. People have used the dregs remaining after sesame oil is pressed to fertilize a bamboo grove, and the bamboo withered the next year. That is the evidence."

I, Li Shizhen have often seen how common physicians treat smallpox. More often than not they advise their patients to drink a bamboo shoot decoction, and they state that "it will help to effuse the pox." The fact is, they do not know that to cure smallpox sores it is not appropriate to smooth and free the large intestine. Bamboo shoots are named "comb scratching the intestines," and it is not known how many people were unknowingly injured with such a therapy. Be cautious! Be cautious!

Tendrils, flower of bottle gourd
Lagenaria siceraria (Molina) Standl. Vol. VI, 28-03-03

It serves to resolve fetal poison as a preventive measure. In the seventh or eighth month, or at the three ten-day periods of the hottest season in a year, or in mid-autumn cut the circularly curled end of the tendrils, dry them in the yin (i.e., shade), boil them in winter on New Year's eve, and with the decoction bathe the child. This can prevent the outbreak of smallpox. Tang Yao, *Tried and Proven Recipes*.

Vine, root of luffa
Luffa cylindrica (L.) Roem. Vol. VI, 28-10-03

To preventively resolve smallpox poison. In the fifth or sixth month gather the curled "beard hair" on a luffa creeper. On the first day of the first month at the *zi* 子 hours (11 p.m. – 01 a.m.) boil two and a half maces in water to obtain a decoction. Let only one of the child's parents, father or mother, know of the treatment. Wash the child with the warm decoction from the top down. This removes the fetal poison and the child will not be affected by an outbreak of smallpox for its entire life. And if there is an outbreak, it will be mild. *Compilation of Applied Benevolence*.

Benincasa hispida (Thunb.) Cogn. White wax gourd
Vol. VI, 28-06-01

Distension of the lower abdomen with water. It frees the flow of urine and ends thirst. *Supplementary Records by Famous Physicians.*

Pounded and the resulting juice ingested, it stops melting with thirst and vexing heart-pressure, and resolves poison. Tao Hongjing.

It boosts the qi and helps to endure aging. It removes heat from the head and the face. Meng Shen.

It dissolves heat poison and obstruction-illness swelling. Cut into slices and rubbed on seething heat rash seeds, it yields very good therapeutic results. Da Ming.

It frees the passage through the large and small intestine, and suppresses the poison of elixir minerals. Su Song.

Poisoning caused by eating fish. Drink wax gourd juice. Good. *Recipes from the Small Essays.*

Cucumber root
Cucumis sativus L. Vol. VI, 28-09-02

Pound it and apply it to a swelling related to a fox urine piercing with poison. Da Ming.

Wood ear mushroom
Auricularia sp. Vol. VI, 28-19

Qi and Flavor. Sweet, balanced, slightly poisonous.

Zhen Quan: As for the fungi ears, those of old *sophora* and mulberry trees are good. Those of silkwormthorn wood are second in quality. Ears from all other trees often excite wind qi and develop obstinacy-illness ailments. They cause tension below one's flanks and injure the conduits, the network vessels, the back, and the arms. They make you depressed.

Chen Cangqi: Wood ears that have been passed over by malign snakes and worms/bugs from below, they are poisonous. Those that have grown on Chinese sweet gum wood, they make you laugh incessantly. Those that have changed their color when you have returned home after collecting them, they are poisonous. Those that radiate a shine in the night and are about to rot but have not yet developed worms/bugs, they are poisonous.

All these poisons are resolved with the juice pressed out of fresh wax gourd creepers.

Li Shizhen: According to Zhang Zhongjing, "wood ears of red color growing upwards, they must not be eaten."

Fragrant mushroom
Lentinus edodes (Berk.) Sing. Vol. VI, 28-22

Wu Rui: Fragrant mushrooms grow on dragon trees, willows, and oriental raisin trees. Those of purple color are called "fragrant mushroom;" those of white color are called "meat mushroom." They all grow steamed by moist qi. Those growing in the mountains at out-of-the-way places are poisonous and kill humans.

Wang Ying: Fragrant mushrooms grow deep in the mountains on rotten Chinese sweet gum wood. They are smaller than *jun*-mushrooms and thin. They are of yellow-black color. Their flavor is very fragrant and delicious. They occupy a most excellent rank.

Smoked plum
Armeniaca mume Sieb. Vol. VI, 29-04-02

They serve to cure depletion exhaustion and bone steaming, and they dissolve the poison of wine. They make you fall asleep easily. Ingested mixed with tea leaves and dried ginger and prepared as pills, they very effectively stop dormant free-flux illness. Da Ming.

They contract the lung and astringe the intestines. They stop long-lasting coughing and outflow with free-flux illness, turned over stomach and gullet occlusion, and eliminate roundworms, with qi recession, vomiting, and free-flow. They dissolve swelling, disperse phlegm, kill worms/bugs, and resolve fish poison and the poison of horse sweat, as well as the poison of sulphur. Li Shizhen.

Harm with poison caused by a mad dog. Ingest two maces of smoked plum powder with wine. *Recipes Worth a Thousand in Gold*.

Diseases caused by poison in water. In the beginning they cause headache and an aversion to cold, heart vexation and contractions. Patients are fine in the morning; their condition worsens in the evening. Pound plum tree leaves to obtain a juice and drink three pints. Good. *Recipes to be Kept Close at Hand*.

15. Raw materials found in nature and objects produced from them

Li Shizhen distinguished himself from the authors of previous comprehensive *materia medica* works by introducing several innovations that we have encountered and discussed in the preceding sections. Here now, attention is drawn to a further characteristic of his work. Li Shizhen widened the scope of of how natural substances could be used by going beyond their therapeutic applications. In the section on woods/trees especially, the *Ben cao gang mu* offers information on an application in other than medicinal areas. Li Shizhen found relevant data for this in earlier *materia medica* texts and in non-medicinal records. For the most part, however, Li Shizhen did not provide a written or other source when he added data on natural things used as raw materials to produce objects required in daily life. He does quote Chen Cangqi, who knew that the boards of old coffins offered the best wood to make a zither. Chen Cangqi had also informed his readers that *platycarya* shrubs give off an aroma that keeps silverfish away from mounted calligraphies. When the paper is wrapped around rods made of *platycarya* stems at the top and bottom of a calligraphy, the ingredients of the wood create barriers preventing the attacks of silverfish.

In an ancient *Treatise on Bamboo,* Li Shizhen had discovered a special type of bamboo suited to making flutes. "Chinese white birch trees," Li Shizhen had learned elsewhere, "grow in Liao dong, Lin tiao, Hezhou, and various regions of the North-West. The wood can serve to absorb fat and oil. The bark is thick, light, spongy, and soft. Craftsmen use the bark to make the inner linings of shoes and also items such as knife handles. It is called 'warming skin/bark'. The Hu people really appreciate it."

In some instances, Li Shizhen offers data on both the therapeutic use of such everyday articles and their production. The lining worn in shoes for years has absorbed vapors of the feet. Burned to ashes and ingested by a woman, these qi are known to help cure obstructed vessels in the breast resulting in festering ulcers. Similarly, Su Gong reports, mats made of cattail absorb the qi of people resting on them. A widow's qi transform a mat made of straw into a pharmaceutical drug effectively curing cholera in children, with vomiting and diarrhea. Donkey hide glue was already recommended as a pharmaceutical substance in the Han era's "*Materia medica* of Shen nong." Over the centuries, it was attributed an ever more diverse range of medicinal effects.

Li Shizhen not only quoted several authors who had noted these effects and had advised on related recipes, he also gave a very detailed account of the hides guaranteeing the highest quality of glue and the individual steps required in its production: "When a glue of whatever type is produced, this is done between the tenth and the second or third months. The best hides are those of cows, water buffaloes, and donkeys. Those of pigs, horses, mules, and camels are secondary. Old hide and the leather from shoes and sandals is inferior. In general, one soaks fresh hide in water for four or five days, then washes it and scrubs it until it is very clean. This is boiled with constant stirring, while more water is continually added. When the hide has turned into a pulp, filter off the juice and boil the rest again until it forms a glue. Pour this into a basin and wait until it has congealed. That which settles at the bottom of the basin is called 'glue holding things together'. When the water used to boil the glue is salty and bitter, then the effects of the glue are wondrous. Generally, ancient recipes resorted most often to ox hide. In later times, the hide of donkeys was appreciated. Fake donkey hide glues are those prepared from horse hide, old shoes, saddles, or boots. Their qi is turbid and malodorous. They are not suited for medicinal use. Genuine donkey hide glue should be yellow and transparent, like amber. Those with the luster of black jade and lacquer are genuine, too. Genuine donkey hide glue does not smell like hides/leather. Also, in summer it will not turn moist and soft."

At the conclusion of a lengthy monograph elucidating the many different names for bottle gourds, their nature and their therapeutic application, Li Shizhen uses a deprecatory term, common in petitions, to add a few remarks on the gourds unrelated to their depiction as a pharmaceutical drug. It sounds as if he is almost apologizing to his readers for this digression from the actual topic: "I venture to say that bottle gourds can be cooked and dried in the sun, and they can also be made into vessels. Big ones can be made into vessels with a big belly and a small mouth; small ones can be made into ladles for wine vessels. If required, they can float on water as boats, and they can be made into wind instruments for music. The skin and the pulp can be used to feed pigs. The style holding the seeds can be used to light lamps. The benefits of this item are so diverse."

Whether a natural raw material is made into candles, saddle covers, cotton filled mattresses, pillowcases, arrow shafts, flagpoles, axe handles, blocks for printing, or poles to push boats, dog troughs, roof beams, or car wheel rims – Li Shizhen may have added detailed information on such alternative uses for the central reason underlying his grand work. He wished to demonstrate to his readers this very thing: the benefits of all these items for mankind.

Cattail mat
Vol. VIII, 38-51

Tao Hongjing: Cattail mats are used only by boat people; they are formed like cattail sails. Mats used by common people are made of *chloranthus* herb; while straw mats are mostly made of cattail. Recipe experts burn them for medicinal use.

Su Gong: Mats and straw mats serve as a place for people to lie down. Those are fine that have received human qi, regardless of whether these are straw mats or cattail mats. The Wu people use red algae to make mats.

Floss grass. *Imperata cylindrica* (L.) Beauv. var. *major* (Nees) C. E. Hubb
Vol. III, 13-19

Lu Ji in his *Commentary on Herbs and Trees* states: "Five inches down from the surface of the ground, there is a white powder in the root. This part of the root is pliable but tough and can be used to prepare a rope. When it is soaked in water it is even better suited for such a purpose."

Li Shizhen: There are several types of floss grass, they include "white floss grass," *themeda* floss grass, yellow floss grass, fragrant floss grass, and maiden grass. They all have similar leaves. Those of white floss grass are shorter and smaller. White floss grass opens white flowers with spikes in the third and fourth month. They form fine seeds. The root is very long. It is white and soft like a sinew, and has knots. It is of sweet flavor and is commonly called "silk thread floss grass." It can be used to prepare straw mats and covers, and thick sack cloth required for sacrifices. This is the floss grass root described in the *Original Classic*.

King crab
Tachypleus tridentatus Leach. Vol. VIII, 45-17

Li Shizhen: King crabs are shaped like the cap/crown of King Hui wen or a flat iron. They are more than a foot wide. Their carapace is shiny and smooth, and of greenish-black color. Their back is shaped like a flat iron cooking plate for cakes, and they have bone eyes. The eyes are situated on top of their back. Their mouth is underneath their abdomen. Their head resembles that of the dung beetle. They have twelve feet, similar to softshell crabs, situated on both sides of their abdomen, with a length of five to six inches. Their tail reaches a length of one to two feet. It has three edges, like the stem of a coir palm tree. On their back they have a bone like a horn. It is seven to eight inches high and it is shaped like a coral. When king crabs pass through the sea, they carry one another on their back, driven by the wind. They are commonly called "king crab sail," and also "king crab raft." Their blood has the color of green jade. In their abdomen they have eggs like millet grains that can be prepared to a minced/pickled product. Their tail has beads like millet grains. When they move, females generally carry males on their back. Once they have lost their female, males will not move any more. When fishermen catch them, they must obtain them as a pair. The males are small and the females are big. When placed into water, the males float on the surface and the females sink into the depth. Hence the people in Min resort to them during their wedding ceremonies. They hide underneath sand and they also fly and jump. Their skin-shell is very hard, and can serve to make a cap. It can also be bent to make a ladle. When it is added to fragrant objects, it will emit fragrant qi itself. Their tail can be made into a small S-shaped baton. By burning their fat, one can attract mice/rats.

Scaly snake
Vol. VIII, 43-12

Wang Ji in his *Classic of Wild Animals* states: "There are many pythons in the mountains of Hengzhou. Large specimens reach a length of more than ten fathoms. They eat roebucks and deer, and even the bones and antlers of these animals are decomposed. The local people stuff grass-cloth (kudzu) vine into their caves. When the python snakes smell them they collapse. Then the locals open the caves and remove them. Their meat is very fat and delicious, and their skin can be used to make drums and also to decorate weapons and musical instruments."

Fan Chengda in his *Treatise of the Supervisor and Guardian of the Cinnamon Sea* states: "The soldiers in the military camp catch pythons in that they wear a fanciful flower arrangement covering their head. When a python sees this, it is dumbfounded and does not move. The soldiers approach it and chop off its head. The python wildly jumps at first, and when its strength is exhausted it dies. The soldiers lift it to carry it home, and eat it."

Board used in an ancient coffin
Vol. VII, 37-21

Chen Cangqi: This is wood of a coffin in an ancient tomb. The older it is, the better. Those made from Chinese cedar are excellent. Those a thousand years old enable communication with the spirits. Such boards are suitable for preparing the base of a Chinese zither.

The *Commentary on the Examples of Refined Usage* states: "In coffins made from Chinese cedar wood, the buried corpse does not decay."

"Big and hollow." Unidentified
Vol. VII, 36-51

Su Gong: "Big and hollow" grows in Xiangzhou. It can also be found everywhere in mountain valleys. People in Qinlong call it "solitary and hollow." These are small trees with a bough rising to a height of six to seven *chi*. The leaves resemble those of paper mulberry trees. They are small, round and thick. The bark of the root is red in color.

Li Shizhen: Small trees with big leaves. They resemble the leaves of dragon trees, but they are not pointed. They are deep-green and have a wrinkled line design. The bark of the root is spongy and soft. Mountain people collect it to kill lice with a most wondrous effect. They pound the leaves and spread them in their vegetable gardens to kill worms/bugs.

Chinese White birch
Betula platyphylla Suk. Vol. VII, 35-40

Li Shizhen: Painters burn the bark and with the smoke they fumigate paper to let it look like an ancient painting with ancient characters. Hence, the name combining the characters "wood" and "painting." … Breast obstruction-illness with a festering ulcer. Burn Chinese white birch bark that has been used as lining in a boot for years to ashes and let the woman ingest with wine one mace. To be ingested once a day. Tang Yao, *Tried and Proven Recipes*.

Safflower
Carthamus tinctorius L. Vol. IV, 15-27

Su Song: Today it can be found everywhere. Households plant it in gardens. The seeds are spread on fertile ground in winter; by the time of spring a seedling grows and in summer flowers appear. Below the flowers a ball-shaped cluster is formed with many thorns. The flowers emerge from above this ball. The gardeners collect them when they are covered with dew. When they are removed, new flowers appear. This is repeated until they are exhausted and decay. The fruits are formed inside the balls. These are white seeds the size of rice beans. The flowers are dried in the sun; they serve as a red dye. Also, they are made to rouge.

Bamboo
Phyllostachys nigra (Lodd. ex Lindl.)
Munro var. *henonis* (Mitf.) Stapf ex Rendle. Vol. VII, 37-13

According to the *Treatise on Bamboo*, "white-sheathed bamboo is hard and has nodes situated close to each other. The trunk is round and sturdy, with a bark as white as frost. Big specimens can be used to make poles to push boats. Fine ones can be made to flutes. Bitter bamboo may be white and it may be purple. Sweet bamboo resembles thicket-bamboo, but is more flourishing. It is bland bamboo. Still, today mostly *cassia* bamboo poles are used to push boats. There is one separate kind that is made to bamboo flutes; it, too, is not called white-sheathed bamboo.

Bamboo from Jiangguang is four to five fathoms long, with thin meat. It can be made to pillars in a house. *Han* 箮 bamboo reaches a size of several handspans. Its meat is thick and it can be made to ridgepoles. *Han* 漢 bamboo from Yong chang can be made to buckets and *dou* measures. *Xun* 箰 bamboo can be used to build boats.

Rough twigs can be woven into armor. Smooth twigs can be used to make mats. Sturdy ones can be used to make spears, knives, and arrows. They are called "spear bamboo," "arrow bamboo," "sinew bamboo," and "stone hemp." Soft twigs are used to make ropes. They are called "vine bamboo," "bow bamboo," "bitter bamboo," and "a grab of hair."

Among further kinds is "spine bamboo," also named "spike bamboo." They are densely covered with awn-like spines. Big ones have a circumference of two feet and can serve to ward off thieves and robbers. "Windmill palm tree bamboo" is also named "solid bamboo." Its leaves resemble those of windmill palm trees and they can be made to walking sticks. "Loving bamboo" is also called "righteous bamboo." It grows as dense clusters, the individuals do not disperse. People plant it to enjoy themselves. People in Guang use the threads of "sinew bamboo" to make bamboo cloth. It is very brittle.

"Numinous longevity tree." Unidentified
Vol. VII, 36-48

According to the *History of the Han,* "when Kong Guang had reached old age, he was given a stick with numinous power to grant longevity."

Yan Shigu in his comment states: "This tree resembles bamboo with its knots. It is no longer than eight or nine *chi,* with a circumference of three or four *cun.* Nature itself shapes it as a walking stick; there is no need to further work on it. Made to a walking stick, it lets one extend the years of life and boosts longevity."

Li Shizhen: The *Commentary on the Meanings in the Book of Songs* states: "*Ju* 椐 is *Gui* 櫃, with swelling at the knots. It resembles a stick that helps old people to walk. It is today's "numinous longevity" wood/tree. People use it to make walking/flogging sticks and horse whips. The tree can be found in the mountains north of Hong nong prefecture.

Silver vine
Actinidia polygama (Sieb. et Zucc.) Maxim. Vol. VII, 36-45

Su Song: Silver vine today comes from Xinyang. The trees are two to three *zhang* tall. They open flowers similar to silkworm thorn flowers in the third and fourth month. The seeds/fruits are collected in the fifth month. They are shaped as balls, similar to those of Indian mallow. They can be stored and are prepared to edible fruits.

Li Shizhen: Even though there are three kinds of silver vine, their therapeutic potentials and usages are similar. The fact is, they are of one group. The seeds can be used to light lamps; the seedlings are edible. Hence, Lu Ji states: "Lamps lighted with silver vine oil are as bright as those lighted with sesame oil."

Box tree
Buxus sinica (Rehd. et Wils.) M. Cheng. Vol. VII, 36-42

Li Shizhen: Box trees grow everywhere in the wild in the mountains. People often plant them by inserting twigs into the ground. Twigs and leaves grow upward gathering closely together. The leaves resemble those of young Chinese scholar tree seedlings, but are greenish and thick. They have neither flowers nor fruits, and they do not wither throughout the four seasons. By their nature they grow slowly. It is commonly said that they grow by one inch per year and recede in a leap year. This has been studied now, and it was found only that in leap years they do not grow. The wood is hard and greasy and very suitable for processing into combs and seals.

Silk-cotton tree
Bombax malabaricum DC. Vol. VII, 36-40

Li Shizhen: There are two kinds of silk-cotton trees: herbs and trees. In Jiao and Guang silk-cotton trees are as big as trees that can be embraced with two arms. The twigs resemble those of dragon trees. They have big leaves, similar to the leaves of walnut trees. Early in autumn they open flowers; they are as red in color as *camellia* tree flowers, with yellow stamina holding filaments. The petals are very thick. Their housings/seedpods are very numerous; they cling together with their short margins. They form fruits the size of a fist. Inside the fruits is white cotton wool, and inside this cotton wool are the seeds.

Li Yanshou in his *History of Southern Dynasties* mentions "old cowry flowers coming from Linyi and some other countries. Inside is a goose down. The threads are taken out and spun into cloths."

Zhang Bo in his *Records of Wu* mentions "silk-cotton trees in Jiaozhou and Yangchang that are taller than a house. If their fruits are not exchanged for ten years or more, they develop to the size of cups. Inside the flowers is a soft, white cotton that can be used as silk wadding or coarse cotton."

All these are references to the tree kinds of silk-cotton trees.

Also, the *Records of Nanyue* states: "The Man in Nanzhao do not raise silkworms. They simply remove the white wadding from within the seeds of *suoluo* trees and spin it to silk threads that are then woven into fabrics. They are called '*suoluolong* pieces'."

Zhu Mu in his *An Overall Survey of the Earth* says: "*Suoluo* 娑羅 trees coming from Ping mian are three to five fathoms tall. They form seeds with cotton wool. It can be spun into silk floss that is further processed to felt and cotton bags and nets."

Cotton rose
Hibiscus mutabilis L. Vol. VII, 36-35

Li Shizhen: Cotton rose trees are present everywhere. Stick a twig bough into the ground and it comes to life. These are small trees. The trunk grows in clusters, similar to chastetree. Tall specimens reach a height of more than one fathom. The leaves are as big as those of dragon trees. Some have five, others have seven pointed ends. They wither in winter and flourish in summer. In mid autumn the flowers begin to blossom. The flowers are in one group with those of various *paeonia* herbs. Some are red, some are white, some are yellow, some have a thousand leaves. They are extremely resistant to cold and do not fall off. They do not bear fruit. People in the mountains take the bark to make thick ropes.

Chinese chastetree
Vitex negundo L. var. *cannabifolia* (Sieb.et Zucc.) Hand.-Mazz
Vol. VII, 36-28

The Chinese chastetree rods that are made to canes of flogging, they are present everywhere. The fruits are fine and yellow in color. The stem is sturdy and grows as a tree.

In the Treatise on Sacrifices in the Suburbs of the *History of the Han* it is recorded that Chinese chastetree stems are used to make flagpoles.

Li Shizhen: Chinese chastetrees are present everywhere in the wild of the mountains. They are gathered as firewood. If they are not used as firewood for years, the trees grow to the size of a bowl. The core of the tree is square and the twigs grow opposite to each other. One twig has five or seven leaves. The leaves are similar to Siberian elm leaves; they are long and pointed, with a sawtooth margin. At the end of the fifth month flowers open; they form spikes and are red-purple in color. The seeds are as big as coriander seeds and they are enclosed by a white membrane skin.

Su Song states that "the leaves resemble castor oil plant leaves." That is wrong. There are two kinds, one greenish, one red. The tender boughs can be used to make rice baskets. In ancient times, poor women used chastetree 荆 to make hairpins.

According to Pei Yuan's *Records of Guangzhou*, "chastetree comprises three kinds. 'Gold chastetree' wood can be made into pillowcases. 'Purple chastetree' wood can be made into beds. 'White chastetree' wood can be made into shoes.

Silky spicebush
Lindera erythrocarpa Makino. Vol. VII, 34-17

Chen Cangqi: Silky spicebush grows in the mountain valleys of Nanhai. In boat building it ranks second after camphor wood.

Platycarya strobilacea Sieb. et Zucc
Vol. VII, 34-20

Chen Cangqi: *Platycarya* grows in the high mountains. The leaves resemble those of old varnish trees. Pound it into a powder and toss it into the headwaters of a river. All fish die with bulging gills. If the wooden sticks holding a calligraphy are of this wood, the calligraphy will not be damaged by silverfish.

Phoenix tree
Firmiana platanifolia (L.f.) Marsili. Vol. VII, 35-12

The *Essential Arts of the Common People* states: "Musical instruments made with phoenix trees that have grown amidst the rocks of mountains, they sound even better."

Vernicia tree
Vernicia fordii (Hemsl.) Airy-Shaw. Vol. VII, 35-13

Li Shizhen: Hill ridge dragontrees are white dragon trees with purple flowers. The twigs, trunk, flowers, and leaves of *vernicia* trees are all in one group with hill ridge dragon trees, but they are smaller. The growth of the tree, too, is slower. The flowers, too, are pink. But the fruits are big and round. Inside each fruit are two or four seeds, similar in size to chaulmoogra seeds. Their meat is white in color; their flavor is sweet and causes vomiting. Some call them "purple flower dragon trees." People often plant and transplant them to get their seeds. They sell them for a production of oil that is used by painters and for boats. It is a daily necessity. People often fake it. To test it dip a ring into the oil and lift it. If the oil covers it like the surface of a drum, only then it is genuine.

Reng tong. Unidentified
Vol. VII, 35-13-A01

Chen Cangqi: These trees grow in mountain valleys. They are shaped like greenish dragon trees. The leaves are forked. People gather the bark and macerate it to generate threads. The bark has a sweet flavor, is warm and nonpoisonous. To cure an illness caused by the poison of silkworm bites that has entered the abdomen, grind the bark into a powder and ingest it. When chicken and dogs eat silkworms and come close to dying, boil the bark in water and force-feed them with it. Once the threads have decayed, they are cured.

Indian coral tree
Erythrina variegata L. Vol. VII, 35-14

Su Song: Indian coral trees grow in Nanhai and Leizhou. They are also found in provinces and prefectures close to the sea. The leaves are as big as a hand, with three pointed ends. The bark is similar to the white bark of yellow *catalpa* trees, but it is hard and pliable and can be processed to ropes that do not rot in water.

Bilobed *grewia*
Grewia biloba G. Don. Vol. VII, 35-18

Su Gong: The leaves of bilobed grewia resemble the leaves of *hibiscus* trees and Siberian elm trees. These are small trees; their seeds are similar to those of scabrious *deutzia*. The leaves grow opposite to each other in pairs of two; they are red in color and their flavor is sweet.

Lu Ji in his *Commentary on the Book of Songs* states: "Bilobed *grewia* trees are in one group with sandalwood trees and Siberian elm trees." They are found everywhere in mountain valleys.

Chen Cangqi: They grow in mountain forests on northern soil. The bark is suitable for a production of ropes.

Persian lilac tree
Melia azedarach L. Vol. VII, 35-15

Li Shizhen: Persian lilac trees grow very fast. After three to five years they can be made into rafters.

Sandalwood
Santalum album L. Vol. VII, 35-17

According to Su Gong, sandalwood resembles Chinese ash tree bark. The leaves are suitable for drinks. The trees have a fine physical body; it is suitable for making axe-handles. ... Sandalwood is suitable for a production of tools such as pestles, poles, and hammers.

Chinese ash tree bark
Fraxinus rhynchophylla Hance. Vol. VII, 35-19

Supplementary Records by Famous Physicians: Chinese ash tree bark grows in the river valleys of Lujiang and close to waters in Yuanju. The bark is collected in the second and eighth month; it is dried in the yin (i.e., shade).

Tao Hongjing: It is commonly said to be Chinese ash tree bark. When it is soaked in water and the liquid is mixed with ink, the color of writing does not fade and is slightly greenish.

Su Gong: This tree resembles sandalwood trees. It has fine leaves. The bark has white dots; it is not as coarse. When the bark is soaked in water, the water assumes a jade-bluish color.

Mimosa
Albizzia julibrissin Durazz. Vol. VII, 35-20

Su Gong: The leaves of mimosa trees resemble those of Chinese honey locust tree and Chinese scholar trees. They are very fine. Flowers develop in the fifth month; they are red-white in color and have a silk thread-like pilose hair on their surface. In autumn, the fruits form pods with extremely thin, fine seeds. They are found everywhere in mountain valleys. Nowadays they are also planted amidst the ponds and mountains of private residences in the eastern and western capital.

Su Song: Today, they are found everywhere in Bian and Luo. People often plant them in their gardens.

Mimosa wood bark
Vol. VII, 35-20-01

It kills worms/bugs. Pounded into a powder and mixed with the soot accumulated under a flat pan and fresh oil, it is applied to sores caused by spider bites. The leaves are used to wash the dirt off of clothes. Chen Cangqi.

Golden raintree
Koelreuteria paniculata Laxm.. Vol. VII, 35-24

Supplementary Records by Famous Physicians: Golden raintrees grow in river valleys of Hanzhong. The flowers are collected in the fifth month.

 Su Gong: The leaves of this tree resemble those of *hibiscus* trees, but they are thin and fine. The flowers are yellow, similar to those of Chinese scholar trees, and a little longer and bigger. The seed shells resemble those of Chinese lantern plants. Inside of them are fruits similar to heat prepared peas. They are round, black, and hard, and can be made to strings of beads. The flowers can be picked in the fifth and sixth month. People in the South use them to dye fabrics yellow. The color achieved is very fresh and clear. They are also used to heal red and festering eyes.

Su Song: Today, they are also found in the South and in some parks in Bianzhong.

Kou Zongshi: They are also found in the mountains of Chang'an. The seeds are taken to the capital where they are made to strings of beads. They have not been seen to be added to medication.

Weeping willow
Salix babylonica L. Vol. VII, 35-29

Supplementary Records by Famous Physicians: Weeping willows grow in the river marshlands of Lang ye.

Su Song: Today, they are present everywhere. This is a group with various kinds. The twigs of weeping willows are pliable but sturdy and can be made to arrow shafts. Many of them grow in He bei. The *qi liu* willows grow to the side of waters. Their leaves are coarse and white. The inner structure of the wood is pink; it can be made to wheel hubs. Nowadays, people heat the fine boughs close to a fire to soften them and then bend them to make chests. The "cups and bowls made of willows" as mentioned by Meng zi are made from trees found especially often in Lu and in He shuo

Schneider's *zelkova*. *Zelkova schneideriana* Hand.-Mazz
Vol. VII, 35-28

Li Shizhen: Schneider's *zelkova* timber is red-purple. Very excellent items, such as cases and tables, are made of it.

Zheng Qiao in his *Comprehensive Treatises* states: "Schneider's *zelkova* trees are in one group with Siberian elms and are made to shovels. Its fruits, too, are similar to those of Siberian elms, they are shaped like coins. The locals collect the leaves to make sweet tea."

Tamarix chinenis Lour. Tamarisk
Vol. VII, 35-30

Li Shizhen: Tamarisks have a short trunk and weak twigs. Inserted into the ground, a new tree easily grows. The red bark and the fine leaves reminiscent of silk threads are graceful and lovely. They form flowers three times within one year. The flowers have spikes three to four inches long. They are watery red in color similar to the color of knotweed flowers. At the time of Southern Qi, Yizhou submitted as tribute willows from Shu with long boughs shaped like silk thread tassels. These were the tamarisks discussed here.

Kou Zongshi: They are plentiful in Bianjing. The Rong people in Hexi use their smooth twigs to prepare whips.

Purple willow
Salix sinopurpurea C. Wang et Ch. Y. Yang. Vol. VII, 35-31

Su Gong: The leaves of purple willows are round, broad, and pointed. The boughs of the twigs are short and hard, entirely different from those of weeping willows. The leaves of weeping willows are narrow and lengthy; their twig boughs are long and tender.

Su Song: Their twigs are sturdy but pliable and can be made to arrow shafts. The stem can be made to arrows.

Populus davidiana Dode. Poplar
Vol. VII, 35-32

Li Shizhen: Poplar trees are tall and big. The leaves are round, similar to pear leaves, and they are fat, big, and have a pointed end. On their front side they are greenish and shiny; their back is extremely white in color. They have a sawtooth margin. The wood has fine, white muscles; by its nature it is hard and straight. It serves to make roof beams and pillars that never bend.

Large-leafed dogwood
Swida macrophylla (Wall.). Vol. VII, 35-34

Ma Zhi: The leaves of large-leaf dogwood resemble persimmon tree leaves. Two leaves grow opposite to each other. The seeds are fine and round, similar to Japanese buckthorn. They are greenish as long as they grow, and they are black when they have ripened. The wood is hard and heavy; when it is boiled in water the juice assumes a red color.

Guo Pu states: "Large-leaf dogwood timber is used to make car wheel rims."

Siberian elm. *Ulmus pumila* L
Vol. VII, 35-35

The ancients gathered elm wood in spring to make fire. Today, people collect the white bark to make elm flour. They mix it with water and make aromatic preparations that are stickier than glue and lacquer.

Chen Cheng: Elm bark is moistened and pounded into a paste that serves to stick together tiles and stones with utmost strength. In Bian and Luo people use stones to make the "mouth" of treadle-operated tilting hammers for peeling rice and they use this paste to glue the stone to the hammer.

Chinese White birch
Betula platyphylla Suk. Vol. VII, 35-40

Chen Cangqi: Chinese white birches resemble mountain peach trees. The bark is suitable for making candles.

Kou Zongshi: White birch bark that is evenly covered with purple-black dotes is used to cover saddles, bows, and stirrups.

Henry *ormosia*
Ormosia henryi Prain. Vol. VII, 35-42

Chen Cangqi: It comes from Annan and Nanhai. It is used to make beds and small tables. It resembles purple sandalwood, but is red in color. By its nature it is hard and good.

Li Shizhen: The wood is by its nature hard; it is purple-red in color. Some of these trees have a flowery line design. Their wood can be processed into household containers and fan frames, all such items.

Windmill palm
Trachycarpus fortunei (Hook) H.Endl. Vol. VII, 35-43

Chen Cangqi: Ropes prepared from the bark do not rot even when left in the soil for a thousand years. Once someone found such a rope when he opened a tomb. The rope had already developed roots.

Li Shizhen: Windmill palms are very numerous in Chuan and Guang. Today, they are also planted in Jiangnan. Their growth is extremely slow. In the beginning, they develop leaves similar to common *bletilla* leaves. When they have reached a height of two or three feet, numerous leaves the size of a fan develop rising from the top end of the tree. They are split and spread into all four directions. Their stems have three edges, and they do not wither throughout the four seasons. The trunk of windmill palms is straight and has no twigs. Near the location where the leaves are situated the trunk is enclosed by bark; with every layer that develops one additional section forms. The body of the trunk is red-black and it is pervaded by a network of sinews. It is suitable for making bell clappers and can also be processed into utensils. The bark contains thread-like hair, interlocked lengthwise as if woven. The bark is cut open to remove the threads that can be processed into clothing, caps, cotton-filled mattresses, and chairs. It is of great, timely use. … Some say that there are two kinds of this tree in the South. One of them with bark threads that can be processed into ropes. The other kind is small and has no such threads; only its leaves can be made into brooms.

Zheng Qian in his *Comprehensive Treatises* identifies them as broom plants, but that is wrong. In addition there is a plant named "cattail mallow." Its leaves resemble those of the item discussed here, but they are soft and thin. They can be made into fans and and hats.

Tallow tree
Sapium sebiferum (L.) Roxb. Vol. VII, 35-46

Su Gong: Tallow trees grow in the marshland of the plains of Shannan. The trees are several fathoms tall. The leaves resemble those of pear and apricot trees. They open fine flowers in the fifth month, yellow-white in color. The seeds are black in color.

Chen Cangqi: The leaves can be used to dye black. The seeds can be pressed to obtain oil. Lamps lit with it are extremely bright.

Mulberry tree
Morus alba L. Vol. VII, 36-01

Guo Pu: "Mulberry trees that are small and have long boughs are called 'female mulberry trees.' 'Mountain mulberry trees' resemble mulberry trees. Their wood is made to crossbows." Mulberry wood with its threads can be made to string instruments. All these are wonderful timbers, that other woods seldom match.

Dragon tree
Paulownia fortunei (Seem.) Hemsl. Vol. VII, 35-11

Tao Hongjing: Dragon trees comprise four kinds. Greenish dragon trees have greenish leaves and bark. They resemble phoenix trees, but they have no seeds. Phoenix trees have a white bark. Their leaves resemble those of greenish dragon trees, and they have seeds. The seeds are fat and edible. White dragon trees are also named *yi tong*. People often plant them. They do not differ from hill ridge dragon trees, but they have flowers and seeds. They open flowers in the second month; they are yellow-purple in color. They are what the *Record of Rites* calls "dragon trees that begin to have flowers in the third month." They are suitable for making string instruments. Hill ridge dragon trees have no seeds; they are the wood that is made to string instruments.

Lu Ji in his *Commentary on Herbs and Trees* says that "white dragon tree wood is suitable for making string instruments. People in Zang ge in Yunnan take the fine white hairs in the flowers, soak them in water and twist them into threads to weave cloths resembling cotton cloths. They call them 'flower cloths'."

Big fruit elm
Ulmus macrocarpa Hance. Vol. VII, 35-37

Supplementary Records by Famous Physicians: Big fruit elms grow in the river valleys of Mount Jinshan. The fruits are collected in the third month; they are dried in the shade.

Tao Hongjing: Today, they only come from Gao li. They are shaped like elm pods. Their qi are as malodorous as those of raccoon dogs. All the people there make soup out of them and eat it. By their nature they kill worms/bugs, and when placed into items they also repel moths. They are simply plagued by their malodorous smell.

Japanese oak
Lithocarpus glaber (Thunb.) Nakai. Vol. VII, 35-45

Li Xun: According to the *Records of the Guang Area*, "Japanese oaks grow in the mountain valleys of Guangnan. People in Persia use the wood to build boats and ships."

Silkworm thorn
Maclura tricuspidata Carr. Vol. VII, 36-02

The interior of silkworm thorn wood has a line design; it is also suitable for making vessels. The leaves can be used to feed silkworms. They are called "silkworm thorn silkworms." Still, their leaves are hard and they are not equal to mulberry tree leaves. For use as a pharmaceutical drug those are good that have no thorns.

Li Shizhen: They are present in the mountains everywhere. They tend to grow as clusters; their trunks are thin and straight. The leaves abound and are thick; they are round with a pointed end. The leaves are used to feed silkworms; with the silk threads produced by these silkworms processed to the strings of musical instruments. Their sound is clearer than normal. The "spine cocoons" mentioned in the *Examples of Refined Usage* are these silkworms.

The *Records of the Investigation of Crafts* states: "Archers use the timber of silkworm thorn trees as it is the best to make bows. Their fruits are shaped like mulberry seeds, but they are round kernels similar to prickly ash. The wood serves to dye items yellow-red; it is called 'silkworm thorn yellow.' The Emperor wears it."

The *Records of the Mutual Influences of Various Categories of Things* states: "Apply lime mixed with wine and vinegar to silkworm thorn wood for one night. The next day a line design of Ceylon ebony wood appears." Things subdue each other by their nature.

Paper mulberry tree
Broussonetia papyrifera (L.) Vent. Vol. VII, 36-04

Supplementary Records by Famous Physicians: Paper mulberry tree fruits grow on Mount Shao shishan. There they can be found everywhere. The fruits are collected in the eighth and ninth month. They are dried in the sun and are ready for use after 40 days.

Tao Hongjing: People in Wuling produce paper mulberry bark clothing. It is very firm and good.

Su Gong: There are two kinds of it: One kind has a bark with a design of flowery dots. It is called "spotted paper mulberry." It is the one used today to make hats. The other kind has a white bark without flowery design.

Li Shizhen: According to Xu Shen's *Explaining Single and Analysing Compound Characters*, *chu* 楮 and *gou* 榖 are one item. They should not be separated. All that is to be distinguished is whether they are female or male. Males have a spotted bark and the leaves are not forked. They open flowers with long spikes in the third month, similar to willow flowers. They do not form fruits. In times of famine, people collect the flowers and eat them. Males have a white bark and their leaves are forked. They, too, open fragmentated flowers and they form fruits similar to red bayberry fruits. When they are half ripe they are soaked in water to remove the seeds. Then they are boiled with honey and prepared to edible fruits. The trees of both kinds grow easily. Their leaves have many unsmooth hairs. People in the South cut off the bark, pound it, boil it in water, and prepare paper, and they also prepare it to fabrics. But they are not firm and easily deteriorate.

Pei Yuan in his *Records of Guangzhou* says: "Man and Yi people boil the root until done, pound it, and make fabrics to imitate felt. They are very warming."

White juice in the bark of paper mulberry trees
Vol. VII, 36-04-05

Li Shizhen: Paper mulberry tree juice is very sticky. People today use it to glue gold foil. An ancient method to glue the classical books was to mix paper mulberry tree juice with common *bletilla* root and wheat flour to make a paste. Paper glued together with it never fell apart again. It is better than to glue with lacquer.

Jujube
Zizyphus jujuba Mill. var. *spinosa* (Bunge) Hu ex H. F. Chow
Vol. VII, 36-08

Song yangzi states: "My home is in Huatai. Today's "Jujube" county actually belongs to Huatai. The trees are several staves tall, with a perimeter of one to two feet. The wood has an extremely fine structure. It is hard and at the same time heavy. It can be made to car wheels, spoons and chopsticks.

Thorny lime bush
Poncirus trifoliata (L.) Raf. Vol. VII, 36-06

Li Shizhen: Thorny lime bush trees can be found everywhere. The tree and the leaves are identical to those of tangerines, but the stem has many thorns. White flowers open in the third month. They have greenish stamina holding filaments and are not fragrant. They form fruits the size of bullets. They are shaped like bitter orange fruits but have a thin shell, and they are not fragrant. People often collect and plant them as a fence. Or they collect the small fruits and sell them falsely declared as bitter orange fruits and greenish tangerine peel. It is essential to differentiate them.

Chinese holly
Ilex cornuta Lindl. ex Paxt. Vol. VII, 36-18,

Su Song: Many Chinese holly trees grow in the region of Jiangsu and Zhejiang. People in the South take the wood to make excellent boxes and vessels.

Li Shizhen. Similar to privet trees, Chinese holly trees have a very white muscle structure. The leaves are two to three inches long. They are greenish-emerald green, thick and hard, and they have five thorny horns. They do not wither throughout the four seasons. The trees open fine, white flowers in the fifth month. They bear fruits similar to privet fruits and Chinese *sarsaparilla* fruits. In the ninth month they ripen and assume a bright red color. Their bark is thin and has a sweet flavor. The seed kernels are covered by four petals. People collect the tree bark and boil it to a paste that is used to glue birds. They call it "sticky paste."

Red sandalwood bead tree
Adenanthera pavonina L. var. *microsperma*. Vol. VII, 35-49

According to Song Qi's *Records of Local Products from Yi*, "the leaves of red sandalwood bead trees are similar to those of evergreen trees, but they are round and moist. In spring they open white flowers, and they form pods between the twigs. The seeds appear in clusters similar to beads stitched together. They are similar to flat soybeans. Their skin is red and their meat is white. Their name reflects this appearance. People in Shu display them as decorative fruits."

Prayer bead tree
Abrus precatorius L. Vol. VII, 35-50

Li Shizhen: Prayer beads grow in Lingnan. The trees are more than a stave tall and their bark is white in color. The leaves resemble those of Chinese scholar trees; the flowers resemble those of soapbean trees. The pods resemble Egyptian kidney beans. The seeds are big, similar to rice beans. They are red on one side, and black on the other side. The locals integrate them into their jewelry.

Duan Gonglu in his *Records from Beihu* says that "they are creepers. It is advisable to store the seeds together with borneol lest it loses its fragrance."

Ailanthus altissima (Mill.) Swingle. Varnish tree
Vol. VII, 35-07

Li Shizhen: *Kao* 栲 trees are varnish trees growing in the mountains. Their wood is also loose with big trunks; people who cut blocks for printing sometimes use the wood. However, when it is scratched it reacts like rotten wood. Hence, people in antiquity did not resort to it as lumber. This is different from *chun* 椿 wood which is hard and solid and can be used to make ridgepoles and beams.

Hardy rubber tree
Eucommia ulmoides Oliv. Vol. VII, 35-06

Su Song: Today it comes from the big mountains near Shangzhou, Chengzhou, and Xiazhou. The leaves are also in one group with silkworm thorn leaves. When the bark is broken, interconnected, white threads appear. In the beginning of their growth the leaves are tender and edible. The flowers and the fruits are bitter and astringent; they are also suitable for adding to medication. The wood can be made into sandals; they are good for the legs.

Eupatorium
Eupatorium fortunei Turcz. Vol. III, 14-44.

The *Investigation of the Woes of Departure*, a poem by Zhu Xi, says: "Its green leaves, purple stem, and plain twigs can be tied to bundles, can be worn as ornaments, can be made to ceremonial mats, can be made to ointments, and can be made into bath liquids." Now, *eupatorium* has leaves but no twigs. It can be enjoyed by looking at it, but it cannot be tied to bundles, worn as an ornament, made to ceremonial mats, and processed into a bath liquid. It cannot be held in the hands, or used as an ointment or burned to effuse fragrant fumes. Hence Mr. Zhu Xi in his *Investigation of the Woes of Departure* says: "In antiquity, fragrant herbs definitely had fragrant flowers and leaves, and the fragrance did not change under dry or moist conditions. Hence one could cut it and wear it as an ornament. Today's *eupatorium* has only fragrant flowers; the leaves have no such qi. Their material substance is weak and easily decays. They cannot be cut to be worn as ornaments. Hence it is very clear that they are not the items referred to by the ancients.

Cuttlefish
Sepiella maindroni de Rochebrune. Vol. VIII, 44-50

Li Shizhen: Cuttlefishes have no scales, but they have palpi. Their skin is black, and their meat is white. Large specimens resemble cattail leaf fans. Eaten fried in a pan with ginger and vinegar they are crispy and delicious. The bone in their back is named "ocean mantis egg capsule;" its physical appearance is reminiscent of the pieces used in board games, but is longer. Its two ends are pointed. It is white, crispy like *tetrapanax* pith, and covered by a line design layer after layer. It is soft enough to be scratched to powder with one's fingernails. The people also carve them to prepare medals and ornaments.

Decayed writing brush
Vol. IX, 51-33

Li Shizhen: In high antiquity, books were written on bamboo slips. Then Meng Tian was the first to use the hair of hares/rabbits to prepare writing brushes. In later times, they were also produced from the fur of goats/sheep and mice. Only those made from the fine hair of hares/rabbits, though, are used for medicinal purposes.

Japanese rough potato
Metaplexis japonica (Thunb.) Makino. Vol. V, 18-50

Li Shizhen: These are the seeds of *metaplexis japonica*. It grows a seedling in the third month, extending as a vine on fences. It multiplies most easily. The root is white and soft. The leaves are long, with a broad basis and a pointed end. When the root, the stem, and the leaves are broken, they all show a white milk similar to the juice of paper mulberry trees. *Metaplex-*

is japonica opens small, lengthy flowers in the sixth and seventh month, similar to bells. They are purple-white in color and they form fruits two or three inches long, the size of *aristolochia* fruits, but with a pointed tip. Their shell is greenish and soft. Inside is white down and a thick juice. After frost they wither and crack open, and the seeds fly away. These seeds are light and thin. They, too, are similar to those of *aristolochia*. Merchants collect the down and use it to make padded mattresses, replacing the cotton with the *metaplexis japonica* down. They say it is very light and warm.

Aloes wood containing resin
Aquilaria agallocha (Lour.) Roxb. Vol. VII, 34-10

Kou Zongshi: Aloe trees are found in all the prefectures of Lingnan. There are especially many close to the sea. The trunks are connected and their twigs intertwine. They spread across hills and mountains without interruption for a thousand miles. The leaves are similar to those of evergreen trees. Big ones have a size of numerous armspans; their wood is spongy and soft. The mountain people use it to build their thatched cottages or bridges, or make rice steamers or dog troughs. Not even one or two out of a hundred trees has a fragrance.

Camphor
A product prepared from *Cinnamomum camphora* (L.) Presl. trees. Vol
VII, 34-31

Li Shizhen: Camphor is pure yang; its nature is identical with that of nitrokalite. It generates fire in water. Its own blaze serves to increase the blazing of other items. Today, specialists operating stoves to prepare elixirs and those who make fireworks often use it. It is acrid, hot, fragrant, and scurrying. Endowed with the qi of dragon fire it eliminates moisture and kills worms/bugs. This is what it is good at. Hence, it is burned to fumigate clothing, baskets, and mats. It can repel bedbugs and moths causing damage.

Li Shi in his *Xu Monograph on a Wide Range of Things* states: "Patients with weak legs soak their feet in a bucket made of Chinese cedar wood. Place camphor between their two thighs and fasten them with a silk ribbon. If this is done for a month or more, the effects are wondrous."

Wang Xi in his *Collected Essentials from the Forest of Medicine* recommends to cure leg qi with a painful swelling as follows. Grind two ounces of camphor and three ounces of *aconitum* main tuber into a powder and with vinegar and wheat flour paste form pills the size of a bullet. Each time place one pill under the sole of the affected foot and tread on it. The ground below is warmed with a fire. The patient is covered with clothes. When sweat appears resembling saliva, a cure is achieved.

16. Explanation of names

By the 16th century, the Chinese empire, founded in 221 BCE, had integrated numerous regions inhabited by people with their own languages and cultures. Naturally, they also knew their plants, minerals, and animals and had their own terms to designate them. Li Shizhen in his *Ben cao gang mu* quotes numerous authors living in earlier times, when some of these ethnic groups were still considered neighbors rather than inhabitants of China. These authors wrote about and described natural substances that had been brought to China from distant regions in the south, the west and the north. This means that in addition to a terminology originating in China, foreign terms were also introduced, and an already complex native Chinese terminology became more and more diverse.

The origins of the plant, animal, and mineral terminology in China date from prehistoric times. Apparently, single-word names for pigs, lions, and sparrows, for iron, silver, and gold, and for pines, leeks, and onions established the beginning of a terminology and have survived to this day. Eventually, with ever more data available, with trade increasing the number of items used, and with writing necessitating specific characters, it was the botanical terminology especially which soon expanded. For items newly introduced, new characters were designed, often with the generic characters for "herb" and "tree/wood" added as "radicals." These signaled to readers that the item so named was a plant or a tree. New terms for minerals and metals were given either the characters "gold/metal" and "jade" (abbreviated to "king") as radicals, or a description with several characters ending with the character "stone."

Hitherto unfamiliar objects were often given names calculated to produce a comparison with known items. Binomial names were created to say something about the appearance of a plant, indicating, for instance, its size, color, or shape. Others were named for the habitat they were taken from and the season in which they flowered or when they were harvested. Often enough, three or even more characters were combined, becoming a familiar name for an item.[33]

The founding of the empire opened up many of the borders which had more or less separated the formerly Warring States. The exchange of goods for daily use increased enormously with the First Qin Emperor's policies

---

[33] Additional reading: Joseph Needham, Lu Gwei-Djen and Huang Hsing-Tsung, Science and Civilisation in China. Vol. 6, Biology and Biological Technology, Part I: Botany, pp. 142 ff.

of standardizing weights and other measures, and equalizing track widths throughout the country. As a result, fusions of provincial usage and dialectical variations resulted in a heterogeneous terminology that required as much standardization as weights, measures, and track widths. As early as during the late Zhou and even more so during the Qin and Han dynasties, word lists were compiled out of a necessity to manage the many names in use. Authors soon began to comment on these lists and add further data.

Conventions emerged as to what name should be recognized as the standard designation, aside from what became known as "alternative names" and "commonly used names." The similarity of certain plants suggested that they were somehow related. Families of names were conceptualized with one identical character forming a link among all members. A nomenclature did not result, however, in the strict sense of an artificial system of designations superimposed on the entirety of plants, distinguishing different levels of relationship, and integrating all plants into one system of interrelated items. Throughout the following two millennia, the dynamics of terminology building never stopped.

The length of documented Chinese pharmaceutical history, the sheer size of the country with its many regional cultures and languages, and the different kinds of sources quoted by Li Shizhen appear to have inspired him to list and discuss the various names of the substances he describes. Not infrequently, Li Shizhen saw a need to explain differing names in the North and South of China assigned to an identical substance. Over the centuries, names once accepted as the standard designation for an item had been replaced by another, now standard, name. In chapter 9, for example, Li Shizhen goes into an extensive discussion intending to end an apparently millennia-old confusion concerning the substance gypsum. It was then known as "stone fat," "finely structured stone/mineral," and "cold water stone/mineral." Some authors identified it as "stone/mineral that splits into rectangular pieces," and as "lengthy stone/mineral." But these names had also been applied to other minerals. Li Shizhen assembles all the relevant quotes and eventually offers his conclusion.

Li Shizhen could have contented himself with enumerating the individual names and distinguishing between standard names and alternative names. In chapter 1 of the *Ben cao gang mu* he lays out the criteria he has applied in this regard. He refers to the proper names as *gang*, "major ordering principle," and to alternative names as *mu*, "specific ordering principle." Chapter 2 begins with a list of five items also known by the same name, followed by lists of four, three, and two items known by the same name. A fifth list enumerates all the names that hint at a similarity with other items. For example, the Japanese plant dock is also known as "rhubarb root resembling an ox tongue."

But Li Shizhen went beyond simply listing and ranking names. For reasons he himself does not openly state, wherever possible he added philological explanations. He took into account, for example, local dialects and the composition of characters. Numerous plant names, for instance, might be mistaken for animal substances. An herb named "grandma's needle thread bag," may not have been correctly identified by many as the Japanese *metaplexis* herb, and a black dragon tail needs to be explained if it is to be understood as dust hanging down from a beam in one's home. Substances imported from foreign countries were often given names in China by transcribing their original pronunciation. Wherever feasible, Li Shizhen included information on the origin of such names, for example, when they were thought to reflect a Sanskrit term. Furthermore, many names were written with characters possibly unfamiliar to the *Ben cao gang mu*'s readers. Hence, Li Shizhen explained their pronunciation by either adducing homophones or resorting to the split-reading approach. And finally, when he felt at his wits' end, he freely acknowledged his inability to explain a certain name.

Crabs
Eriocheir sinensis H. Milne-Edwards. Vol. VIII, 45-16

Heng xing jie shi 橫行介士, "armed warrior moving sideways," *Crab Treatise*.

Wu chang gong zi 無腸公子, "prince without intestines," *The Master Embracing Simplicity*.

Males are called *lang yi* 蜋螘. Females are called *bo dai* 博帶, *Expanded Examples of Refined Usage*.

Kou Zongshi: These items appear at the beginning of autumn when they slough off their shell like cicadas do. This is the meaning underlying their name *xie* 蟹 (i.e., a combination of *jie* 解, "to dismiss," and *chong* 虫, "worms/bugs").

Li Shizhen: According to Fu Gong's *Crab Treatise*, "crabs are water worms/ bugs. Hence the character *xie* 蟹 is based on the character *chong* 虫, 'worms/bugs'. They also belong to the group of fishes. Hence in ancient scripts, the character *xie* 蟹 was written with the radical *yu* 魚, 'fish'. Because they move sideways, they are called *pang* 蟧 (i.e., a combination of pang 旁, 'side', and *chong* 虫, 'worms/bugs') crabs. Because of the sounds they make when they move they are called *guo suo* 郭索. Because of their external bone they are called *jie shi* 介士, 'armed soldier'. Because they are hollow inside, they are called *wu chang* 無腸, 'without intestines'."

Pill bug
Armadillidium vulgare Latreille. Vol. VIII, 41-23

(Note: The standard Chinese name of pill bug is written using to homophonic character: *shu fu* 鼠婦, "mouse/rat wife," and *shu fu* 鼠負, "carried by the mouse/rat.")

Tao Hongjing: *Shu fu* 鼠婦 is written in the *Examples of Refined Usage* as *shu fu* 鼠負, because mice/rats, *shu* 鼠, in ditches often carry, *fu* 負, them glued to their back. Hence they are called *shu fu* 鼠負, "carried by mice/rats." When nowadays this is written with the character *fu* 婦, "wife," instead of *fu* 負, "carried," then this is contrary to the original meaning.

Han Baosheng: They are often found at the bottom of porcelain containers and in earth pits, and they are generally attached to the back of mice/rats. Hence their name. They are also commonly called *shu nian* 鼠粘, "glued to mice/rats." This is just like the name *yang fu lai* 羊負來, "comes carried by goats/sheep" of *xanthium* stem and leaves.

Li Shizhen: According to Lu Dian's *Increased Examples of Refined Usage*, "when men eat pill bugs, they love to have sex. Hence they are named *fu* 婦, 'wife'. They are also named *shu gu* 鼠姑, meaning the same as *shu fu* 鼠婦. *Shu nian* 鼠粘 is the same as *shu fu* 鼠負." The meanings of both *fu* 婦 and *fu* 負 make sense. Since they come to life through the transformation of moisture, they are commonly called *shi sheng chong* 濕生蟲, "bugs born from moisture." When they are called *di ji* 地雞, "ground chicken," and *di shi* 地虱, "ground louse," then this is a reference to their physical appearance.

Flounders
Pleuronichthus cornutus Temminck et Schlegel. Vol. VIII, 44-47

(Note: The standard Chinese name of flounder is *bi mu yu* 比目魚, literally, "fish with eyes close to each other.")

Li Shizhen: *Bi* 比 is *bing* 並, "side by side," "together." Each of these fishes has one eye. When they move, they place each other side by side. This is what the *Examples of Refined Usage* means when it states: "In the East there are the fishes with their eyes side by side, *bi yu* 比目魚. If they are not side by side, they do not move. They are called *die* 鰈."

Mr. Duan Gonglu in his *Records from Beihu* calls them *jian* 鰜, read *jian* 兼.

The *Rhapsody on the Capital of Wu* calls them *jie* 魪, read *jie* 介.

The *Rhapsody on the Upper Forest* calls them *xu* 鮥, read *xu* 墟.

Die 鰈 is like *xie* 屧, "shoes." *Jian* 鰜 is *jian* 兼, "concurrently." *Jie* 魪 is *xiang jie* 相介, "situated together." *Qu* 魼 is *xiang qu* 相胠, "side by side." They are commonly called "shoe sole fishes."

The *Records from Linhai* calls them *bei xi yu* 婢屣魚, "a servant girl's straw sandal fishes."

The *Records from the Waters and Lands of Lin hai* calls them *nu jue yu* 奴屩魚, "a slave girl's straw sandal fishes."

The *Records of Nanyue* calls them *ban yu* 版魚, "board fishes."

The *Records of Extraordinary Things from the Southern Regions* calls them *ruo ye yu* 箬葉魚, "broad-leaved bamboo leaf fishes."

All these names refer to the physical appearance of flounders.

Tamarisk
Tamarix chinenis Lour. Vol. VII, 35-30

(The standard Chinese name of tamarisk is *zhen liu* 檉柳.)

Li Shizhen: According to Luo Yuan's *Wings to the Examples of Refined Usage*, "When heaven is about to send down rain, tamarisks are the first to know it. They raise qi in response, and when covered by frost and snow they do not wither. They are the sages, *sheng* 聖, among trees. Hence, the character *zhen* 檉 is derived from the character *sheng* 聖. Another name is *yu shi* 雨師, 'rain authority'."

It is also said: "When tamarisks are exposed to rain the twigs droop like 'silk threads,' *si* 絲. *Yu shi* 雨師, 'rain authority' should be written *yu si* 雨絲, 'rain threads'."

Also, the *Tales from the three Capital districts* states: "In the garden of Han emperor Wu di a willow was shaped like a human being. It was called *ren liu* 人柳, 'human willow'." Each day it rose three times and fell asleep, *mian* 眠, three times. That is, tamarisk sages do not only know rain and shoulder snow! Today, they are commonly called *chang shou xian ren liu* 長壽仙人柳, "longevity hermit/immortal willow." They are also called *Guan yin liu* 觀音柳, "Guanyin willow." That is to say, Guanyin uses tamarisk twigs to spray water.

Kou Zongshi: Today, people call them *san chun liu* 三春柳, "triple spring willow," and they are named so because they bloom three times within one year.

Chinese white pine
Pinus armandi Franch. Vol. VII, 34-02

(Chinese standard name: Song 松.)

Li Shizhen: According to Wang Anshi's *Elucidation of Characters*, "pines, *song* 松, and arborvitae, *bai* 柏, trees are the chiefs of the hundreds of woods/trees. *Song* 松 is like *gong* 公, 'duke'. *Bai* 柏 is like *bo* 伯, 'count'. Hence, the character *song* 松 is derived from the character *gong* 公, and the character *bai* 柏 is derived from the character *bai* 白."

"Water from wells and springs."
Vol. II, 05-15

(Chinese: *jing quan shui* 井泉水.)

Li Shizhen: The character *jing* 井, "well," reflects the physical appearance of an artificially constructed well. The character *quan* 泉, "spring," reflects the physical appearance of a hole/cave from which water flows.

"Fire needle."
Vol. II, 06-08

(Chinese: *huo zhen* 火鍼.)

Li Shizhen: The "fire needle" is identical to the "heated needle" and the "scorched needle" mentioned in the *Basic Questions*. Zhang Zhongjing names them "burned needle." The people in Chuan and Shu name them "heated needle." The method of applying them in a medical therapy is as follows. Fill a cup with sesame oil. Then place two times seven *juncus* stalks as lamp wicks into the oil and light them as a lamp. Dip the needle several times into the sesame oil, heat it over the lamp until it has become red, and then use it for its therapeutic purpose. If it is not red, or if it is even cold, then, contrary to one's intentions, it will cause injury and the disease will not be removed. To be of excellent quality, the needle is to be prepared from iron tempered by fire. The needle insertion hole is to be marked with ink to clearly show its position. If this is missed, the treatment will have no effect.

Chalk. Kaolin
Vol. II, 07-01

(Chinese standard name: *bai e* 白堊).

Alternative Names: *Bai shan tu* 白善土, "white, good soil," *Supplementary Records by Famous Physicians. Bai tu fen* 白土粉, "white soil powder," *Yan yi. Hua fen* 畫粉, "powder for drawings."

Li Shizhen: Since the proper color of soil is yellow, white, *bai* 白, soil is a bad, *e* 惡, soil, (*tu* 土). Hence the name *bai e* 堊, "white bad soil." In later times, the people placed a taboo on this negative designation and they named it "white good soil," *bai shan tu* 白善土, instead.

Ink stick
Vol. II, 08-51

(Chinese standard name: *mo* 墨.)

Li Shizhen: The ancients used black soil as ink. Hence, the character *mo* 墨, "ink" is based on the characters *hei* 黑, "black," and *tu* 土, "soil."

Xu Shen in his *Explaining Single and Analysing Compound Characters* states: "Ink is produced from soot left by smoke. It is a type of soil. Hence the character *mo* 墨, 'ink' is based on the characters *hei* 黑, 'black', and *tu* 土, 'soil'."

Liu Xi in his *Explanation of Names* states: "Mo 墨 is *hui* 晦, 'dark'."

Native gold
Vol. II, 08-81

(The standard Chinese name for gold, *jin* 金, also refers to "metal" as a whole. An alternative name for gold is "ivory," Chinese: *huang ya* 黃牙, literally, "yellow tooth.")

Li Shizhen: According to Xu Shen's *Explaining Single and Analysing Compound Characters*, among the five metals, the yellow metal, i.e., gold, is the chief. Even when buried for a long time it will not take on a layer of corrosion. Even when smelted in a fire a hundred times it will not become lighter. It is obedient to any processing. It grows in the soil (*tu* 土), hence its written character *jin* 金 has marks on its left and right to reflect the physical appearance of gold in the soil.

The *Examples of Refined Usage* states: Yellow metal/gold is called *dang* 璗. Beautiful specimens are called *liu* 鏐. Gold shaped like a flat pie is called *ban* 鈑. Gold with a superb luster is called *xi* 銑. Dugu Tao states: Natural ivory is called "yellow ivory." In Sanskrit texts it is called *sufaluo* 蘇伐羅.

Tao Hongjing: In the recipes of the hermits/immortals, gold is called *tai zhen* 太真, "superb authenticity."

Red copper. Copper
Vol. II, 08-06

(Chinese standard name: *chi tong* 赤銅, "red copper.")

Tao Hongjing. Names of copper fragments: *Tong luo* 銅落, "copper chips;" *tong mo* 銅末, "copper powder;" *tong hua* 銅花, "copper blossoms;" *tong fen* 銅粉, "copper powder;" *tong sha* 銅砂, "copper sand." Li Shizhen: Copper and gold are identical. Hence the character *tong* 銅, "copper," is derived from the characters *jin* 金, "gold," and *tong* 同, "identical."

Golden eye grass
Curculigo orchioides Baertn. Vol. III, 12-22

(Chinese standard name: *xian mao* 仙茅, "the immortals' floss grass.")

Li Xun: Its leaves resemble those of floss grass, *mao* 茅. Ingested over a long time they relieve the body of its weight. Hence the name 仙茅 *xian mao* "hermit's/immortal's floss grass." In Sanskrit texts it is called *ashuqiantuo* 阿輸乹陁, a transcription of the Sanskrit sound with Chinese characters.

Su Song: The root grows "independently," *du* 獨. The beginnings of its use in China date back to a Brahman, *poluomen* 婆羅門, priest from the Western lands who presented a recipe to Tang Emperor Xuan zong. Hence in today's Jiangnan it is called *poluomen shen* 婆羅門參, the "Brahman's ginseng root." That is to say, its therapeutic potential as a supplementing medication resembles that of ginseng root.

Wrinkled giant hyssop
Agastache rugosa (Fisch. et Mey.) O. Kuntze. Vol. III, 14-42

(Chinese standard name: *huo xiang* 藿香.)

Li Shizhen: The leaves of soybeans are called *huo* 藿. Because the leaves of wrinkled giant hyssop resemble them, the present substance is called *huo xiang* 藿香, ("soybean leaf aromatic").

The *Surangama Sutra* states: "Prior to altar services, take a bath in water in which *douloupo* aromatic was boiled." This is the item discussed here.

The *Lotus Sutra* calls it *moluoba* aromatic 摩羅跋香. The *Jin guang ming jing* calls it *bodaluo* aromatic, 鉢怛羅香.

All these are pronunciations of the two characters *dou lou* 兜婁 in Sanskrit.

The *Nirvana Sutra* calls it *jiasuan* aromatic 迦算香.

Silk-cotton tree
Bombax malabaricum DC. Vol. VII, 36-40

(Chinese standard name: *Mu mian* 木綿, "tree silk.")

Li Shizhen: There are two kinds of *mu mian* 木綿. Those resembling trees, they are called *gu bei* 古貝. Those resembling herbs, they are called *gu zhong* 古終. When it is sometimes written *ji bei* 吉貝, it is an erroneous modification of *gu bei* 古貝. In Sanskrit texts they are called *shanpo* 睒婆 and also *jiuluopojie* 迦羅婆劫.

Amber
Vol. VII, 37-02

(Chinese standard name: *hu po* 琥珀.)

Li Shizhen: When a tiger, *hu* 虎, dies its essence and *po* 魄-soul enter the ground and transform to stones. This item resembles them. Hence, it is called *hu po* 虎魄, a "tiger's *po*-soul." In common writings, the character *po* 珀 is derived from the character *yu* 玉 as amber is in one group with *yu* 玉, jade. In Sanskrit texts it is called *ashimojiepo* 阿濕摩揭婆.

Ginseng root
Panax ginseng C. A. Meyer. Vol. III, 12-03

(Chinese standard name: *ren shen* 人參)

Li Shizhen: When ginseng gradually develops over many years it forms a root with a physical appearance resembling a human person, *ren* 人, endowed with a spirit, *shen* 神. Hence it is called *ren shen* 人薓 and *shen cao* 神草, "spirit herb." The character *shen* 薓 is based on the character, meaning "gradual immersion." is *jin* 浸, "to immerse." Because this character is so complicated, in later times it was replaced with the character *shen* 参, referring to one of the 28 constellations, to simplify its writing. This error has lasted for a long time now, and cannot be changed again. Only Zhang Zhongjing in his *Shang han lun* still writes the character *shen* 薓.

The *Supplementary Records by Famous Physicians* has *ren wei* 人微 as an alternative name. *Wei* 微 is an erroneous version of the character *shen* 薓. Ginseng is present in different classes. Hence it is called *ren jian* 人衔, "human rank." This herb turns its back on the yang and reaches out toward the yin. Hence it is called "demon's canopy," *gui gai* 鬼盖. As there are five different herbs called *shen* 参, ginseng root with its yellow color associated with the phase soil, and supplementing spleen and stomach and generating yin blood, is called *huang shen* 黄参, "yellow *shen*," and *xue shen* 血参, "blood *shen*." It is endowed with the miraculous essence power of the earth, hence it is called *tu jing* 土精, "essence of the soil," and *di jing* 地精, "essence of the earth."

The *Expanded Records of the Five Phases* states: "At the time of Emperor Wen of the Sui dynasty, in Shangdang people heard voices behind their house during the night. They searched but did not find anything. More than one *li* away from the house, they observed abnormal ginseng branches and leaves. When they dug into the ground five *chi* deep, they found a ginseng root entirely shaped like a human body, with four complete limbs. From then on, the voices fell silent." In view of this, the name "essence of the soil" appears to be more than appropriate.

In *The Majestic Presence of the Big Dipper in the Record of Rites* it is stated: "Where there is a ginseng root below, there are purple qi above."

The *Chun qiu yun dou shu* states: "Light dispersed by the *yao guang* star becomes ginseng root. When the rulers of mankind disregard mountains and channels, the *yao guang* star loses its brightness, and ginseng does not grow." Seen from this, the name "spirit herb" is legitimate.

Atractylodes macrocephala Koidz. Largehead *atractylodes*
Vol. III, 12-15

(Chinese standard name: *zhu* 术.)

Li Shizhen: According to *The Original Meanings of the Six Categories of Characters*, the character *zhu* 术 is seal script reflecting the physical appearance of the herb's root, stem, branches, and leaves. In Wu Pu's *Ben cao*, it is also named *shan jie* 山芥, "mountain mustard," and *tian ji* 天薊, "heavenly thistle," because its leaves resemble those of thistles, *su* 薊, and the flavor resembles that of ginger, *jiang* 薑, and mustard, *jie* 芥. In the western regions they call it *chi li jia* 吃力伽. This is why the *Arcane Essential Recipes from the Outer Censorate* lists a "powder with *chi li jia* 吃力伽."

Much white *zhu* grows in the region of Yangzhou. Its shape resembles a drumstick, *bao* 枹, hence it is named *yang bao* 楊枹, "poplar drumstick," and *bao ji* 枹薊, "drumstick thistle." Nowadays, the people call it *wu zhu* 吳术, "*zhu* from Wu." Bao 枹 is the name of drumsticks. Ancient recipes resorted to the two kinds of *zhu* alike. Later people began to distinguish between a *cang* 蒼, "dark green/grey," and a *bai* 白, "white," type.

Indian mulberry
Morinda offi cinalis How. Vol. III, 12-18

(Chinese standard name: *ba ji tian* 巴戟天.)

Alternative Names: *Bu diao cao* 不凋草, "an herb that does not wither," *Rihua*. *San man cao* 三蔓草, "triple creeper herb."

Li Shizhen: The meaning of the name *ba ji tian* 巴戟天 is totally incomprehensible.

Wild leek
Allium thunbergii G. Don. Vol. VI, 26-02

(Chinese standard name: *shan jiu* 山韭, "mountain leek.")

Alternative Names: *Yu* 蒮, read *yu* 育. *Xian* 韱, read *xian* 纖. The meaning of both these names remains unclear.

Chinese senega
Polygala tenuifolia Willd. Vol. III, 12-19

(Chinese standard name: *yuan zhi* 遠志, "Expansion of consciousness.")

The seedlings are named *xiao cao* 小草, "little herb," *Original Classic*.

Xi cao 細草, "delicate herb," *Original Classic*.

Ji wan 棘菀, "thorny luxuriance," *Original Classic*.

Yao rao 葽繞, "circling *yao* herb," *Original Classic*.

Li Shizhen: To ingest this herb can boost wisdom and strengthen the mind, *zhi* 志. Hence its designation as *yuan zhi* 遠志, "extending the mind."

The *Tales of the World* records a saying of Xie An: "If you stay home, you will be someone with a farreaching mind. When you leave, you will be a small herb."

In the *Pearls of Recorded Things* it is called *xing xin zhang* 醒心杖, the "cane to arouse the heart."

Horny goat weed
Epimedium brevicornum Maxim. Vol. III, 12-21

(Chinese standard name: *yin yang huo* 淫羊藿, "soybean leaves for horny goats.")

Tao Hongjing: When this is ingested, it lets people find more pleasure in yin and yang exchange (i.e., sexual intercourse). In the northern region of Xichun there are randy sheep, *yin yang* 淫羊, that mate a hundred times a day. The fact is, this is a result of their eating soybean leaves, *huo* 藿. Hence this herb is called *yin yang huo* 淫羊藿, "randy sheep soybean leaves."

Li Shizhen. The leaves of soybeans are called *huo* 藿 and the leaves of this plant resemble them. Hence, they, too, are called *huo* 藿. *Xian ling pi* 仙靈脾, "an hermit's/immortal's magic spleen," *qian liang jin* 千兩金, "leaves worth 1,000 *liang* of gold," *fang zhang* 放杖, "leaves setting free one's stick," and *gang qian* 剛前, "leaves hardening one's front," are references to the therapeutic potential and strength of these leaves. *Ji jin* 雞筋, "chicken sinews," and *huang lian zu* 黃連祖, "*coptis'* ancestor," refer to the physical appearance of the root.

The *Literary Collection of Liu Zihou* writes the name as *xian ling pi* 仙靈毗. The human navel is called *pi* 毗. This item serves to supplement qi in the lower body region. Hence the reason for naming it is all the more understandable.

Artemisia scoparia Waldst. et Kit. Virgate wormwood
Vol. IV, 15-07

(Chinese standard name: *yin chen hao* 茵蔯蒿.)

Although this item belongs to the wormwood, *hao* 蒿, group, it does not die throughout winter. Rather, it comes to life again "ensuing from/relying on" (*yin* 因) old seedlings. Hence it was called *yin chen* 因陳, "following from/relying on (*yin* 因) the old (*chen* 陳)." Later, the character *hao* 蒿 was added.

Li Shizhen: According to Zhang Yi's *Expanded Examples of Refined Usage* and the *Materia Medica of Wu Pu*, it is written *yin chen* 因塵, "ensuing from dust." I have no idea what that could mean.

Datura metel L. Downy thorn apple
Vol. IV, 17-34

(Chinese standard name: *mantuolo hua* 曼陀羅花.)

Alternative Names: *Feng qie er* 風茄兒, "wind eggplant," *Gang mu.*

Shan qie zi 山茄子, "mountain eggplant."

Li Shizhen: The *Lotus Sutra* says that when Buddha recited his sutras, *mantuoluo* 曼陀羅 flowers rained from heaven. The Daoists hold that the Big Dipper has sent a *tuoluo* 陀羅 star emissary, holding this plant in his hand. Hence, later on, people named this flower after him. *Mantuoluo* 曼陀羅 in Sanskrit means "multi-colored." The name *qie* 茄, "eggplant," refers to the shape of the leaves.

In Yao Bosheng's "categories/ranks of flowers," it is called *e ke* 惡客, "malicious visitor."

Artemisia sieversiana Ehrhart ex Willd. Sievers wormwood
Vol. IV, 15-10

(Chinese standard name: *bai hao* 白蒿, "white wormwood.")

Li Shizhen: There are two kinds of *bai hao*. One "water" *bai hao* and one "land" *bai hao*. The *Examples of Refined Usage* calls both of them *fan* 繁, because they multiply, *fan yan* 繁衍, easily. When it is said "*fan* 繁 is *po hao* 皤蒿," then this is today's *ai hao* 艾蒿, common mugwort, growing on land. It is acrid and has a bad smell. When it is said "*Fan* 繁 is *you hu* 由胡," then this is today's *lou hao* 蔞蒿, growing in waters. It is acrid and has a nice fragrance. When it is said "The unsightly kind of *fan* 繁 turning into *hao* 蒿 in autumn," then this is a reference to both the water and the land kinds. That is, in spring they have individually descriptive names, and by autumn, when they turn old, they all alike are called *hao* 蒿. *Lai* 籟, *xiao* 蕭, and *qiu* 萩 are designations of old *hao* 蒿. They reflect the solemn, *su* 肅, and trustworthy, *lai* 賴, qi of autumn, *qiu* 秋.

Pedicularis resupinata L
Vol. IV, 15-13

(Chinese standard name: *ma xian hao* 馬先蒿.)

Li Shizhen: The qi of this kind of *hao* resembles the smell of horse dung, *ma shi* 馬矢, hence the name. *Ma xian* 馬先 is an erroneous writing of *ma shi* 馬矢. *Ma xin* 馬新, in turn, is an erroneous writing of *ma xian* 馬先.

Tao Hongjing: *Lian shi cao* 練石草, "white silk stone herb," alternatively named *lan shi cao* 爛石草, "rotten stone herb," is a less offensive writing of *ma shi cao* 馬矢蒿, "horse dung *hao*." In commonly resorted to pharmaceutical recipes it is no longer used.

Mei xian. Unidentified
Vol. IV, 15-19

(Chinese standard name: *mei xian* 薇銜.)

Su Gong: The people in the South call it *wu feng cao* 吳風草, and also *lu xian cao* 鹿銜草. That is to say, when deer, *lu* 鹿, have an illness they use this herb as a bit, *xian* 銜, and it will be healed.

Li Shizhen: According to Su Gong, *mei xian* 薇銜 and *mi xian* 麋銜 should be written *lu xian* 鹿銜. Deer, *lu* 鹿, and *mi* 麋, Pére David's deer, belong to the same group.

According to Li Daoyuan in his *Shui jing zhu*, "plenty of *wei xian cao* grows on Mount Xishan in Weixing. When wind blows it does not lie down. When there is no wind, *wu feng* 無風, it sways by itself." Hence *wu feng* 吳風 should be written *wu feng* 無風, "in the absence of wind." That makes sense.

Chen Cangqi: It is also called *wu xin cao* 無心草, "herb without 'heart'." But this is not an herb "without heart." It is seldem resorted to in medicinal recipes.

Ramie plant
Boehmeria nivea (L.) Gaud. Vol. IV, 15-35

(Chinese standard name: *zhu ma* 苧麻.)

Li Shizhen: The first character *zhu* 苧 of *zhu ma* 苧麻 is also written *zhu* 紵, because *zhu ma* can be used to weave "sack cloth," *zhu* 紵. Hence this herb is called *zhu ma* 紵麻, "sack cloth bast fibers. All fine fibers and silk threads are *quan* 絟, "fine cloth." Coarse ones are *zhu* 紵, "sack cloth.""

Tao Hongjing: "*Zhu* 苧 is the ramie, *zhu ma* 苧麻, used for weaving today." The character *ma* 麻 is a combination of *yan* 广, "thatched hut," and 林, read *pai* 派. It is to reflect the fitting underneath a roof by means of bamboo shingles, *lin* 林, and bast fibers, *ma* 麻. 广 is read *yan* 掩.

St. Paulswort
Siegesbeckia orientalis L. Vol. IV, 15-44

(Chinese standard name: *xi xian* 豨薟.)

Li Shizhen: According to rhyme books, in Chu people call *zhu* 豬, "pigs," *xi* 豨, and they refer to the acrid and poisonous qi of herbs as *xian* 薟. This herb has malodorous qi similar to pigs and the flavor is poisonous and stinging, *xian shi* 薟螫. Hence, it is called *xi xian* 豨薟. "Pig paste," *zhu gao* 豬膏, "tiger paste," *hu gao* 虎膏 and "dog paste," *gou gao* 狗膏, are all based on the similarities of their qi. Also, this herb serves to cure harm caused by tigers and dogs. *Huo xian* 火枚 should be *hu xian* 虎薟: This is a common mispronunciation. In recent times, people have mistakenly converted *xi xian* 豨薟 to *xi xian* 希仙, "invisible hermit/immortal."

The *Materia Medica for Famine Relief* says: "Heat its tender leaves until done and soak them to eliminate the bitter flavor. Then eat them mixed with oil and salt. Hence it is commonly said to be a 'vegetable sticky like a paste,' *nian hu cai* 粘糊菜."

Musa sapientum L. Banana
Vol. IV, 15-47

(Chinese standard name: *gan jiao* 甘蕉.)

Li Shizhen: According to Lu Dian's *Increased Examples of Refined Usage*, "the leaves of banana trees do not fall off. When a new leaf unfolds, an old leaf is 'scorched,' *jiao* 焦. Therefore the plant is called *jiao* 蕉. Dry items are commonly called *ba* 巴. *Ba* 巴, too, has the meaning of *jiao* 蕉, 'scorched plant'." The *Rhapsody Examining the Sagely* states: "When bamboo displays fruits, the root turns bitter. When *jiao* 蕉 unfolds flowers, its stem withers." *Ba ju* 芭苴 is a modified reading of *ba jiao*. In Shu, people call it *tian ju* 天苴, "celestial hemp plant."

Cao Shuya in his *Records of Extraordinary Things* states: "The fruits formed by *ba jiao* have a skin as red as fire and the flesh is sweet, *gan* 甘, like honey. Four or five can fill a person. Its flavor remains between the teeth for a long time. Hence it is called 'sweet *jiao*,' *gan jiao* 甘蕉."

Chinese ephedra
Ephedra sinica Stopf. Vol. IV, 15-49

(Chinese standard name: *ma huang* 麻黃.)

Alternative Names: *Long sha* 龍沙, "dragon sand/droppings," *Original Classic*.

Bei xiang 卑相, *Supplementary Records by Famous Physicians*.

Bei yan 卑鹽, *Supplementary Records by Famous Physicians*.

Li Shizhen: These names cannot be explained. Some say, the flavor of *ma huang* is "numbing," *ma* 麻, and its color is "yellow," *huang* 黃. Could this be so?

Zhang Yi in his *Expanded Examples of Refined Usage* states: "*Long sha* 龍沙 is *ma huang* 麻黃; *gou gu* 狗骨, 'dog bone,' is the root of *ma huang* 麻黃."

It is not clear how these names can serve to distinguish these items from others.

Dodder
Cuscuta chinensis, Lam. Vol. V, 18-01

(Chinese standard name: *tu si zi* 菟絲子)

Zhang Yuxi: According to the *The Spring and Autumn Annals of Mr. Lü*, "it is also called *tu si* 菟絲, an herb without root. The root does not touch the ground. It is *fu ling* 伏苓, *poria*."

The *Master Embracing Simplicity* states: "Below the herb *tu si* 菟絲 is *fu tu* 伏菟 as its root. If there is no such *fu* 伏 *tu* 菟, *tu* 菟 *si* 絲 cannot grow above it. However, fact is that they are not linked to each other. When the *fu tu* 伏菟 is removed, the *tu si* 兔絲 dies."

It is also said: "The root of *tu si* 菟絲 in an early stage of its growth is shaped like a rabbit, *tu* 兔. When it is dug out and its 'blood' is ingested mixed with an elixir, an immediate change or transformation to an immortal is possible." That is why *tu si* 菟絲 was given its name.

Tao Hongjing: In former times it was said: "Below is *fu ling* 伏苓, above is *tu si* 菟絲." But this is not necessarily so.

Su Song: What the *Master Embracing Simplicity* describes is no longer seen today. Perhaps this is something different.

Sun Yan in his comments on the *Examples of Refined Usage* states: "It is *tang* 唐, it is *meng* 蒙, it is *nü luo* 女蘿, it is *tu si* 兔絲 – one item, four names." But the *Ben cao* mentions *tang meng* 唐蒙 as an alternative name.

The *Book of Songs* states: "*Niao* 蔦 with *nü luo* 女蘿."

Mao Chang states in his commentary: "*Nü luo* 女蘿 is *tu si* 兔絲." But the *Ben cao* does not mention *nü luo* 女蘿 as a name of *tu si* 兔絲. Only *song luo* 松蘿 is said to be also named *nü luo* 女蘿. How can it be that there are two different items that are both parasites and have the same name, but this is overlooked by the *Ben cao*?

Zhu Zhenheng: *Tu si* 兔絲 is in no way related to *fu ling* 伏苓, poria. *Nü luo* 女蘿 grows attached to pines. They have nothing in common. These are erroneous sayings that have been transmitted for long.

Li Shizhen: Mao Chang's commentary on the *Book of Songs* says: "*Nü luo* 女蘿 is *tu si* 兔絲." The *Materia Medica of Wu Pu* says: "*Tu si* 兔絲 is also named *song luo* 松蘿."

Lu Dian says: "When it is a tree, it is *nü luo* 女蘿; when it is an herb, it is *tu si* 兔絲." These are two entirely different items. They are identified as one and the same item since that erroneous commentary to the *Examples of Refined Usage.*"

Zhang Yi in his *Expanded Examples of Refined Usage* states: "*Tu qiu* 兔丘 is *tu si* 兔絲. *Nü luo* 女蘿 is *song luo* 松蘿."

When Lu Ji in his *Commentary on the Book of Songs* says: "*Tu si* 兔絲 is a creeper on herbs. It is yellow-red, similar to gold. *Song luo* 松蘿 is a creeper on pines, *song* 松. It has twigs that are really greenish, unlike other vines," then everything should be clear. For details see the entry *song luo* 松蘿, in the section "trees." As to what is said about *tu si* 兔絲 and *fu ling* 伏苓, see the entry *fu ling* 伏苓.

Korean bramble
Rubus coreanus Miq. Vol. V, 18-04

(Chinese standard name: *fu pen zi* 覆盆子.)

Li Dangzhi: The seeds, *zi* 子, are shaped like an upturned pot, *fu pen* 覆盆. Hence the name.

Kou Zongshi: The seeds boost the qi of the kidney long-term depot. They restrain urination. When they are ingested, the chamber pot can be up-turned, *fu* 覆. This is where they got their name from.

Aristolochia contorta, Bunge. Northern pipevine
Vol. V, 18-10

Kou Zongshi: It grows as a creeper and rises attached to trees. When the leaves fall off, the fruits still hang like a bell, *ling* 鈴, at the neck of a horse, *ma* 馬. Hence the name.

Li Shizhen: The root causes vomiting and free flow. It has slightly fragrant qi. Hence names such as *du xing* 獨行, "moving alone," and *mu xiang* 木香, "tree fragrance." People in Lingnan use it to cure *gu* poisoning. They camouflage it with the name "pharmaceutical drug worth three hundred *liang* of silver," *san bai liang yin yao* 三百兩銀藥.

The *Recipes to be Kept Close at Hand* writes *du lin* 都淋. The fact is, this is an erroneous transmission.

Pharbitis nil (L.) Choisy
Vol. V, 18-13

(Chinese standard name: *qian niu zi* 牽牛子, "to bring an ox.")

Tao Hongjing: This pharmaceutical drug was first named *qian niu zi* 牽牛子, "the one to lead forward an ox" when a person from the wild lead forward, *qian* 牽, an ox, *niu* 牛, to express his gratitude, *xie* 謝, for obtaining this pharmaceutical drug. Hence the name.

Li Shizhen: Today people avoid its name and call it *hei chou* 黑丑, "black *chou*," instead. White ones are called *bai chou* 白丑. The fact is, the earthly branch *chou* 丑 is associated with oxen as its emblematic animal. *Jin ling* 金鈴, "golden bell," refers to the shape of the seeds. *Pen zeng* 盆甑, "basin," "jar," and *gou er* 狗耳, "dog's ear," refer to the shape of the leaves.

Duan Chengshi in his *A Miscellany from Youyang* states: "*Pen ceng* herb is a creeper similar to Chinese yam. When its fruits are formed and broken off, they are shaped like a basin or jar."

Hedge bindweed
Calystegia sepium (L.) R. Br. Vol. V, 18-14

(Chinese standard name: *xuan hua* 旋花, "twisted flower/blossom.")

Su Gong: *Xuan hua* 旋花 is the *xuan fu* 旋葍 of the marshlands in the plains. Its roots resemble sinews, *jin* 筋, this is why it is also called "sinew root," *jin gen* 筋根.

Xiao Bing: *Xuan fu* 旋葍 should be written *fu xuan* 葍旋, read *fu xuan* 福鏇. The root is added to medication. There is also a *xuan fu* 旋覆, read *xuan fu* 璇伏; its flowers are added to medication. Today, it is called *xuan fu* 旋葍, but that is wrong.

Su Song: The *Supplementary Records by Famous Physicians* says that the root controls the reconnecting of sinews. Hence people in the South call it the "root to reconnect sinews," *xu jin gen* 續筋根. Another name is *tun chang cao* 狘腸草, "piglet intestine herb," a reference to its shape.

Kou Zongshi: It is commonly called "bugle flower," *gu zi hua* 鼓子花, because its flowers resemble bugles.

Li Shizhen: The flowers do not have petals. They look like bugles, *gu* 鼓, blown in the military. Hence it has names such as *xuan hua* 旋花, "whirling flower," and *gu zi* 鼓子. There is one kind with a thousand leaves. Its color resembles that of a pink *paeonia*. It is commonly called "intertwined branches *paeonia*," *chan zhi mu dan* 纏枝牡丹.

Chinese radish
Raphanus sativus L. Vol. VI, 26-16.

(Chinese standard name: *lai bei* 萊菔)

Han Baosheng: *Lai bei* 萊菔 is commonly called *luo bei* 蘿蔔.

According to the *Examples of Refined Usage*, "*Tu* 葖 is *luo bei* 蘆萉."

Sun Yan in his comment states: "This is *zi hua song* 紫花菘, commonly called *wen song* 温菘. It resembles rape turnip, with a big root. It is commonly called *bao tu* 雹葖." An alternative name is *lai bei* 蘆菔.

Su Song: *Zi hua song* 紫花菘 and *wen song* 温菘 are names given to *lai bei* in the South. People in Wu call it *Chu song* 楚菘; "celery cabbage from Chu;" people in Guangnan call it *Qin song* 秦菘, "celery cabbage from Qin."

Li Shizhen: According to Sun Mian's *Expanded Book on Rhymes*, "people in Lu call it *la da* 菈薘, read *la da* 拉荅. People in Qin call it *luo bei* 蘿蔔."

Wang Zhen in his *Nong shu* says: "In the North the one kind of *luo bei* 蘿蔔 is known by four names. In spring it is called *po di zhui* 破地錐, the 'awl that breaks up the ground'. In summer it is called *xiao sheng* 夏生, 'summer growth'. In autumn it is called *luo bei* 蘿蔔. In winter it is called *tu su* 土酥, 'butter of the soil'. That is to say, it is as spotlessly white as butter."

I, Li Shizhen comment: *Song* 菘 is the name of a vegetable because it endures winter similar to the pines, *song* 松, and arborvitae trees, *bai* 柏. *Lai bei* 萊菔 is the name of the root. In high antiquity it was named *lai bei* 蘆萉. In the meantime the name was changed to *lai bei* 萊菔, which later times erroneously modified to *luo bei* 蘿蔔. People in the South call it *luo bao* 蘿瓟. *Bao* 瓟 is identical with *bao* 雹. See Jin Zhuo's *Annotations to the History of the Han*.

Lu Dian says: "*Lai bei* 萊菔 can check the poison of flour." That pertains to an ingestion, *fu* 服, of *lai mou* 來麰. *Bei* 菔 was read *fu* 服, "to ingest."

The fact is, the idea of *lai bei* being able to check the poison of flour resulted from the meaning of that writing.

Mr. Wang Gun in his *Recipes of Universal Benefit* refers to dried *luo bei* 蘿蔔 as "the bones of an hermit/immortal." That is another one of those baseless names of recipe masters.

Chinese small onion
Allium fistulosum L. Vol. VI, 26-03

(Chinese standard name: *cong* 葱.)

Li Shizhen: *Cong* 葱 is derived from *cong* 怱, "rushed and abrupt." It is straight on the outside and hollow inside. The name reflects the image of *cong tong* 怱通, "rapid penetration." *Kou* 芤 is to say that this herb is hollow inside. Hence, the character *kou* 芤 is derived from *kong* 孔, "hole." It reflects the image of *kong mai* 芤脉, "hollow vessels." When onions, *cong* 葱, have just begun to grow they are called *cong zhen* 葱針, "onion needle." The leaves are called *cong qing* 葱青, "onion greenish." The "clothing" is called *cong pao* 葱袍, "onion gown." The stem is called *cong bai* 葱白, "onion white." The mucus inside the leaves is called *cong ran* 葱苒. It is appropriate for combinations with all other items. Hence it is called *cai bo* 菜伯, "venerable senior among vegetables," and *he shi* 和事, "the herb that harmonizes the affairs."

Trachycarpus fortunei (Hook) H.Endl. Windmill palm
Vol. VII, 35-43

(Chinese standard name: *zong lü* 椶櫚.)

Li Shizhen: Inside the bark are hair threads similar to a horse mane, *zong lü* 駿鬣. Hence, the name. *Zong* 椶 is commonly written *zong* 棕. The character 鬣 is read *lü* 閭; it is *lie* 鬣, "mane." *Bing* 枅 is read *bing* 并.

Prayer bead tree. *Abrus precatorius* L
Vol. VII, 35-50

(Chinese standard name: *xiang si zi* 相思子, "seeds of mutual yearning.")

Li Shizhen: According to the *Gu jin shi hua*, "prayer beads are round and red. According to an old saying, 'in ancient times someone died at the frontier. His wife longed for him (*si* 思). She rested crying under a tree and died there.' Hence, the tree was named 'longing for each other,' *xiang si* 相思. This is different from the *xiang si* 相思 trees described by Han Ping as growing in graveyards. They are two *catalpa* trees growing together as one." Some say that they are in one group with red sandalwood bead trees. It is not clear whether this is so or not.

Mulberry tree. *Morus alba* L
Vol. VII, 36-01

(Chinese standard name: *sang* 桑.)

Li Shizhen: Xu Kai in his *Explaining Single and Analysing Compound Characters* states: "The character 叒 is read *ruo* 若. It is the name of a tree that is divine by nature in the East. The character reflects its shape. Mulberry trees, *sang* 桑, are divine trees the leaves of which are eaten by silkworms. Hence, the character *mu* 木, 'wood,' 'tree,' was added below *ruo* 叒 to distinguish them."

Zizyphus jujuba Mill. var. *spinosa* (Bunge) Hu ex H. F. Chow
White spine tree. Vol. VII, 36-09

(Chinese standard name: *bai ji* 白棘.)

Li Shizhen: Those that grow alone and on tall trees, they are jujubes. Those that grow in a row and on low bushes, they are white spines. Hence, two characters *ci* 朿, one on top of the other, form the character *zao* 棗, jujube. Two characters *ci* 朿 side by side form the character *ji* 棘, spine. A look at the names of these two items allows to distinguish them. The character *ci* 朿 is an abbreviated character *ci* 刺, "thorn."

Rhamnus utilis Decne. Japanese buckthorn
Vol. VII, 36-15

Li Shizhen: *Shu li* 鼠李 in a local reading is also written *chu li* 楮李. The meaning of the name is not clear. As it can be used to dye green it is commonly called *zao li* 皂李, "black plum," and *wu chao* 烏巢, "black nest." *Chao* 巢, *cuo* 槎, and *zhao* 趙 are all mistaken modifications of the character *zao* 皂. There is a *ku qiu* 苦楸 which is also named *shu zi* 鼠梓. It is different from the item discussed here. See under the entry *zi* 梓, yellow catalpa tree. (35-09)

Lycium chinense Mill. *Lycium* seeds/root bark
Vol. VII, 36-24

(Chinese standard name: *gou qi* 枸杞.)

Alternative Names: *Xian ren zhang* 仙人杖, "an hermit/immortal's cane."

Supplementary Records by Famous Physicians. Xi wang mu zhang 西王母杖, "the Queen Mother of the West's cane."

Li Shizhen: *Gou* 枸 and *qi* 杞 are the names of two trees. This item has thorns similar to the thorns of *gou* 枸, it is has a stem similar to the boughs of *qi* 杞. Hence, the two characters are combined to name the present tree. In Daoist texts it is said that a *qian zai gou qi* 千載枸杞, "*gou qi* of a thousand records," was shaped like a dog, *gou*, and for this reason was named *gou* 枸. Whether this is so or not has not been investigated.

Su Song: There are three kinds of *xian ren zhang* 仙人杖, "an hermit/ immortal's cane." One is *gou qi* 枸杞. One is in the group of vegetables, with leaves resembling those of sow thistle. One is the black stem of dead bamboo.

Chinese chastetree
Vitex negundo L. var. *cannabifolia* (Sieb.et Zucc.) Hand.-Mazz.
Vol. VII, 36-28

(Chinese standard name: *mu jing* 牡荆.)

Tao Hongjing: This is *mu jing* 牡荆, "male chastetree." There should be no character *zi* 子 added to the name. *Xiao jing* 小荆 should be *mu jing* 牡荆. The seeds/fruits of *mu jing* 牡荆, Chinese chastetree trees, are bigger than those of *man jing* 蔓荆, leaf chastetree trees, but contrary to the relative sizes of the seeds, Chinese chastetree shrubs are called *xiao jing* 小荆, "small chastetree." Maybe this is related to the size of the trees. I do not know whether leaf chastetree trees are tall and big, too.

Su Gong: *Mu jing* 牡荆, Chinese chastetrees, grow as trees; they do not grow as creepers. Hence, they are called *mu* 牡, "male." This is not to say that they do not bear fruit. *Man jing* 蔓荆, "leaf chastetree," seeds are big; *mu jing* 牡荆, "Chinese chastetree," seeds are small. Hence, the trees are called *xiao jing* 小荆, "small chastetree."

Li Shizhen: In ancient times, chastetrees, *jing* 荆, were used as canes to carry out punishments, *xing* 刑. Hence the character *jing* 荆 is derived from the character *xing* 刑. Chastetree trees grow as clusters, but are scattered. Hence, they are also called *chu* 楚, a character derived from the two characters *lin* 林, forest, and *pi* 疋. *Pi* 疋 is identical with the character *shu* 疏, "scattered." The name *chu* 楚 is based on the meaning of *ji chu* 濟楚, "to come to an end of being scattered." The region *Jing chu* 荆楚 got its name because of the great amount of chastetree produced there.

Hibiscus syriacus L. Syrian *hibiscus*
Vol. VII, 36-33

(Chinese standard name: *mu jin* 木槿.)

Li Shizhen. This flower opens at dawn, *zhao* 朝, and falls off at dusk, *mu* 暮. Hence, it is named *ri ji* 日及, "catching up with the sun." Names such as *jing* 槿 and *shun* 蕣 express the meaning that their flourishing is only ephemeral.

The *Examples of Refined Usage* states: "*Tuan* 椵 is *mu jing* 木槿. *Chen* 櫬 is *mu jing* 木槿."

Guo Pu commented: "These are two alternative names of one item." He states: "White ones are called *tuan* 椵. Red ones are called *chen* 櫬."

In Qi and Lu they are called *wang zheng* 王蒸. That is to say, they are beautiful and plentiful. When the *Shi* states "a lady with a countenance like the flower of the *shun* 舜 tree," this is the item discussed here.

Brocade
Vol. VIII, 38-01

(Chinese: *mu jin* 木槿.)

Li Shizhen: The ornamental design of brocade is woven from silk threads of all five colors. Hence the character *jin* 錦 is composed of the two characters *bo* 帛, "silk," and *jin* 金, "gold." It is a pictographic character with one element indicating meaning and the other sound. It also serves to reflect its value.

"Sweatshirt." Undershirt
Vol. VIII, 38-07

(Chinese: *han shan* 汗衫.)

Alternative Names: *Zhong dan* 中單, "inner unlined garment," *Gang mu. Liang dang* 裲襠, "garment attached to both front and back," *xiu tan* 羞袒, "garment to cover the upper part of the body one feels ashamed to display."

Li Shizhen: In ancient times, an unlined short garment, *ru* 襦, was called *shan* 衫. Today long garments, too, are called *shan* 衫. Wang Rui in his *Zhi gu zi* states: "When King Han fought with Xiang yu, the sweat seeped through his *zhong dan* 中單, 'inner unlined garment'. Hence its name was changed to 'sweat shirt,' *han shan* 汗衫."

Liu Xi in his *Explanation of Names* states: "The 'sweat garment,' *han yi* 汗衣, was called *ze yi* 澤衣, 'moist garment,' in the *Book of Songs*, and also *bi tan* 鄙袒 and *xiu tan* 羞袒.

It is prepared from a piece of fabric of six *chi*, and this is sufficient to cover the chest and the back. The names *bi tan* 鄙袒 and *xiu tan* 羞袒 are to say that this shirt covers the upper part of the body, *tan* 袒, one feels ashamed to display, *xiu bi* 羞鄙. Hence this garment covers this region. Also, in the front it lies close, *dang* 當, to the chest; and behind it lies close, *dang* 當, to the back. Hence it is also called *liang dang* 裲襠."

"Head scarf."
Vol. VIII, 38-11

(Chinese: *tou jin* 頭巾.)

Li Shizhen: In ancient times a piece of cloth of one *chi* length was wrapped around the head, *tou* 頭, to serve as scarf, *jin* 巾. In later times, tulle and gauze, bast fibers and grass-cloth were sewed together. When the headgear is rectangular, it is called *jin* 巾, "scarf." When it is round, it is called *mao* 帽, "cap." When it is lacquered, it is called *guan* 冠, "crown." Also, silk fabric used to fasten the hair is called *xu* 縭. The scarf used to cover the hair is called *ze* 幘. A net spread over the hair is called *wang jin* 網巾, "net scarf." Such products are of recent origin.

Hemp shoe
Vol. VIII, 38-20

(Chinese: *ma xie* 麻鞋.)

Li Shizhen: *Xie* 鞋 in ancient times was written *xie* 鞵; it means *lü* 履, "shoes/to stride." In ancient times they used straw to make sandals, *ju* 屨, and they used silk fabric to make shoes, *lü*履. The Zhou used hemp to prepare shoes, *xie* 鞋.

Liu Xi in his *Explanation of Names* states: "*Xie* 鞋 is *jie* 解, 'to resolve/untie.' When they are fastened on their top, they are easily untied, *shu jie* 舒解. *Lü* 履 is *li* 禮, 'etiquette.' To decorate the feet is part of the 'etiquette.' *Xi* 靸 is *xi* 襲, 'to cover.' The shoes cover the entire foot. Those with a leather sole are called *fei* 屝. The *fei* 屝 are *pi* 皮, 'leather shoes.' Those with a wooden sole are called *xi* 舄. They keep the feet dry. Therefore, moisture will not jeopardize them." For medication, one must use those made of yellow hemp and of ramie.

Mantis egg capsules
Tenodera aridifolia Stoll. Vol. VIII, 39-14

(Standard Chinese names: *tang lang* 螳螂, *dang lang* 蟷蜋. Composed of genus reference *chong* 虫, "worm, insect," and pronunciation indicating characters *tang* 堂, *dang* 當, *liang* 良. *Sang piao xiao* 桑螵蛸. Compounded from *sang* 桑, "mulberry tree," genus reference *chong* 虫, "worm/insect," and pronunciation indicating characters *piao* 票 and *xiao* 肖).

Li Shizhen: The mantis have two arms like hatchets. When one confronts them on the wheel tracks, they do not go out of the way. Hence they are named *dang lang* 當郎, "gentlemen standing up in front of one." A common designation is *dao lang* 刀蜋, "beetle armored with blades." The people in Yan call them *ju fu* 拒斧, "those who resist with hatchets." They also name them *bu guo* 不過, "not to be surpassed." The people in Dai speak of them as *you ma* 天馬, "celestial horse," because their head resembles that of a prancing horse. In the region of Yan and Chao they are called *shi you* 蝕肬, with the character *you* 肬 standing for *you zi* 疣子, "warts," i.e., small flesh growths.

When the people of today suffer from warts, they often resort to these creatures and eat them. This has a long tradition. Their larvae are called *piao xiao* 螵蛸 because their appearance reminds one of the light weight of raw silk, *xiao* 飄, fluttering, *piao* 飄, in the air. The villagers roast and scorch them and feed them to their children, and they state that this is to end bedwetting. Hence, names such as *bo jiao* 蟭蟟 and *zhi shen* 致 神, are all related to these habits. The *A Miscellany from Youyang* names them *ye hu bi ti* 野狐鼻涕, "nasal mucus of wild foxes," a reference to their physical appearance.

Dragonfly spec
Vol. VIII, 40-03.

(Chinese standard name: *qing ling* 蜻蛉. Composed of genus reference *chong* 虫, "worm/insect," and pronunciation indicating characters *qing* 青 and *ling* 令). Alternative names: *Qing ding* 蜻虰, read *ding* 丁; *qing ting* 蜻 蜓, also written *ting* 蝏; *ding xin* 虰蛵, read *xin* 馨; *fu lao* 負勞, Examples of Refined Usage.)

Cong 蟌, read *cong* 怱; *zhu cheng* 諸乘, "riding on everything," Tao Hongjing.

Li Shizhen: *Qing* 蜻 and *cong* 蟌 are designations referring to the greenish, *qing* 青, color of onions, *cong* 葱. *Ling* 蛉 and *ding* 虰 refer to their solitary appearance, *ling ding* 伶仃. Some say that *ding* 虰 refers to their tail that is shaped like a "pin," *ding* 丁. Still others say that it is because of their tails being "flat," *ting* 亭, and "straight," *ting* 挺, that they are called *ting* 蜓 and *ting* 蝏. They are commonly called *sha yang* 紗羊, "gauze goats/sheep," because their wings are thin like "gauze," *sha* 紗.

According to Cui Bao's *Notes on Things Old and New*, "those that are big and of greenish color, they are called *qing ting* 蜻蜓. Those that are small and of yellow color, they are called *hu li* 胡黎 in Jiang dong, *kan yi* 蜫蚐 in Huainan, and *jiang ji* 江雞, 'river chicken,' in Bo yang. Those that are small and red, they are called *chi zu* 赤卒, or *jiang zou* 絳緅, or *chi yi shi zhe* 赤衣使者, or *chi bian zhang ren* 赤弁丈人. Those that are large and of dark-purple color, they are named *gan fan* 紺蟠 in Liao hai, and also *tian ji* 天雞, 'heaven's chicken'."

When Mr. Tao Hongjing says that the *hu li* 胡黎 are the dragonflies, *qing ling* 蜻蛉, he did so because he had not investigated this sufficiently.

Whooper swan
Cygnus cygnus L. Vol. IX, 47-10

(Chinese standard name: *hu* 鵠. Composed of original pronunciation indicating character *gao* 告 and genus indication *niao* 鳥, "bird.")

Li Shizhen: According to Shi Kuang's *Bird Classic*, "swans cry *hao hao* 喵 喵. Hence their name is written 鵠."

Seng Zanning, a Buddhist monk in Wu, stated: "All items that are big are named with the character *tian* 天, 'heaven'. The character *tian* 天 is to say *da* 大, 'big'." The meaning of the name *tian e* 天鵝, "heavenly/big goose," corresponds to this.

When Mr. Luo stated that "*hu* 鵠 is identical with *he* 鶴," he was wrong.

Great bustard
Otis tarda L. Vol. IX, 47-11

(Chinese standard name: *bao* 鴇. Composed of pronunciation indicating character *bao* 乇, and genus reference *niao* 鳥, "bird.")

Li Shizhen: According to Luo Yuan, "bustards are covered with the dots of a leopard. Hence they are called *du bao* 獨豹, 'lonely leopards'. This has been mistakenly changed to *bao* 鴇."

Lu Dian states: "Bustards naturally flock together. Like wild geese they move in a certain order. Hence the writing of their name with the element 乇. 乇 is read *bao* 保. Its meaning is: to follow one another."

When the *Book of Songs* speaks of "the movement of bustards," this is what was meant.

Domestic duck
Anas domestica L. Vol. IX, 47-12

(Chinese standard name: *wu* 鶩, read: *mu*. Alternative: *ya* 鴨.)

Li Shizhen: *Mu* 鶩 is often written *mu* 木. Ducks are of the nature of wood; they have no second thoughts in their heart. Hence, the masses present them as a valuable gift.

The *Record of Rites* states: "The masses cherish pairs, *pi* 匹." *Pi* 匹 means "a pair of ducks." *Pi* persons, *pi fu* 匹夫, are people of low status. Hence the *Expanded Examples of Refined Usage* speaks of ducks as *mo pi* 鶩鴄, i.e., "insignificant birds."

The *Bird Classic* states: "Ducks cry *ya ya* 呷呷, as if calling their own name. Wild ducks, *fu* 鳧, can fly high, while common ducks, *ya* 鴨, are easygoing and cannot fly. This is why they are called *shu fu* 舒鳧, 'easygoing wild ducks'."

Little egret
Egretta garzetta L. Vol. IX, 47-18

(Chinese standard name: *lu* 鷺. Composed of pronunciation indicating character *lu* 路, "way," and genus indication *niao* 鳥, "bird.")

Li Shizhen: The *Bird Classic* states: "When the 'eagles,' *shuang* 鷞, fly, there will be 'frost,' *shuang* 霜. When the 'egrets,' *lu* 鷺, fly, there will be 'dew,' *lu* 露." This is where their names have originated. They step in shallow waters, and they tend to lower and raise their head, just like a pestle and a hoe are lowered and raised. Hence they are also called *chong chu* 舂鋤, "pestle and hoe."

Lu Ji in his *Commentary on the Book of Songs* states: "In the region of Qing and Qi they are called *chong chu* 舂鋤, while in Liaodong, Wu and Yang they are called *bai lu* 白鷺, 'white egret'."

Cotton rose leaf and flower
Hibiscus mutabilis L. 36-35-01

(Chinese standardname: *mu fu rong* 木芙蓉, "tree-lotus.")

Li Shizhen: Flowers and leaves of cotton rose have balanced qi and are neither cold nor hot. Their flavor is slightly acrid, and by their nature they are as sticky as smooth saliva. Their ability to cure obstruction-illness and impediment-illness is divinely effective. In recent times, ulcer specialists have camouflaged their name as *qing liang gao* 清凉膏, "paste to clear and cool," *qing lu san* 清露散, "clear dew powder," and *tie gu san* 鐵箍散, "iron hoop powder." They all refer to this item.

Storax
Liquidambar orientalis Mill. Vol. VII, 34-27

(Chinese standard name: *su he xiang* 蘇合香, "compound of multiple flavoring agents.")

Tao Hongjing: Legend has it that storax consists of lion's droppings. In foreign countries they say that this is not the case. Today, all storax that comes from Xi yu is no longer added to medication. It is only used to compose good aromatics.

Su Gong: These are absurd sayings of the Hu people. Tao Hongjing was unaware of this.

Chen Cangqi: Storax is yellow-white in color. Lion's droppings are red-black in color. The two items resemble each other, but they are not the same. Lion's droppings are extremely malodorous.

Some say: "Lion's droppings are prepared from herbs and tree bark in western countries. This item is brought here by Hu people. As they wish to obtain high prices they give it a decorative name."

Common pheasant
Phasianus colchicus L. Vol. IX, 48-02

(Chinese standard name: *zhi* 雉. Composed of pronunciation indicating character *shi* 矢, "arrow," and genus indication *zhui* 隹, "bird with short tail.")

Kou Zongshi: Pheasants fly like arrows; once they head for somewhere, they drop down there. Hence the character *zhi* 雉 is based on the character *shi* 矢, "arrow." Today, the people attach the tails of pheasants to their boats and carts, hoping that they move as fast as that bird. The queen mother Lü of the Han was named "Pheasant," Zhi 雉. This is why Emperor Gao zu changed the name of pheasants in common use to "wild chicken." Pheasants are indeed a type of chicken.

Li Shizhen: The *Huang shi yun hui* states: "*Zhi* 雉 means 'structure,' because pheasants have a decorative structure. Hence the *Documents of the Elder* speaks of them as *hua chong* 華蟲, 'worms/bugs of extravagance.'

The *Record of Rites* calls them *shu zhi* 疏趾, 'scattered toes'. There are many different kinds of pheasants, and they are named differently with respect to their shapes and colors."

The *Bird Classic* states: "Pheasants are upright birds. Those with a colorful plumage on a white body, they are called *hui zhi* 翬雉, 'variegated pheasants'. Those with a colorful plumage on a greenish body, they are called *yao zhi* 鷂雉, 'hawkish pheasants'. Those with a red and yellow plumage are called *bi zhi* 鷩雉, 'sultry-bird pheasants'. Those with a white plumage are called *zhao zhi* 鵫雉, 'erect-bird pheasants,' with the character *zhuo* 鵫 read here as *zhao* 罩. Black ones are called *hai zhi* 海雉, 'sea pheasants'."

The *Examples of Refined Usage* states: "*Yao zhi* 鷂雉 have a greenish body with colorful plumage. *Bu zhi* 鳪雉 are yellow pheasants named after their own cries. *Di zhi* 翟雉, 'plume-bird pheasants,' are mountain pheasants. They have a long tail. *Jiao zhi* 鷮雉, 'tall-bird pheasants,' have a long tail, and they walk and cry at the same time. *Zhi zhi* 秩秩 are a kind of sea pheasants."

In the Brahman texts, pheasants are called *jiapinsheluo* 迦頻闍羅.

Eupatorium
Eupatorium fortunei Turcz. Vol. III, 14-44

(Chinese standard name: *lan cao* 蘭草, "orchid herb.")

Ma Zhi: The leaves are similar to those of *ma lan* 馬蘭 (lit.: "horse/big orchid"), purple *chrysanthemum*. Hence it is called *lan cao* 蘭草, "orchid herb." The leaves are forked, and hence it is called "swallow tail fragrance," *yan wei xiang* 燕尾香. Now the people boil it in water and bathe in it to heal wind intrusion. Hence it is also called "fragrant water orchid," *xiang shui lan* 香水蘭.

Chen Cangqi: *Lan cao* grows at the side of marshlands. Women apply it mixed with oil to give their head glossiness, *ze* 澤. Hence they call it "orchid glossiness," *lan ze* 蘭澤.

Sheng Hongzhi in his *Jingzhou ji* states: "In Duliang 都梁 at the foot of a mountain is a clear, shallow water in which *lan cao* 蘭草 grows. Hence it is called *du liang xiang* 都梁香, 'Du liang fragrance'."

Li Shizhen: Duliang is today's Wugangzhou. There is also a Duliang mountain in Xuyixian in Linhuai where this fragrant herb is produced. *Lan* 蘭 is a fragrant herb. It is able to repel the inauspicious.

Lu Ji in his *Commentary on the Book of Songs* says: "In Zheng it is common that in the third month a male and a female holding *xian* 蕳 in their hands go to the water's edge to repel evil. The fact is, it is named *lan* 蘭 because it serves as a fence, *lan* 闌, against the evil. It is called *xian* 蕳 because it serves as a barrier, *xian* 閑, against the evil. The meaning is the same in both cases."

The Master of Huainan: "When males plant *lan* 蘭, it will be beautiful but remains without fragrance. Hence *lan* 蘭 should be planted by females." This is the origin of the name *nü lan* 女蘭, "girls' orchid." The leaves are similar to those of *chrysanthemum*, and girls and children love to wear them. This is the origin of names such as *nü lan* 女蘭 and *hai ju* 孩菊, 'child's orchid'."

Tang Yao in his *Tried and Proven Recipes* says: "In Jiangnan people plant it. They collect it in the summer months and put it in their hair to prevent their heads from becoming sticky. Hence they call it 'herb to safeguard the head,' *sheng tou cao* 省頭草."

This statement perfectly agrees with the meaning underlying the name *jian ze* 煎澤, "boiled for glossiness." The ancients called both *lan* 蘭 and *hui* 蕙 *xiang cao* 香草, "fragrant herb," similar to *ling ling xiang* 零陵香草, "fragrant herb from Ling ling," and *du liang xiang cao* 都梁香草, "fragrant herb from Du liang." In later times, people abbreviated these names and always referred to them simply as *xiang cao* 香草, "fragrant herb." Nowadays, only *lan hua* 蘭花, "orchid flower," is known, but not *lan cao* 蘭草, "orchid herb." Only Xugu, Fang Hui, in his research decidedly points out that "the *lan cao* 蘭草 of ancient times is today's *qian jin cao* 千金草, 'herb worth thousands in gold,' which is commonly called *hai er ju* 孩兒菊, 'children's *chrysanthemum*'." This is reliable. For details see below "Correction on Errors."

17. "Further research is required": Controversy and judgment

Perhaps the most notable innovation introduced by Li Shizhen was the transition from earlier *materia medica* works which had merely propagated alleged facts as simple assertions to an encyclopedia based on argumentation. Li Shizhen was the first to collect in a *materia medica* work the statements of earlier authors and systematically discuss them in search of what he considered facts and truth. Earlier writers had already contradicted views they failed to agree on. But Li Shizhen vastly extended this approach and made it his basic principle. He did not simply reject earlier views and statements. Rather, he discussed their origins and shortcomings, eventually deciding who was right and who was wrong, or presenting his own dissenting view. This is a principle followed throughout the entire *Ben cao gang mu*. It is not least because of this feature of the *Ben cao gang mu* that Li Shizhen deserves a pre-eminent place in the history of Chinese natural science.

By assembling the statements of previous authors, Li Shizhen opened heated discussions that lasted for many centuries. They cast a unique light on a continuing quest for accuracy, both in the description and identification of natural substances, and, closely related, in the determination of their usefulness as *materia medica*. In a controversy concerning which region produces the best virgate wormwood, Su Song (1019 – 1101) concludes with a statement whose concerns permeate the debate right up to Li Shizhen: "Such statements, too, have no basis to rely on. ... Such evidence cannot be taken from the *materia medica* literature. For its application in medical recipes, further research is required."

With Song neo-Confucianism, the study of the "classics" had received a new impetus. The thoughts of scholars concerned about a continuation of genuine Confucianism moved in various directions. The search for a principle, *li*, behind the natural order and human morality, the question of how to reduce this principle to a single basic precept, and the significance of the study of literature and of entering the real world to uncover the principle *li*, all this occupied philosophers and resulted in multiple positions.

Half a century before Li Shizhen sat down to compile the *Ben cao gang mu*, Chen Xianzhang (1428 – 1499) made himself an enduring name as a Confucian with statements that appear, at first glance, reminiscent of demands voiced by Renaissance writers in Europe: "The organizational principle inherent in things can be recognized only through personal experience, direct observation, and eventual reflection. Personal experience is more important for the formation of knowledge than the wisdom provided in the ancient classics." And then he urged his fellow scholars: "Have doubts and do research! Do research and arrive at knowledge! Reach true knowledge and then form your convictions. To have doubts is the starting point on the path leading to the WAY!" We should not, of course, think that Chen Xianzhang had in mind a program of opening labs or sending students into the workshops of the craftsmen. We do know that in his youth he had combined agricultural work with the study of books. He knew what labor was required to keep his family's farmland productive, and he knew what previous authors had written about the supposed forces that were believed to exist behind natural and social developments.

It may well be that, during his preparation for the exams, Li Shizhen came into contact with the ideas of Chen Xianzhang. Chen, too, had several times failed in the exams. Still, his writings and his teachings had made him a widely read and honored scholar. In one of his poems he frankly states his dual status: "On market days at Jiang Men, I buy hoes and I buy books. Ploughing the fields and reading the books, I am half farmer and half scholar." The question was to what degree knowledge acquired from books was enough to enable one to make the fundamental principles of all existence one's own. Was man a toy, or in the words of the time: a "straw puppet," at the mercy of these principles, or could man with the knowledge of these principles take fate into his own hands? Li Shizhen never went that far in his quest for knowledge. We do not know to what extent he entertained such philosophical musings. He studied texts that gave him knowledge from times past. He travelled to acquire knowledge he could not find in the texts. And instead of "buying hoes at the market and ploughing the fields," Li Shizhen accepted patients and practiced hands-on medicine to both apply his knowledge and to expand it.

Kou Zongshi in the 12th century was the first author of a *materia medica* text signaling the advent of so-called Neo-Confucianism in the theoretical foundations of medicine. He was aware of his pioneer role and gave his work the title *Extended Meaning of Materia Medica*. He had read everything written on colored arsenolite in previous centuries, and he concludes with a sigh: "There has never been an examination as to whether these are facts, and there has never been research on their underlying principles." Often enough, as a result of his review of the existing literature, Li Shizhen agreed with Kou. At the end of his monograph of a major yang stone/

mineral, the identity of which is unknown today, he writes: "The major yang stone/mineral, the major yin stone/mineral, and others resorted to in this recipe have generally not been researched and identified. The listing here is tentative." Ginseng root is one of the best described substances used in Chinese *materia medica*, and yet, Li Shizhen still finds errors in illustrations of its appearance: "They were drawn without detailed research."

Research is a central requirement in the formation of new knowledge. Ancient texts reflecting the knowledge of past experts are an important source of information. But they do not suffice. Similarly, the expansion of Han-Chinese rule into new regions opened up access to things that had been unfamiliar before. Hence, "when our present dynasty recaptured Lingnan, researchers were sent out to question the local population." Li Shizhen in his *Ben cao gang mu* chiefly compares written evidence when reaching a judgment. His conclusions are based on the logic he sees in an argument, on the proximity of a writer's locality to the locations where the objects discussed have actually been seen, on a majority opinion set against that of a minority, and also on insights gained from his own personal study and experience. The following selections are examples of a fascinating historical process of information gathering and knowledge formation.[34]

Chinese licorice
Glycyrrhiza uralensis Fisch. Vol. III, 12-01

Li Shizhen: According to Shen Gua's *Brush talks*, "The comment in the *Materia Medica* to the quote '*ling* is very bitter' from the *Examples of Refined Usage*, stating that this is a reference to Chinese liquorice is wrong. Guo Pu's comment refers to *polygonum* root. It is of an extremely bitter flavor. Hence the *Book of Songs* identifies it as 'very bitter'. This is not Chinese liquorice. Both the twigs and the leaves of Chinese liquorice resemble those of *sophora japonica* trees with a height of five to six feet. However, the leaves of Chinese liquorice are round with only a slightly pointed tip and a coarse surface as if it were covered by white hair. Its fruits are beans, like the beans of rosary peas. They grow as one stalk and taproot. When they are ripe, the beans split open. Their seeds are flat like red mung beans. They are extremely hard and even when bitten with one's teeth they will

---

34 Additional reading: Wm. Theodore de Bary and the Conference on Ming Thought, Self and Society in Ming Thought. Columbia University Press. New York and London, 1970.

not break open. Today they originate in the western border region of He dong."

Mr. Kou Zongshi, too, in his *Extended Meanings of Materia Medica* has adopted these statements, but he fails to point out that the "very bitter" flavor does not refer to Chinese liquorice. Judged with reason, the physical appearance and shape described by Guo Pu do not agree with those of Chinese liquorice, while Shen Gua is close to the facts. Nowadays, the people consider only those as fine that have a diameter of one inch, are hard, and have a ruptured structure, and they call them "powder herb." Those that are light, porous, fine, and small, they do not reach them in quality. Liu Ji in his *Records of Swirling Snow Flakes* states: "In Annan Chinese liquorice specimens may be as large as columns. The locals use them to build the frames of their houses." I have no idea whether this is so or not.

Apricot leaf ladybell
Adenophora trachelioides Maxim. Vol. III, 12-05

Tao Hongjing: Both the root and stem of *Adenophora trachelioides* resemble those of ginseng, but the leaves are smaller and look different. The flavor of the root is very sweet; it can kill poison. Since it is found in the same locations as poisonous medicinal herbs, its nature is used to kill all poisons. Recipe experts do not use it regularly. It is also said that when Emperor Wen said that "apricot leaf ladybell is confused with ginseng," he was referring to the substance discussed here. The leaves of apricot leaf ladybell are very similar to those of balloon flower. However, there is one difference. The leaves of the apricot leaf ladybell are shiny, smooth, and moist on their underside and have no hairs. Also, unlike those of ginseng, they do not grow opposite to each other.

Su Gong: The seedlings of ginseng resemble those of apricot leaf ladybell shrubs, but are wider and shorter. The trunk is round with three to four branches. There are five leaves at the ends of the branches.

What Tao Hongjing tells with regard to confusing apricot leaf ladybell with ginseng is wrong. Besides, some kinds of apricot leaf ladybell and balloon flowers have different leaves, and there are some with three or four leaves facing each other. Both have a stem that grows straight up. If the leaves of the apricot leaf ladybell can be confused with those of ginseng, the only real difference is that the root of the apricot leaf ladybell has no core.

Su Song: Nowadays, they can be found in Chuan, Shu, Jiang, and Zhe. In spring, apricot leaf ladybell develops seedlings and stems. Both are similar to those of ginseng, but the leaves are smaller and look different. The roots resemble those of the balloon flower, but differ from them because they have no core. They are ubiquitous especially in Runzhou and Shaanzhou. People collect them as fruits or preserve them as delicacies. Their taste is very sweet and delicious, and they can be shipped long distances. The roots are harvested in the second and eighth month and dried in the sun.

Chen Cheng: Nowadays, many people steam them and press them flat to mistakenly offer them as ginseng root. But their taste remains bland.

Kou Zongshi: Tao Hongjing speaks of the root. Therefore, he says that the roots of apricot leaf ladybell are confused with the ginseng root.

Su Gong speaks of the seedlings. Therefore, he thinks that Tao Hongjing's statement is wrong.

Wang Ji: The seedlings and stems of apricot leaf ladybell resemble those of balloon flower. The root is mistakenly thought to be that of ginseng. Today, when it is said that both the seedlings and the stem resemble those of ginseng, it is completely wrong. It is important to carefully study all three, ginseng, apricot leaf ladybell flower and balloon flower, so that the differences and similarities become clear.

Li Shizhen: The seedlings of apricot leaf ladybell resemble those of balloon flower. The root resembles that of *Adenophora tracheloides stricta*. Therefore, fraudulent traders repeatedly offer *Adenophora stricta* and *Adenophora tracheloides* falsely as ginseng root. The apricot-leaved *Adenophora tracheloides* mentioned by Su Song in his *Illustrated Classic of Materia Medica* and the apricot-leaved *Adenophora tracheloides* mentioned by Zhou Xian wang in his *Materia medica for Famine Relief* are both the apricot leaf ladybell discussed here.

The *Illustrated Classic of Materia Medica* states, "The apricot leaf ladybell grows in the open country of Zizhou. Its root resembles that of a small vegetable. The natives collect the seedlings and the leaves in the fifth month to cure coughs with rising qi."

The *Materia medica for Famine Relief* states, "The apricot leaf ladybell is also called 'white-flour root'. The seedlings reach a height of one to two feet. The stems are greenish-white in color. The leaves resemble apricot leaves, but are smaller. They are slightly pointed and their back is white.

At their edges they are forked like teeth. The flowers open at the tips of these teeth. They have five petals and are shaped like cups. The appearance of the root resembles that of wild carrots. It is quite thick. The skin is ash-black, the inside is white. The taste is sweet and they are slightly cold. There are also varieties that open bluish-green flowers. The tender leaves are fried in fat, rinsed in water and eaten with oil and salt. If the root is boiled in water changed several times, it can also be eaten. People boil them in honey and serve them as fruit."

In his commentaries on the balloon flower herb, Tao Hongjing also says that "the leaves are called 'latent endurance'. They can be boiled for consumption and are used to cure *gu* poisoning."

According to the examples of refined usage, "*bang* 蒡" means "latent endurance." In his commentary, Guo Pu states, "The apricot leaf ladybell resembles *perilla* and has hair. People in Jiang dong use it to prepare vegetables. After it is cooked, it is edible."

Ge Hong writes in his recipes to keep on hand, "The herb 'latent endurance' has seedlings similar to those of balloon flower herb, and all people eat it. They pound it and drink the juice. It is used to cure *gu* poisoning."

Chinese *pulsatilla*. *Pulsatilla chinensis* (Bge.) Rgl
Vol. III, 12-29

Supplementary Records by Famous Physicians: Chinese *pulsatilla* grows in the valleys of high mountains and also in the open country.

Su Gong: Its leaves resemble those of *paeonia* herbs, but are bigger. It develops one stem, and one purple flower at the end of the stem, similar to the flowers of *hibiscus* herb. Its fruit may be as big as chicken eggs. It has white hair and is more than one *cun* long. It looks like a head draped over with a banneret, just like the white head of an old man. Hence the name.

Tao Hongjing says "close to the root it has white hairy regions." Apparently he did not know the root. The creeper kept in the Imperial court's storage facility of pharmaceutical substances is in fact the *clematis* creeper. The root of Chinese *pulsatilla* resembles *dipsacus* root, but is flat.

Han Baosheng: It can be found everywhere. It has fine hair. It is not smooth and moist. The stamen is yellow. The flowers are collected in the second month; the fruits are collected in the fourth month; the root is collected in the eighth month. All are dried in the sun.

Su Song: It can be found everywhere. It develops seedlings in the first month; they grow as clusters. They are shaped like those of *cynanchum atratum* herbs, but are soft, delicate, and a little longer. The leaves grow at the end of the stem, similar to apricot leaves. They have fine, white hair on their surface and are neither smooth nor moist. Close to the root is a white hairy region. The root is of purple color. It reaches into the depth like a turnip. The seedling remains unmoved when there is wind. It sways when there is no wind. This is similar to *gastrodia* herbs and *angelica biserrata* herbs. Tao Hongjing failed to describe the stem and the leaves. Su Gong in his comment says that "the leaves resemble those of *paeonia* herbs," and that "the fruits are as big as chicken eggs and have white hair more than an inch long." This is all wrong.

Kou Zongshi: Chinese *pulsatilla* grows in the border region of Luo yang in Henan and it has repeatedly been seen in the wilderness of the mountains in Xin an. Just as Su Gong says. The mountain people there sell "the white head old man's pills" to this day. They say that to ingest them extends life, but this does not agree with the meaning of the name given to this substance by the ancients. What Tao Hongjing says lacks a careful examination; it needs to be contradicted.

Wang Ji: Kou Zongshi believes that Su Gong is right. Su Song believes that Tao Hongjing's statement is right. Generally speaking, the root of this item is used for medicinal purposes. Its name reflects its appearance. The description in Su Song's *Illustrated Classic of Materia Medica* is reliable. The item described by Su Gong may be something different.

Black cardamom. *Alpinia oxyphylla* Miq
Vol. III, 14-21

Li Shizhen: The spleen controls wisdom. This item can boost spleen and stomach qi, hence its name: "wisdom boosting seeds." The underlying meaning is the same as that when longan seeds are called "wisdom boosting seeds."

According to Su Shi's records, "black cardamom grows in Hainan. Its flowers and fruit are situated on a long spike that is divided into three sections. The upper, middle, and lower section are observed to predict early, mid-term, or late ripening of grain as auspicious and inauspicious signs. In the case of future massive abundance they will all have fruit. In the case of misfortune, none will have fruit. Only rarely all three sections ripen at the same time."

Black cardamom as a pharmaceutical drug only serves to cure illnesses related to water, and it does not boost wisdom at all. Having this name, how could it foretell the harvest? This is one of those sayings that are contrary to all principles.

Chen Cangqi: Black cardamom comes from the country of Kunlun and from Jiaozhi. Today it can be found at many places in the *zhou* and prefectures of Lingnan.

Gu Wei in his *Records of Guangzhou* states: "Its leaves resemble those of *zingiber* herb, they are more than one stave long. On its root are small branches, reaching a height of eight to nine inches. There is no calyx. The stem resembles a bamboo arrow shaft. The seeds come out of its center. One branch develops a tussock of ten seeds, the size of small Chinese dates. Within a white skin is a black kernel. Those with small kernels are fine. When they are held in the mouth they stimulate some foul salivation. It is also possible to break the seed into four pieces and remove the kernel. Then boil the outer skin in water with honey and use this to make rice dumplings for food, with an acrid flavor." During the Jin dynasty, Lu Xun submitted to Emperor Liu Yu "wisdom boosting dumplings." These were the dumplings just referred to.

Su Gong: Black cardamom seeds resemble *forsythia* seeds with a tip that has not yet opened. Its seedling, leaves, flowers, and root are not different from *alpinia katsumadai* seeds. Only the seeds are smaller.

Li Shizhen: According to Ji Han's *Forms of Herbs and Trees from the Southern Regions*, black cardamom flowers open in the second month, and the fruits follow. They ripen in the fifth and sixth month. The seeds look like the tip of a brush, with both of their ends pointed. They are seven to eight tenths of a mace long. Mixed with any of the five flavors they lend fragrance to wine drinking. They can also be processed with salt and dried in the sun to prepare rice dumplings for food. With this in mind, Gu Wei's statement that they lack a calyx is wrong. Today's *black cardamom* seeds are shaped like a date kernel, and both the skin and the seed kernel are similar to *alpinia katsumadai* seeds.

Siberian motherwort
Leonurus japonicus Houtt. Vol. IV, 15-17

Supplementary Records by Famous Physicians: Siberian motherwort grows in ponds and marshlands at the seaside. It is collected in the fifth month.

Tao Hongjing: Today it can be found everywhere. The leaves are similar to those of *perilla*. The stem is square. The seeds are fine and lengthy, with three edges. Siberian motherwort, too, is seldom used in pharmaceutical recipes.

Su Song: Today it can be found very often in gardens and in the open country.

Guo Pu in his comment on the *Examples of Refined Usage* states: "The leaves are similar to *perilla* leaves. The stem is square and has white flowers. The flowers grow from between the nodes. Every two nodes grow a flower. The fruits are similar to cockscomb seeds; they are black. The stem is rectangular with four edges. It is collected in the fifth month."

It is also said: "Collect the fruit in the ninth month." Physicians seldom use the fruits.

Kou Zongshi: When Siberian motherwort grows in early spring, it can be soaked and washed. It is washed in a pan and its bitter flavor is discarded with the water. Then it is boiled and eaten as a vegetable. It does not wither in winter.

Li Shizhen: Siberian motherwort grows very strongly in waters and moist locations nearby. In early spring a seedling grows similar to tender wormwood. By summer, it reaches a height of three to four feet. The stem is square like a yellow hemp stem. The leaves resemble mugwort leaves with a greenish back. One stalk has three leaves, and the leaves have pointed ends. The nodes are situated in a distance of about one inch. Spikes develop between two nodes, forming clusters embracing the stem. In the fourth and fifth month, small flowers open in the spikes; they are of red-purple color. There are also some of a pale white color. Each calyx includes four fine seed kernels. These kernels have the size of garden daisy seeds. They have three edges and are brown. Apothecary's shops often substitute them with sesame seeds. When the herb grows it emits malodorous qi. After Summer Solstice it withers and the root is white.

When Su Song in the *Illustrated Classic of Materia Medica* says: "Its leaves are similar to *perilla* leaves, its seeds are black, similar to cockscomb seeds.

The fruits are collected in the ninth month," and when Kou Zongshi in his *Extended Meanings* says: "They do not wither in winter," they are both wrong. This herb has two kinds of flowers, white flowers and purple flowers. Stem, leaves, seeds, and spike are the same. However, the white ones can enter the qi section, while the red ones enter the blood section, and their application should differ accordingly.

According to the *Arrangements for the Ladies' Chambers*, "those with white flowers are called "benefitting mothers;" those with red flowers are called "wild heaven's hemp." A commentary to the *Straightforward Guide to Recipes* recipe of the "elixir to let the *hun*-soul return" states: "Those with purple flowers are called 'benefitting mothers;' those with white flowers are not."

Chen Cangqi in his *Ben cao* states: "Siberian motherwort grows in the open country. People call it 'pent-up malodorous stench herb'. 'Heaven's hemp' grows in the plains, in marshlands. It resembles vervain. Always between two nodes purple flowers grow, and in these flowers are seeds, similar to *celosia* herb seeds."

Sun Simiao in his *Recipes Worth a Thousand in Gold* states: "Heaven's hemp herb has a stem like hemp herbs. It grows a seedling in winter and develops red flowers in summer, similar to the flowers of Japanese *salvia*."

Apparently, all these statements suggest that Siberian motherwort and "heaven's hemp" are two items. The fact is, they do not know that these are two kinds of one item. Many items have red and white flowers, such as tree *paeonia*, *paeonia*, and *chrysanthemum* flowers.

Also, as Guo Pu in his commentary on the *Examples of Refined Usage* states: "*Tui* 蓷, read *tui* 推, is Siberian motherwort, alternative name: 'benefitting mothers'. The leaves are similar to *perilla* leaves. It has white flowers. The flowers grow between the nodes."

It is also stated: "*Tui* 蕡, read *tui* 推, has a square stem. The leaves are long and pointed. It has spikes. Flowers are situated between the spikes; they are of a purple, indistinct color. They can be prepared to a beverage. In Jiang dong it is called 'ox *tui* 牛蘈'."

That is, the names *tui* 蓷 and *tui* 蕡 are basically identical; the plants differ only in terms of the color of their flowers. Hence it is without doubt that they are one and the same item. In the *Ben cao* newly revised by Song people, heaven's hemp herb is erroneously commented upon as *tian ma* 天麻. This is a particularly gross mistake.

The *Materia Medica of Chen Cangqi* also mentions a "chisel vegetable," stating that "it grows at yin (i.e., shady) places in Jiangnan and is similar to 'benefitting mothers'. It has a square stem and white flowers growing facing each other at the nodes, and controls blood diseases following birth." This is a Siberian motherwort with white flowers. Hence they have the same therapeutic potential of controlling blood disease.

St. Paulswort
Siegesbeckia orientalis L. Vol. IV, 15-44

Su Gong: St. Paulswort is known to everybody in the open country. Another name is "fire pillow." The leaves are similar to those of Chinese lantern plants, but they are narrower and longer. The flowers are yellow-white. Seedling and leaves are collected in the third and fourth month. They are dried in the sun.

It is also said: "Lard berry" grows in the plains in marshlands, on low-lying, moist ground. It can be found everywhere. Another name is "tiger paste," and yet another name is "dog paste." The leaves are similar to those of cocklebur. The stem is round and has hair.

Su Song: St. Paulswort can be found everywhere. It grows a seedling in spring. The leaves resemble black mustard leaves, but are narrower and longer, with a coarse line design. The stem is two to three *chi* tall. At the beginning of autumn flowers similar to *chrysanthemum* flowers appear. At the end of autumn they form fruits, quite similar to those of *carpesium* herbs. The leaves are collected in summer. They are dried in the sun before they are used.

Chen Cangqi: The leaves of St. Paulswort are similar to those of *perilla* herbs, but they have hair.

Han Baosheng: The leaves of "lard [herb]" resemble those of *carpesium* herbs. Always two branches grow facing each other. Stem and leaves have yellow-white hair. The seedling is collected in the fifth and sixth month. It is dried in the sun.

Li Shizhen: According to Su Gong's *Materia Medica of the Tang*, St. Paulswort is similar to Chinese lantern plant, while *zhu gao mei* is similar to cocklebur herbs. So, these are two different kinds.

Cheng Na submitted a "St. Paulswort pill memorandum," saying that "this drug differs from the description in the *Ben cao*. It often grows on fertile land and is more than three feet tall. The leaves at the nodes grow facing each other."

Zhang Yong in his "St. Paulswort pill memorandum" says: "This herb has gold edges and silver threads, a plain stem and a purple root. The leaves grow facing each other at the nodes. In Shu it is called 'fire pillow'. Stem and leaves are similar to those of cocklebur."

Also, according to Shen Gua's *Brush talks*, "the common people erroneously identify *carpesium* herb as 'fire pillow'. There exists a therapeutic method of ingesting *huo xian* as a single substance, but this refers to *carpesium* herb; it is not suitable to resort to 'fire pillow'. 'Fire pillow' is named 'lard berry' in the *Materia Medica*, but this was unknown to people of later times and they established a separate entry."

Now, all these many statements differ, and when today people with wind blockage of joints often use St. Paulswort pills, which of them should they follow? I, Li Shizhen have gathered all types of these herbs and have studied them. Now, "lard [herb]" has a plain stem with a straight edge, covered with many dots. The leaves are similar to those of cocklebur, but they are a little longer. They resemble those of *carpesium* but are a little thinner. They grow facing each other at the nodes. Stem and leaves have fine hair. On fertile land one stem develops several tens of branches. In the eighth and ninth month small flowers open; they are of a deep yellow color. In their midst they have lengthy seeds similar to garden daisy seeds. On the outside of the calyx are many fine thorns that let them cling to humans.

Carpesium herb has a greenish stem. It is round and has no edges, no dots and no hair. The leaves are wrinkled like those of pak choi and black mustard, and they do not grow facing each other at nodes. This view on these two items is in agreement with the statements by Cheng Na and Zhang Yong. Today, in Chenzhou of Henan *St. Paulswort* is collected and then served as a local item. It is shaped like "lard [herb]," and when Mr. Shen Gua states that St. Paulswort is in fact "lard berry," this is not to be doubted. That which Su Gong says is similar to Chinese lantern plant is common nightshade. It is not St. Paulswort.

The fact is, his identification is wrong. However, when Mr. Shen Gua says that "'fire pillow' is commonly ingested as a single substance and that this is *carpesium*, and that it must not be substituted by 'lard berry,'" then this contradicts the statements of Cheng Na and Zhang Yong. According to the *Materia Medica* entries on *St. Paulswort* and "lard berry," none of them serves to cure wind intrusion. Only the *Original Classic*, in its *carpesium* entry, says: "It removes blockage of joints and eliminates heat. Ingested over a long time it relieves the body of its weight and helps to endure aging." That is, to cure wind intrusion it seems as if one had to resort to *carpesium*. Still, the recipes submitted to the Emperor by Cheng Na and Zhang Yong are definitely not based on a principle of omission and error. But maybe the two substances have a potential of curing wind intrusion nevertheless? Today, the application of *St. Paulswort* as "lard berry" regularly yields good effects, but such effects are not observed when *carpesium* is ingested. Hence it is without doubt that *St. Paulswort* is "lard berry."

Yellow day lily
Hemerocallis citrina Baroni. Vol. IV, 16-06

Su Song: Yellow day lily can be found everywhere in the open country. It is commonly named "deer's onion." The flowers are collected in the fifth month. The root is collected in the eighth month. Today many people collect its tender seedlings and the flowers to prepare a pickled vegetable food.

Li Shizhen: Yellow day lily grows on low-lying, moist ground. In the winter months it grows as clusters. The leaves are similar to those of cattail and garlic, but they are even softer and weaker. New leaves replace old leaves, one after another, and they remain greenish through all four seasons. In the fifth month a stem rises and opens flowers. Of six that appear, four hang down. They open in the morning and wither in the evening. Deep in autumn they are all gone. The flowers may be of three colors, red, yellow, and purple. They form fruits with three edges, with seeds the size of *firmiana* seeds inside. They are black and shiny moist. The root is similar to that of *ophiopogon* herb. It is very easy to multiply.

The *Forms of Herbs and Trees from the Southern Regions* says: "In Guangzhong is a kind of water onion shaped similar to 'deer's onion'. Its flowers may be purple or yellow." The fact is, they are of the same group. It is also said: "Deer onion flowers have a dotted line design and they are alive at another time than yellow day lily flowers." This is wrong. When the plant grows on fertile soil, its flowers are thick, the color is deep with a dotted line design and there are many layers of petals. The flowers remain open for several months. Those growing on poor soil have thin flowers with a pale color, and they do not remain open for a long time.

Ji Han in his preface to his article on "flowers making girls attractive for men" states: "In the land of Jing and Chu it is called 'deer onion'. It can be prepared as pickled vegetable." This is most trustworthy. Today, in the East people collect the flowers, dry them and market them. They call them "yellow flower vegetable."

Ducksmeat. Pepperwort
Marsilea quadrifolia L. Vol. V, 19-12

Wu Pu: Ducksmeat, is also named "water cheap." It grows in ponds and on marshland on the water. The leaves are round and small, with one leaf per stem. The root enters the earth at the bottom of the water. White flowers open in the fifth month. It is collected in the third month and dried in the sun.

Tao Hongjing: Big ducksmeat growing in bodies of water has flowers white in color in the fifth month. This is not the ducksmeat growing in ditches. The fruit obtained by the King of Chu when he crossed the river, is the fruit of the item discussed here.

Su Gong: There are three kinds of *ping* ducksmeat. The big ones are called pepperwort. Those of medium size are called *xing* 荇. The leaves of all these varieties resemble each other and are round. The small kind is the "floating ducksmeat" on the water.

Chen Cangqi: The leaves of pepperwort are round, with a diameter of about one inch. On the lower side of the leaves is a spot similar to watery foam. It is also called *fu cai* 苤菜. Dried in the sun it can be added to medication. The small ducksmeat is the one that grows in ditches.

Zhang Yuxi: According to the *Examples of Refined Usage*, "ducksmeat is *ping* 蓱. Big ones are called pepperwort." Also, the *Book of Songs* states: "She gathers the pepperwort by the banks of the stream."

Lu Ji comments: "Crude, big specimens are called pepperwort. Small ones are ducksmeat. It begins to grow in the last month of spring, and can be steamed to serve as an edible vegetable. It can also be soaked in bitter wine as a wine condiment. This pepperwort is used by physicians rarely today. They only use the small ducksmeat.

Li Shizhen. Pepperwort is the "four leaves vegetable." The leaves float on the surface of the water; the root links up with the bottom below the water. The stem is finer than that of water mallow and fringed water lily. The leaves are the size of a fingertip. They are greenish on the front and purple on the back, with a fine line design. They are quite similar to the leaves of fetid *cassia*. Four leaves grow joined together, leaving fissures in the center resembling the character for "ten," *shi* 十. Small, white flowers open in summer and autumn. Hence the plant is called "white pepperwort." The leaves are situated closely together like those of ducksmeat. Therefore, the *Examples of Refined Usage* says that pepperwort is a variety of ducksmeat with big leaves.

When the *Spring and Autumn Annals of Mr. Lü* states: "Among the delicious vegetables is pepperwort from Kunlun," then this is the substance discussed here.

The *Master Han's Outer Commentary to the Book of Song* says: "Those that float are algae. Those in the depth are pepperwort."

Qu Xian says: "Those with white flowers are pepperwort; those with yellow flowers are fringed water lily, i.e., gold lotus."

Su Gong says: "Big specimens are pepperwort, small ones are fringed water lily."

Yang Shen in his *Uncertain Words* says: "The four leaves vegetable is fringed water lily."

Tao Hongjing says: "The one obtained by the King of Chu is pepperwort."

All these sayings differ. The fact is, so far no in-depth research has been conducted; all of them are nothing but guesses put down on paper. I, Li Shizhen have collected and inspected each of these herbs and this enables me to present the facts. Those with leaves of a diameter of one or two *cun*, and with a crevice and a round shape similar to a horse hoof, they are water mallow. Those similar to water mallows but with leaves that are pointed and lengthy are fringed water lily. Both water mallow and fringed water lily have yellow-white flowers. Those with leaves with a diameter of four to five inches, similar to small lotus leaves, and with yellow flowers, and forming fruits similar to small three-edged millet dumplings are least water-lily. The fruits of ducksmeat obtained by the King of Chu are the fruits of this least water-lily. Those with four leaves growing joined together forming one leaf similar in shape to the character *tian* 田, they are pepper-wort. Through this differentiation all uncertainties should be eliminated.

Also, Mr. Xiang says: "White pepperwort grows in bodies of water. Green-ish pepperwort grows on land."

The herb known today as "character *tian* 田 herb" has two kinds, one water and one land variety. That growing on land is often found in pad-dy fields, in damp places. Its leaves consist of four parts joined together, similar to white pepperwort, except for that its stem grows on land, is three to four inches tall and not edible. Recipe masters gather it to calcine sulphur and to boil it with mercury to conglomerate it to sand. They call it "old man in the water fields." The fact is, that is the greenish pepperwort spoken of by Mr. Xiang. Some assume greenish pepperwort to be a water herb, but that is wrong.

Hemp
Cannabis sativa L. Vol. V, 22-03

Original Classic: *Ma ben* 麻蕡 is also called *ma bo* 麻勃, a reference to the "exuberant," *bo bo* 勃勃, flowers of hemp. Specimens collected on the seventh day of the seventh month are good. The seeds of hemp are col-lected in the ninth month. Those that have entered the soil are harmful to humans. It grows in the mountain valleys of Mount Taishan.

Tao Hongjing: *Ma ben* 麻蕡 is *mu ma* 牡麻, "male hemp." *Mu ma* does not bear fruit. Nowadays, people use it to make fabrics and shoes. Su Gong: *Ben* 蕡 are the fruits of hemp, not the flowers.

The *Examples of Refined Usage* states: "*Ben* 蕡 are the fruits of *xi* 枲." The *Ritual and Etiquette* states: "*Ju* 苴 is hemp with *ben* 蕡, 'fruits'." A com-ment states: "Hemp with seeds is *ju* 苴."

All these are references to the seeds. When Tao Hongjing identifies *ben* 蕡 as *ma bo* 麻勃, saying that it grows as exuberant as flowers, and introduces a separate entry of hemp seeds, he is wrong. That is, when *ben* 蕡 is a cereal of upper rank, how can its flowers be edible?

Chen Cangqi: When hemp seeds are planted early in spring, they are "spring *hemp* seeds." They are small and poisonous. When they are plant-ed late in autumn, they are "autumn hemp seeds." When they are added to medication, the effects achieved are excellent. The oil pressed out of them can be used to oil things.

Kou Zongshi: Hemp seeds from Maoluo island in Eastern Sea that have the size of lotus fruits are the best. Those second in quality that come from Shangjun in the northern regions are as big as soybeans. The seeds from the southern regions are small.

Su Song: Hemp seeds are planted everywhere. The skin is twisted to prepare fabrics. Farmers pick seeds with a black spot design. They call them "female hemp." When they are planted they produce abundant seed crops. The other seeds are not the same. The therapeutic control attributed in the *Original Classic* to *ma ben* 麻蕡, "hemp fruits," and *ma zi* 麻子, "*hemp* seeds," is identical, while hemp flowers are items that are not edible. What Su Gong says seems to be adequate. Still, the additions in the *Materia Medica* written in red characters state: "Hemp fruit, flavor acrid; hemp seeds, flavor sweet." Apparently, these are two different items. That is, the statements in the *Materia Medica* on the one side and in the *Examples of Refined Usage* and the *Record of Rites* may differ.

Also, the *Discourse on the Properties of Pharmaceutical Substances* in its use of hemp flowers states: "Flavor bitter, controls all types of wind intrusion, blocked female menstruation." If that is the case, then hemp fruits, the seeds and the flowers are three different items?

Li Shizhen: Hemp is today's "fire hemp," also called "yellow hemp." It is planted everywhere. Hemp is peeled and the seeds are stored. It has female and male variants. The females are *xi* 枲; the males are *ju* 苴. Large specimens are similar to sesame. The leaves are narrow and long; they are shaped like the leaves of *leonurus* herbs, with one twig carrying seven or nine leaves. It opens fine, yellow flowers with spikes in the fifth and sixth month that form fruits soon afterwards the size of coriander seeds. They can be used for oil production. The skin is peeled to prepare hemp. The stalks are white and have edges. They are light and hollow and can serve as wicks.

The *Essential Arts of the Common People* states: "When hemp seeds blossom, remove the male flowers. It they are removed before they blossom, they will not form seeds. Their seeds are black and heavy. They can be pounded and further processed to make candles." That is the item discussed here.

The *Original Classic* lists hemp fruits and hemp seeds in two different entries. It identifies hemp fruits as *ma bo* 麻勃, and says that hemp seeds that have entered the soil kill humans.

Su Gong says "*Ma ben* 麻蕡 is *hemp* seeds not the flowers." Su Song says that "hemp fruit, the seeds and the flowers are three different items."

All these statements fail to clarify these issues.

According to *Wu Pu's Materia Medica*, "*ma bo* 麻勃 is also called *ma hua* 麻花, '*hemp* flower'. Flavor acrid, nonpoisonous. *Ma lan* 麻藍 is also called *ma ben* 麻蕡 and *qing ge* 青葛, flavor acrid, sweet and poisonous. The leaves of hemp are poisonous. When they are eaten they kill one. The kernel in the hemp seeds is not poisonous. But when they have been in the ground first and are eaten then, they kill one."

Based on these statements, *ma bo* are the flowers; *ma ben* 麻蕡 are the fruits; *ma ren* 麻仁 are the kernels in the fruits. Wu Pu was a contemporary of the Three Kingdoms. That was not distant from antiquity and the differentiation he points out is very clear.

The *Divine Farmer's Classic of Materia Medica* identifies the flowers as *ben* 蕡, stating that they kill humans when they have been kept in the ground or had entered the ground. Such wordings are transmissions of texts marred by omissions and errors.

Mr. Tao Hongjing and all the experts of the Tang and Song era, instead of doing sufficient research they all have voiced their personal estimates. They may be said to have been irresponsible. This is corrected in the following based on Mr. Wu Pu.

Small toad
Rana limnocharia Boie. Vol. VIII, 42-02

Su Song: Even though small toads and toads belong to the same group, their therapeutic functions are slightly different. They must not be used indiscriminately.

Li Shizhen: Ancient recipes often recommended to use small toads; in recent times, they mostly recommend to use toads. The fact is, the ancient people named all small toads toads. Recent research has shown that the therapeutic functions of these two items are not far apart from each other. That is, what the ancient people used were mostly toads. Furthermore, today the people only resort to toads as an effective substance, while small toads are no longer added to medication.

18. Sample text and plant monograph:
Chai hu, sickle-leaved hare's ear

It is not known whether Li Shizhen saw the *Materia Medica Written on Imperial Order, Containing Essential Data Arranged in Systematic Order* of 1505 before he set out to compile the *Ben cao gang mu*. Out of his own personal interest, Qiu Jun (1420 – 1495), a scholar official, had devised a scheme to overcome the unwieldy nature of the final texts from the main tradition of *materia medica* literature. He restructured the individual substance monographs and removed the critical obstacle to practical use of the former, comprehensive *materia medica* texts. He dismissed the idea that newer *materia medica* works were simply emendations of the *Original Classic* with whatever new knowledge had become available. Qiu Jun divided each monograph into 13 characteristics of a substance he had taken from previous works.

As a result, a reader interested in the origin, the pharmaceutical processing or the therapeutic indications of a particular substance found relevant data collected under a respective heading. To find the information they sought, users of the new text were no longer required to read through all the historical layers that had accrued among the texts in the main tradition of *materia medica* works. Qiu Jun died after finishing only one chapter, however. Following hectic intrigue and conflicts of interest, Liu Wentai (fl. 1503), an official in the Imperial Medical Office, and a team of collaborators were ordered by Emperor Xiao zong (1470 – 1505) in 1503 "to prepare a new *material medica* edition so as to simplify the consultation of these works." They adopted Qiu Jun's structural proposals but expanded the number of subheadings in each substance monograph from 13 to 24.

The new work was completed only two years later. Pleased, the emperor personally gave it the title *The Essentials of Materia medica with the Data on Items Arranged According to their Similar Nature, compiled on Imperial Order*. Soon afterward, the emperor died. The manuscript was never published, possibly because of the exquisite color illustrations added to each entry. In the 16th century no technology was available to print such a work. Nevertheless, several manuscript copies were prepared, and a few have ended up in libraries in Japan, Rome, and Berlin. In 1701 a revised and amended version without the illustrations was prepared by order of Emperor Kang xi (1654 – 1722). And in 1937 it was finally published by Shanghai Commercial Press.

Li Shizhen chose a structure for his *Ben cao gang mu* entries similar to that of the substance monographs adopted in the 1505 work. However, rather than dividing the data of each entry into 24 categories, he decided to limit their subheadings, where required, to the following ten:

1. Corrections of Erroneous Listings of Substances

2. Explanation of Names

3. Collected Explanations

4. Pharmaceutical Preparation

5. Discussion of Uncertain Issues

6. Correction of Errors

7. Qi and Flavor

8. Therapeutic Control

9. Explication

10. Added Recipes

What follows is an example of an average length substance description of an herb known by its standard name: *Chai hu* and listed in chapter 13. Scientific identification: *Bupleurum falcatum* L. English vernacular name: Sickle-leaved hare's ear. Vol. III, 13-05.

Chai hu
First Appearance: The Original Classic. Upper rank

Explanation of Names

Di xun 地薰, "ground fragrance," *Original Classic.*

Yun hao 芸蒿, *Supplementary Records by Famous Physicians.*

Shan cai 山菜, "mountain vegetable," Wu Pu.

Ru cao 茹草, Wu Pu.

Su Gong: *Ci* 茈 is the ancient writing of *chai* 柴. When the *Rhapsody on the Upper Forest* speaks of *ci jiang* 茈薑, and the *Examples of Refined Usage* speaks of *ci cao* 茈草, they always use the character *ci* 茈. The root of this herb is of purple, *zi* 紫, color. It is today's commonly used *ci hu* 茈胡. Then the radical *cao* 艸 was replaced by the radical *mu* 木 and ever since it was called *chai hu* 柴胡. I have examined all *materia medica* works, but this name is used nowhere.

Li Shizhen: The character 茈 may be read *chai* 柴 and *zi* 紫. The 茈 in *zi jiang* 茈薑 and *zi cao* 茈草 is always read *zi* 紫, while the 茈 in *chai hu* 茈胡 is read *chai* 柴. *Chai hu* 茈胡 grows in the mountains. As long as it is tender, it can be eaten as a vegetable, *ru* 茹. When it is old, it is collected to serve as firewood, *chai* 柴. Hence the seedlings are called *yun hao* 芸蒿, *shan cai* 山菜, and *ru cao* 茹草, while the root is called *chai hu* 柴胡. Su Gong's statement is not clear on this. The ancient versions of Zhang Zhongjing's *Shang han lun* still have the character *ci* 茈.

Collected Explanations

Supplementary Records by Famous Physicians: *Chai hu* leaves are called *yun hao* 芸蒿. They are acrid, fragrant, and edible. They grow in the river valleys of Hongnong, and in Yuanju. Their roots are collected in the second and eighth month. They are dried in the sun.

Tao Hongjing: Today they come from nearby places. They are shaped like *peucedanum* roots, but are sturdier. The *Monograph on a Wide Range of Things* states: "The leaves of *yun hao* resemble those of *libanotis* herb. In spring and autumn they have white roots like rushes. They reach a length of four to five *cun*. They are fragrant and delicious; they are edible. They are present in both Chang an and He nei."

Su Gong: The major and the minor decoctions with *chai hu* for harm caused by cold are important medications for phlegm qi. If they were prepared with *yun hao* root, that would be a grave mistake.

Su Song: Today they are present in places near the region between Guanshan and Jianghu. Those from Yinzhou are best. In the second month the herb develops very fragrant seedlings. The stem is greenish-purple, hard, and solid, with some fine threads. The leaves resemble those of bamboo, but are a little smaller. There are also those with leaves resembling those of *ophiopogon* herbs, but are shorter. In the seventh month they open yellow flowers. The root is of a pale-red color. It resembles *peucedanum* roots, but is sturdier. Those growing in Danzhou, they form greenish seeds. They differ from those from other places. Their root resembles the tip of reed. It has red hair, like the tail of a mouse/rat. Those with a long root consisting of only one single stalk are good.

Lei Xiao: *Ci hu* comes from Pingzhou and Pingxian; these are today's Yinzhou and Yinxian. At the places where they grow on the Western banks, there are many white and green cranes. They fly circling above this region where the fragrance of *ci hu* ascends into the clouds. It appears as if the cranes came to smell all these pleasant qi.

Chen Cheng: The best *chai hu* are those from Yinxia. The root resembles the tail of a mouse/rat. It is one to two *chi* long, and its fragrant smell is very fine. Based on the record in today's *Illustrated Classic of Materia Medica*, the genuine ware is commonly not recognized. The vendors on the market replace it with ware from Tong and Hua. But these specimens are still better than those from other places. The fact is, the region of Yin xia has much sand. The roots coming from Tong and Hua also grow in sandy gardens.

Wang Ji. To resolve and disperse one resorts to *chai hu*. For depletion heat tender *chai hu* roots from Hai yang are good.

Li Shizhen: Yinzhou is today's Shen muxian in Yan'anfu. Its remains are found in Wuyuancheng. The *chai hu* root grown there is more than a *chi* long and of a pale white color; it is tender. It is not easily obtainable. Those from the northern regions, they also resemble those of *peucedanum*, but are softer. They are the ones called by the people "northern *chai hu*" today. They, too, are good medication. The roots of those grown in southern soil do not resemble those of *peucedanum*. They are like the roots of common mugwort. They are sturdy and solid, and are not suited for therapeutic use. The seedlings of some have leaves resembling those of Chinese leek and others resembling those of bamboo leaves. Those with bamboo leaves are best. Those resembling *libanotis* herb are of lowest rank. According to the *Monthly Ordinances from the Small Calendar of Xia*, "Yun 芸 begins to grow in the middle period of spring." The *Cang Jie jie gu* states: "Yun 芸 is *hao* 蒿. It resembles *xie hao* 邪蒿, *libanotis* herb, and is edible. It is of the same group as *chai hu*, but does not lend itself very well for therapeutic application." This is why Su Gong states that it is not genuine *chai hu*. Today there is a variety with a white and big root resembling those of *platycodon* herb and *adenophora stricta* herb. The vendors on the market sell them as fake Yinzhou *chai hu* roots, but they lack qi and flavor. It is essential to distinguish between genuine and fake specimens.

Root of *chai hu*

Pharmaceutical Preparation

Lei Xiao: Whenever *chai hu* collected in Yinzhou is obtained, the hair and the tip of the root are to be removed. Then scratch off, with a silver knife, a little of the red, thin skin and rub it clean with a coarse cloth. Chop it and use it. Do not allow it to be offended by fire. It would be ineffective immediately.

Qi and Flavor

Bitter, acrid, nonpoisonous.

Supplementary Records by Famous Physicians: Slightly cold.

Wu Pu: Shen nong, Qi Bo, Lei gong: Bitter, nonpoisonous.

Da Ming: Sweet.

Zhang Yuansu: Its qi and flavor are all light; it is a yang substance. It rises in the body. It is a pharmaceutical drug for the minor yang conduits. It leads stomach qi to rise. Its bitter flavor and cold qi effuse and disperse heat from the body's outer regions.

Li Gao: It rises. It is a yang in yin substance. It is a pharmaceutical drug for the four hand and foot minor yang and ceasing yin conduits. In the long-term depots it controls the blood. In the conduits it controls the qi. If one wishes it to rise, he resorts to the root soaked in wine. If one wishes it to act in the center and to descend, use the smaller parts of the root.

Xu Zhicai: *Pinellia* root serves as its guiding substance. Ingested together, it abhors *gleditsia* pods/seeds, and fears *turczaninowia* root and *veratrum* root.

Li Shizhen: When it is supposed to move to the hand and foot minor yang conduits, it is assisted by *scutellaria* root. When it is supposed to move to the hand and foot ceasing yin conduits, it is assisted by *coptis* rhizome.

Control

Bound qi in heart, abdomen, intestines, and stomach. Accumulations of beverages and food. Alternating sensations of cold and heat resulting from an intrusion of evil qi. It pushes away what is old and lets arrive what is new. Ingested for a long time, it relieves the body of its weight. It clears the eyes and boosts the essence/sperm. *Original Classic*.

It removes vexing heat from below the heart in association with harm caused by cold, all bound and solid accumulations of phlegm and heat, evil qi in the chest, qi roaming in between the five long-term depots, accumulations stagnating in the large intestine, water swelling, and cramps and contractions resulting from blockages caused by moisture. It can also be used for a hot bath. *Supplementary Records by Famous Physicians*.

It serves to cure heat exhaustion and vexing pain in the bone joints, heat qi causing pain in the shoulders and the back, as well as emaciation resulting from exhaustion and weariness. It discharges qi and dissolves food. It facilitates the passage of qi and blood. It controls inner and outer heat caused by seasonal ailments that have not been resolved. When it is boiled as a single substance and ingested, this is good. Zhen Quan.

It supplements the five types of exhaustion and the seven types of harm. It eliminates vexation and ends fright. It boosts the strength of the qi. It dissolves phlegm and ends cough. It moistens the heart and the lung, increases essence/sperm and marrow, and acts against forgetfulness. Da Ming.

It eliminates depletion exhaustion, disperses sinew heat, and removes heat waves early in the day. It serves to cure alternating sensations of cold and heat, gallbladder solitary heat-illness, all types of heat of women prior to and following birth, obstacle-illness below the heart, and pain in chest and flanks. Zhang Yuansu.

It serves to cure descending yang qi, and it levels the qi of liver, gallbladder, Triple Burner and heart enclosing network, and the minister fire. Also, it serves to cure headache with vertigo, eyes that are dizzy, red, painful and have screens and shades, sounds in the ears, all types of malaria. Also, fat qi and alternating sensations of cold and heat, in women the intrusion of heat into the blood chamber, with irregular menstruation, in children surplus heat associated with smallpox macula, and the five types of *gan*-illness with emaciation and heat. Li Shizhen.

Explication

Xu Zhicai: *Chai hu* boiled down to four *sheng* in one *hu* of water together with *platycodon* root, rhubarb root, gypsum, hemp seeds, *glycyrrhiza* root, and *cassia*, with the amount of nitrokalite held by a three square inch spoon added, heals alternating sensations of cold and heat and headache associated with harm caused by cold, and a vexing feeling of fullness below the heart.

Su Song: In his therapy of harm caused by cold, Zhang Zhongjing resorted to the major and the minor decoction with *chai hu*, and to decoctions of *chai hu* with dragon bones, as well as of *chai hu* with mirabilite. Hence, to people in later times, when they cured harm caused by cold these were the most essential medications.

Li Gao: It can lead clear qi to move into the yang paths. Apart from harm caused by cold, for all types of heat *chai hu* is added. If no heat is present, it is not added. Also, it is able to lead stomach qi to move upward. When the order of spring lets yang qi vigorously ascend, it should be added. Furthermore, for all types of malaria, *chai hu* is the ruler substance in a recipe. It is to be assisted by conduit guiding pharmaceutical drugs as required by the location of a disease in a conduit in accordance to the time of its effusion. For sores caused by impediment-illness in any of the 12 conduits, *chai hu* is to be applied to disperse all types of conduit blood and of bound qi amassments. The potential is identical with that of *forsythia* fruit.

Wang Haogu: *Chai hu* is able to remove from inside and outside of the long-term depots and short-term repositories all types of weariness, and it is able to guide clear qi to ascend and follow the yang paths. Also, it enters the foot minor yang conduits. In the conduits it controls the qi. In the long-term depots it controls the blood. When a disease progresses, patients abhor heat. When it retreats, patients abhor cold. Hence only medications with slightly cold qi and a weak flavor are able to pass through the conduits. When *chai hu* root is assisted by substances such as *sparganium* root, zedoary root, and *croton* seeds, it is able to dissolve hard accumulations. This is its control of blood. For a woman whose menstruation at times comes and at times is interrupted, and for various diseases of harm caused by cold, Yi lao always uses the "minor decoction with *chai hu*." If substances of the group of the "decoction with four items" or substances such as gentian root and *paeonia* root bark are added, then these are preparations to regulate menstruation. It is also said that it is a pharmaceutical drug that must be used by women with blood heat following birth.

Kou Zongshi: The *Original Classic* has not a single character devoted to *chai hu's* ability to cure exhaustion. In the recipes of the people today aimed at curing exhaustion, it is rarely resorted to. Alas! This has led to so much malpractice in the world! Given that the original disease was exhaustion, there is one type where a depletion injured long-term depot repeatedly has received evil heat. Because of the already existing depletion, this resulted in exhaustion. That is, *lao* 勞, "exhaustion," is *lao* 牢, "distressed." In such a situation, *chai hu* may be used only after careful consideration. The cure of exhaustion heat by means of an *Artemisia carvifolia* decoction as recommended in the *Tried and Proven Recipes* is quite appropriate. Its ingestion is always effective. Once the heat is eliminated the treatment must be ended immediately. If it is ingested once there is no heat, the original disease will become more serious. But even if it ends in death, the people do not complain. I have witnessed very many such cases.

Rihua zi says that it serves to supplement the five types of exhaustion and seven types of harm.

The *Discourse on the Properties of Pharmaceutical Substances*, too, says that "it cures exhaustion, weariness, and emaciation." If such diseases are not associated with a repletion heat and physicians nevertheless resort to *chai hu*, how could it be that patients will not die? Of the commentaries in the *materia medica* works, not a single character must be ignored. Otherwise for ten thousand generations to come, innumerable errors will be committed. How can one not be careful! For example, when Zhang Zhongjing cures malaria-like alternating sensations of cold and heat, he uses decoctions with *chai hu* in exactly the right way.

Li Shizhen: There are five types of exhaustion; the disease is in the long-term depots. If an exhaustion is associated with heat in the liver, the gallbladder, the heart, and the heart enclosing network, or if there is alternating cold and heat in the minor yang conduits, then *chai hu* is a pharmaceutical drug that must be used to approach the hand and foot ceasing yin and minor yang conduits. If an exhaustion is associated with heat in the spleen and the stomach, and if yang qi descend, then *chai hu* is a pharmaceutical drug that must be used to guide clear qi and push back the heat. Only in the case of exhaustion affecting lung and kidneys, it cannot be used. Still, Mr. Li Dongyuan says that "it is appropriate to add *chai hu* to medication for all cases with heat, and that it should be omitted if there is no heat." He also says that "in recipes for all types of malaria in the conduits, *chai hu* should be the ruler drug. For sores resulting from impediment-illness affecting any of the 12 conduits, *chai hu* must be used to disperse collections of bound qi." That is, it can be used for all cases such as lung malaria and kidney malaria as well as sores related to the 12 conduits as long as they are associated with heat. However, if one intends to use *chai hu*, it is essential to consider the origin of the disease and to decide which substance can be added or omitted, which serves as assistant and which as guide.

Mr. Kou Zongshi does not distinguish whether there is heat or not in the long-term depots, the short-term repositories, the conduits, and the network vessel. He says that "*chai hu* does not cure exhaustion and weariness." But this is to be rejected; it is certainly not a commonly accepted position. For example, when the *Recipes from the Pharmaceutical Bureau* recommends to cure all types of blood disorders in the upper and lower sections of the body, the "pills with borneol and Japanese betony" use *chai hu* from Yinzhou that has been soaked to prepare a juice that was then boiled to prepare a paste. Only a few people today are familiar with the underlying meaning of this method.

According to Pang Yuanying's *Tan sou*, "Zhang Zhige for a long time suffered from malaria. At times, his heat was hot like fire. After more than a year, he was emaciated to the bone. The physicians resorted to a stag's pilose antlers and to *aconitum* accessory tubers, but the heat just got bigger. Eventually, the medical official Sun Lin was consulted to examine him. Sun Lin gave him a dose of a decoction with *chai hu*, and the heat decreased by 90%. After three ingestions the patient was free from all worries. Sun Lin: 'This is called exhaustion-malaria. The heat comes out of the marrow. If violent preparations are added, qi and blood will increasingly be harmed. How could this not result in emaciation?!' The fact is, when heat is in the skin, in the longterm depots and short-term repositories, and in the bone marrow, only *chai hu* can help. If one resorts to Yinzhou *chai hu*, only one ingestion is required. *Chai hu* from the South is weaker. Hence three ingestions are necessary to reach an effect." This shows the wondrous potential of an adequate application of pharmaceutical drugs. What Mr. Kou Zongshi said is not entirely reliable.

Added Recipes

One of old. Five newly recorded.

Remaining heat associated with harm caused by cold.
When following a harm caused by cold, evil qi enter the conduits and network vessels, the body will lose weight, and the muscles become hot. To push back the old and let the new arrive, to resolve harm caused by cold, seasonal epidemic qi, and hidden summerheat, to cure all these different ailments, regardless of the patient's age, the following recipe will help. For each dose four ounces of *chai hu* and one ounce of *glycyrrhiza* root are boiled in one bowl of water and ingested. Xu xueshi, *Recipes Based on Facts*.

Bone heat of children aged 15 or younger.
The entire body is hot like fire. Day after day they increasingly assume a yellow complexion and lose weight. They suffer from robber sweating,

cough, and vexing thirst. Grind four ounces of *chai hu* and three ounces of cinnabar to powder. Mix this with bile of a castrated pig, steam this above cooked rice until done, and form pills the size of mung beans. Each time ingest one pill, to be sent down with a decoction of peach kernels and smoked plums. To be ingested three times a day. *General Records of Sagely Benefaction.*

Depletion exhaustion and effusion of heat.
Boil equal amounts of *chai hu* and ginseng root, for each dose amounting to three maces, in water together with ginger and Chinese dates and ingest the liquid. *Recipes of the Tranquil Hut.*

Yellow *dan*-illness/jaundice associated with moisture and heat.
Prepare a dose of one ounce of *chai hu* and two and a half maces of *glycyrrhiza* root and boil this in one bowl of water with a handful of *imperata* root down to 70%. Ingest this as you wish from time to time. The total dose should be finished within one day. Sun Shangyao, *Secret and Precious Recipes.*

Dim vision.
Sift a powder of six scruples of *chai hu* and 18 scruples of fetid *cassia* seeds, mix it with human milk sap and apply this to the eyes. If this is continued for long, you will be able to see all five colors at night. *Recipes Worth a Thousand in Gold.*

Discharge with free-flux illness associated with heat accumulation.
Boil a mixture of one half of wine and one half of water down to 70%, steep equal amounts of *chai hu* and *scutellaria* root in the hot liquid until it has become cold, and ingest the liquid on an empty stomach. *Recipes for Aid in Emergencies.*

Seedling of *chai hu*

Control

Sudden deafness. Pound *chai hu* seedlings to obtain a juice and repeatedly drip it into the affected ear. *Recipes Worth a Thousand in Gold.*

Appendix

Dynasties

Shang	ca. 16th – 11th c. BCE
Zhou	1045 – 256 BCE
Warring States Period	403 – 221 BCE
Qin	221 – 207 BCE
Han (western)	206 BCE – 8 CE
Han (eastern)	25 – 220
Six Dynasties	220 – 589
Wei Dynasty	220 – 265
Three Kingdoms	220 – 265
Western Jin	265 – 317
Eastern Jin	317 – 420
Liu Song	420 – 479
Sui	581 – 618
Tang	618 – 907
Five Dynasties/Ten Kingdoms	907 – 960
Later Liang	907 – 923
Later Tang	923 – 936
Later Jin	936 – 946
Later Han	947 – 950
Later Zhou	951 – 960
Song	960 – 1279
Yuan	1271 – 1368
Ming	1368 – 1644
Qing	1644 – 1911

Approximate times of persons and texts mentioned in the anthology

For details, see *Dictionary of the Ben Cao Gang Mu*, Vol. III.

101 Select Recipes (12ᵗʰ c.).

A Miscellany from Youyang (9ᵗʰ c.). *All the Ten-thousand Arts of Huainan* (2ⁿᵈ c. BCE). *An Overall Survey of the Earth* (13ᵗʰ c.). *Annotations to the History of the Han* (post-Han era). *Arcane Essential Recipes from the Outer Censorate* (8ᵗʰ c.). *Arrangements for the Ladies' Chambers* (Yuan era).

Basic Annals of Xuanyuan (Tang era). *Basic Questions* (Han era, BCE). *Bifeng's Impromptu Poem Recipes* (early Ming). *Biographies of Divine Immortals* (Jin era). *Biography of Hua Tuo* (*Biography of Qian Yi* (11ᵗʰ/12ᵗʰ c.). *Bird Classic* (unclear). *Book of Nourishing the Elderly* (Song/Yuan era). *Book of Transformations* (Five Dynasties/Ten Kingdoms era). *Book on Nurturing Life* (Three Kingdoms era Wei). *Brush talks* (11th c.).

Cai Tao's Collected Talks (12ᵗʰ c.). *Categorized Compilation* (Song era). *Categorized Essential Recipes on Harm caused by Cold* (11th c.). *Categorized Stories* (12ᵗʰ c.). Chen Cheng (11ᵗʰ c.). Chen Linqiu (Jin era). Chen Shiliang (10ᵗʰ c.). Chen Yanzhi (Jin era). Chen Zhengmin (12ᵗʰ c.). Chen Ziming (Southern Song era). Chu Yushi (11ᵗʰ c.). *Classic Erudition* (5th c.). *Classic of Changes* (attributed to Zhou era). *Classic of Deities and Extraordinary Things* (Six Dynasties, unclear). *Classic of Difficult Issues* (Han era). *Classic of Mountains and Seas* (Han era BCE). *Classic of Sagely Benefaction* (12ᵗʰ c.). *Classic of Supporting Life* (12ᵗʰ c.). *Classic of the Northern Mountains* (see *Classic of Mountains and Seas*). *Classic of the Numinous Pivot* (Han era). *Classic of Wild Animals* (16ᵗʰ c.). *Collected and Proven Recipes* (unclear). *Collected and Proven Recipes for Childbirth and Nursing* (9ᵗʰ c.). *Collected and Proven Recipes Recorded while Avoiding the Floods* (16ᵗʰ c.). *Collected Essentials from the Forest of Medicine* (15ᵗʰ c.). *Collection from the Reign Period 'Long-lasting Favor Accorded by Our Association with Heaven'* (9ᵗʰ c.). *Commentary on Herbs and Trees* (3ʳᵈ c.). *Commentary on the Book of Songs* (different authors, different times). *Commentary on the Examples of Refined Usage* (4ᵗʰ c.). *Commentary on the Meanings in the Book of Songs* (3ʳᵈ c.). *Compilation for Engendering Life* (unclear). *Compilation from Bozhai* (11ᵗʰ c.). *Compilation of Applied Benevolence* (16ᵗʰ c.). *Compilation of My Studies* (16ᵗʰ c.). *Complete Records from Court and Commonality* (8ᵗʰ c.). *Comprehensive Treatises* (12ᵗʰ c.). *Correct Meanings in the Examples of Refined Usage* (Wei, Three Kingdoms era). *Correction of Errors in the Rhymed Instructions on the Movements in the Vessels* (14th c.). *Crab Treatise* (11th c.). *Crucial Points of the Laws of Life* (13th c.). Cui Bao (Western Jin era).

Da Ming (see Rihua zi). Dai Qizong (Yuan era). *Daoist Canon* (general reference to Daoist books). *Declarations of the Perfected* (5th/6th c.). *Deng Bifeng's Recipes* (see *Bifeng's Impromptu Poem Recipes*). Deng Deming (5th c.). Ding Wei (11th c.). *Discourse on All Diseases from Harm Caused by Cold* (11th c.). *Discourse on Nature* (Song era or earlier). *Discourse on the Properties of Pharmaceutical Substances* (unclear). *Distinguishing Doubtful Points about All Disease Signs* (16th c.). *Documents of the Elder* (Han era or earlier, BCE). *Dogmatic Conversations Among the Learned* (Song to Yuan era). Dong Bing (16th c.). Dong Zhongshu (2nd c. BCE). Dongyuan (see Li Gao). Du Bao (7th c.). Duan Chengshi (9th c.). Duan gonglu (9th c.).

Easy and Simple Recipes for Protecting Life (15th c.). *Easy Recipes for Rescue in Emergencies* (15th c.). *Edited Essentials of Zhu Danxi* (15th c.). *Elegies of Chu* (2nd c.). *Elucidation of Characters* (11th c.). *Essential Arts of the Common People* (6th c.). *Essentials of the Discipline Concerned with External Diseases and Treatments* (12th c.). *Eternal Key Recipes* (14th c.). *Examples of Refined Usage* (ca. 200 BCE). *Exceptional Recipes for Strange Diseases* (16th c.). *Expanded Book on Rhymes* (8th c.). *Expanded Examples of Refined Usage* (Three Kingdoms era). *Expanded Records of the Five Phases* (7th c.). *Explaining Single and Analysing Compound Characters* (2nd c.; by Xu Kai 10th c.). *Explanation of Names* (ca. 200). *Exploring the Profound* (13th c.). *Extensive Records of the Reign Period "Great Peace"* (Song era).

Fan Wang fang (4th c.). Fang Shao (11th c.). *Forgotten Matters of the Reign Periods "Opening a New Era" and "Heavenly Treasures"* (Five Dynasties era). *Forms of Herbs and Trees from the Southern Regions* (4th c.). Fu gong (11th c.).

Gan Bao (4th c.). Gao Yangsheng (Six Dynasties era). Gao You (3rd c.). *Garden of Extraordinary Things* (5th c.). *Gazetteer of the South Central Area* (Jin era). Ge Hong (284 – 364). *General Records of Sagely Benefaction* (12th c.). *Geographical Records of the Reign Period "Great Well-Being"* (Jin era). Gong shi (Ming era). *Good recipes for Women* (13th c.). *Good Recipes of Su Dongpo* (11th c.). *Great Compendium of Medical Recipies* (14th c.). Gu Wei (Jin era). Gu Yewang (519 – 581). *Guo Jizhong's Recipes* (12th c.).

Han Baosheng (Five Dynasties era). *Heart Mirror of Diet Physicians* (9th c.). *Heart Mirror of Healing the Young* (15th c.). *History of Southern Dynasties* (7th c.). *History of Southern Qi* (Liang era). *History of the Han* (1st/2nd c.).

History of the Jin (4th c.). *History of the Later Han* (Liu Song era). Hong Mai (12th c.). *How Scholars Should Serve Their Parents* (13th c.). Hu Yan (Ming era or earlier). Hu Ying (1375 – 1463). Huang Shangu (11th c.).

Idle Views from a Secluded Study (12th c.). *Illustrated Classic of Materia Medica* (7th c.). *Illustrated Compilation To Benefit the People* (16th c.). *Increased Examples of Refined Usage* (11th c.). *Informal Notes of Hong Rongzai* (12th c.). *Instructions for Ingesting Pepper* (Jin era). *Investigation of the Woes of Departure* (12th c.).

Jade Chapters (6th c.). *Jade Volume from the Years Geng to Xin* (15th c.). *Jewels of Childbirth* (9th c.). Ji Han (263 – 306). Ji Kang (223 – 262). Jin Zhuo (Jin era). Jing Fang (77 – 37 BCE). *Jing Fang's Divination by the Book of Changes* (1st c. BCE).

Kong Pingzhong (1044 – 1111).

Lei Xiao (Liu Song to Song era). *Leisure-hours Conversations of Rustics* (Song era). Li Ao (772 – 841). Li Dongyuan (see Li Gao). Li Gao (1180 – 1251). Li Jiang (764 – 830). Li Lou (16th c.). Li Xun (9th c.). Li Yanshou (570 – 628). Li Yanwen (died 1572). *Literary Collection of Song Qianxi* (Yuan era). *Literary Notes Written During Recuperation* (13th c.). Liu Changchun (1351 – 1432). Liu Jingshu (5th c.). Liu Songshi (died 1545). Liu Xi (ca. 200). Liu Yuxi (772 – 842). *Liuzhou's Recipes for Rescue from the Three Kinds of Death* (9th c.). *Lotus Sutra* (ca. 400). Lu Dian (1042 – 1102). Lu Ji (Three Kingdoms era). Luo Tianyi (13th c.). Luo Yuan (12th c.).

Ma Zhi (10th c.). Mao Chang (Western Han era). *Master Han's Outer Commentary to the Book of Songs* (2nd c. BCE). *Materia Medica for Decoctions* (13th c.). *Materia Medica for Famine Relief* (15th c.). *Materia Medica of Tang Shenwei* (12th c.). *Materia Medica of the Food Mirror* (16th c.). *Materia Medica of the Reign Period "Opening Treasures"* (10th c.). *Materia Medica of Wu Pu* (Three Kingdoms Wei era). *Medical Anecdotes* (13th c.). Meng Shen (621 – 713). *Method for Stone Cooking by the Perfected One Donghua* (Tang era). *Miraculous Recipes to Conserve Life* (16th c.). *Mirror of Medicine* (16th c.). *Miscellaneous Records from the Time of Emperor Ming* (9th c.). *Monograph on a Wide Range of Things* (3rd c.). *Mr. Sun's Collected Efficacious Recipes* (16th c.). *Mr. Wei's Recipes to Obtain Good Results* (14th c.). *Mr. Xu's Recipes for Pregnancy and Birth* (15th c.). *Mr. Xu's Recipes for Pregnancy and Birth* (15th c.). *Mr. Yang's Book on Childbirth and Nursing* (Tang era). Mr. Ye (different texts, different times). *Mr. Zheng's Recipes* (12th c.). *Mr. Zhu's Collected* and Proven Recipes (13ᵗʰ c.). *Mr. Zhu's Records Collecting the Extraordinary* (9ᵗʰ c.). *Mushroom Treatise* (13ᵗʰ c.).

Nagarjuna's Discourse (Song to Yuan era). Nan Gongcong (Ming era). *Nirvana Sutra* (5ᵗʰ c.). *Notes on Discerning Extraordinary Things* (Eastern Jin era). *Notes on Polygonum* (9ᵗʰ c.). *Notes on Things Old and New* (Western Jin era). *Odds and Ends Recorded Vastly as an Ocean* (12ᵗʰ c.).

Offices of Zhou (s. *Rites of Zhou*). *On Recipes for the Three Causes* (12ᵗʰ c.). *Original Classic* (1ˢᵗ/2ⁿᵈ c.).

Pang Anshi (Song era). Pang Yuanying (11ᵗʰ c.). *Patterns and Treatment of Smallpox Papules* (16ᵗʰ c.). *Personally Proven Recipes for Harm Caused by Cold* (4ᵗʰ c.). *Picking up the Green Fragmentary Writings* (Song era). *Poetry from the Brocade Bag* (around 1500). *Precious Classic of the Highest Origin* (Song era or earlier). *Precious Mirror to Protect Life* (13ᵗʰ c.). *Precious Recipes to Be Kept up the Sleeve* (15ᵗʰ c.). *Proper and Essential Things for the Emperor's Beverages and Food* (14ᵗʰ c.). *Proven Recipes Recorded in Ancient and Modern Times* (7ᵗʰ c.).

Qian Yi (1032 – 1113). Qin Yueren (legendary, BCE). *Quick-Working Recipes* (8ᵗʰ c.). Quxian (1378 – 1448).

Recipes Based on Facts (12ᵗʰ c.). *Recipes Collected by Hand from the Ministry of War* (ca. 800). *Recipes for Aid in Emergencies* (Yuan era). *Recipes for Children* (Song era and Ming era texts). *Recipes for Emergencies* (by Zhang Wenzhong, 7ᵗʰ c.). *Recipes for Emergency Rescue* (16ᵗʰ c.). *Recipes for Extensive Assistance* (8ᵗʰ c.). *Recipes for Extensive Assistance of the Reign Period "Opening a New Era"* (8ᵗʰ c.). *Recipes for Protecting Life, Treasured by the Family Recipes for Rescue in Emergencies* (Song era). *Recipes for Supporting Long Life* (16ᵗʰ c.). *Recipes for Universal Benefit* (15ᵗʰ c.). *Recipes from Abroad* (unclear). *Recipes from Lingnan to Protect Life* (13ᵗʰ c.). *Recipes from the Numinous Garden* (11ᵗʰ c.). *Recipes from the Pharmaceutical Bureau fang* (12ᵗʰ c.). *Recipes from the Realm of Longevity* (15ᵗʰ c.). *Recipes from the Small Essays* (Jin era). *Recipes Kept in the Quiver* (11ᵗʰ c.). *Recipes of Bian* Que (unclear). Recipes *of Du Ren* (11ᵗʰ c.). *Recipes of Illumination* (12ᵗʰ c.). *Recipes of Master Mei* (Sui or Tang era). *Recipes of Tan Yeweng* (15ᵗʰ c.). *Recipes of the Big Dipper Gate* (Northern Song era). *Recipes of the Tranquil Hut* (13ᵗʰ c.). *Recipes of Universal Benefit* (11ᵗʰ c.). *Recipes of Universal Benefit* (15ᵗʰ c.). *Recipes of Unusual Illnesses* (Song era). *Recipes to be Kept Close at Hand* (4ᵗʰ c.). *Recipes to benefit Life* (14ᵗʰ c.). *Recipes Transmitted by Immortals* (14ᵗʰ c.). *Recipes with the Superfluous Deleted* (Sui era or earlier). *Recipes Worth a Thousand in Gold* (7ᵗʰ c.). *Recipes Worth More than Gold* (Song era or earlier). Reclusive Scholar Li (unclear). *Record of Rites* (Warring States era, BCE). *Record on the Western Territories* (Five Dynasties era or earlier). *Records Collecting the Extraordinary* (9ᵗʰ c.). *Records from Beihu* (9ᵗʰ c.). *Records from Inside the Mysterious* (pre-Tang era). *Records from Lin hai* (Liu Song era). *Records from Lingbiao* (10ᵗʰ c.). *Records from the Leisure Time at the Prefect's Office* (11ᵗʰ c.). *Records from the Summer Resort* (12ᵗʰ c.). *Records from the Waters and Lands of Lin hai* (Liu Song era). *Records Kept in one's Headrest* (7ᵗʰ c.). *Records Narrating the Extraordinary* (Qi and Liang era). *Records of Customs and Geographical Surroundings* (3ʳᵈ c.). *Records of Entering Heaven* (13ᵗʰ c.). *Records of Entering the Netherworld* (Tang era). *Records of Extraordinary Things* (different texts, different times). *Records of Extraordinary Things from the Southern Regions* (9ᵗʰ c.). *Records of Famous Physicians* (11ᵗʰ c.). *Records of Fan Dongyang* (4ᵗʰ c.). *Records of Guangzhou* (Jin era). *Records of Linchuan* (5ᵗʰ c.). *Records of Local Products from Yi* (11ᵗʰ c.). *Records of Nankang* (5ᵗʰ c.). *Records of Nanyue* (Liu Song era). *Records of Nanzhou* (Tang era or earlier). *Records of Qixie* (Liu Song era). *Records of Retrieved Stories of the Great Inherited Responsibility Reign Period* (Tang era). *Records of Searching for the Supernatural* (Jin era). *Records of Swirling Snow Flakes* (15ᵗʰ c.). *Records of the Annual Seasons in Jing and Chu* (Liang era). *Records of the Core of Classics* (Sui – Tang era). *Records of the Golden Gate* (10ᵗʰ/11ᵗʰ c.). *Records of the Guang Area* (Jin era). *Records of the Immortals of the Clouds* (unclear). *Records of the Investigation of Crafts* (pre-Qin BCE). *Records of the Mutual Influences of Various Categories of Things* (10ᵗʰ c.). *Records of Trivial Things* (12ᵗʰ c.). *Records of Waters and Clouds* (12ᵗʰ c.). *Records of Weary Wanderings* (11ᵗʰ c.). *Records of Wu* (Jin era). *Records of Yong jia* (Liu Song era). *Records Taken while Stopping from Field Work* (14ᵗʰ c.). *Regional Languages* (Western Han) Ren Fang (460 – 508). *Rhapsody Examining the Sagely* (6ᵗʰ c.). *Rhapsody on the Capital of Wu* (Jin era). *Rhapsody on the Upper Forest* (Han era, BCE). *Rhymed Instructions on the Movements in the Vessels* (3ʳᵈ c.). Rihua zi (Five Dynasties era). *Rites of Zhou* (unclear, pre-Han era). *Ritual and Etiquette* (Han dynasty or earlier). *Rong zhai sui bi* (12ᵗʰ c.). *Rural Records from the Western Watchtower* (16ᵗʰ c.). *Rustic Conversations from East of Qi* (13ᵗʰ c.).

Sagely and Benevolent Recipes (10ᵗʰ c.). *Secret and Precious Recipes* (11ᵗʰ c.). *Secret Conversations on the Mysterious Pearl* (Song era). *Secret Records About Children and Mothers* (Song era). *Selected Profound Recipes* (different texts, different times). Shen Gua (1031 – 1095). Shi Yuan (physician: 12th c.; minor official: Tang – Song era). *Simple and Convenient Recipes* (16th c.). *Simple and Convenient Recipes to Benefit the Masses* (11th c.). *Simple Recipes from the Collection of Li Binhu* (16th c.). Song Qi (998 – 1061). Song Qiqiu (10th c.). Song Yangzi (785 – 805). Songhuang (16th c.). *Spirit Book of Gou lou Mountain* (Ming era). *Straightforward Guide to Recipes of Yang Renzhai* (13th c.). Su Dongpo (see Su Shi). Su Gong (7th c.). Su Shi (1037 – 1101). Su Song (1019 – 1101). Sun Mian (8th c.). Sun Shangyao (11th c.). Sun Simiao (581 – 682?). Sun the Perfected One (s, Sun Simiao). Sun Yan (Three Kingdoms era). *Supplementary Amplifications on the Materia Medica* (8th c.). *Supplementary Biography of Liu Gen* (Eastern Jin, BCE). *Supplementary Records by Famous Physicians* (ca. 500). *Supreme Commanders of the Medical Ramparts* (13th c.). *Surangama Sutra* (8th c.).

Tales of the World (5th c.). *Talks from the States* (Han era). Tang Shenwei (11th/12th c.). Tang Yao (unclear). Tao Hongjing (456 – 536). Tao Jiucheng (1316 - ?). *Tested and Proven Recipes* (15th c.). *Tested Efficacious Recipes* (possibly 13th c.). *The Book for Saving People's Lives* (12th c.). *The Book from Nan yang for Saving People's Lives* (12th c.). *The Classic of Movements in the Vessels* (3rd c.). *The Classic of Mysterious Changes up on High* (unclear). *The Divine Farmer's Materia Medica* (Han era). *The Divine Immortal's Classic of Ingesting Essences* (Sui era). *The Divine Immortal's Text on Interactions* (Five Dynasties era). *The Farmer's Classic* (unclear). *Nong shu* (14th c.). *The Heart Mirror of Universal Love* (16th c.). *The Intentions of Written Language* (Sui era). *The Majestic Presence of the Big Dipper in the Record of Rites* (Han era). *The Master Embracing Simplicity* (4th c.). *The Master of Huainan* (2nd c. BCE). *The Original Meanings of the Six Categories of Characters* (14th c.). *The Orthodox Transmission of Medical Studies* (16th c.). *The Orthodox Transmission of Medical Studies* (16th c.). *The Posthumous Works of the Cheng Brothers* (Northern Song era). *The Records of Yijian* (12th c.). *The Spring and Autumn Annals of Mr. Lü* (3rd c. BCE). *Token of the Agreement* (Eastern Han era). *Tradition of Heavenly Aromatic Substances* (11th c.). *Transmitted Core Recipes* (9th c.). *Treasury of the Jade Candle* (Qi/Sui era). *Treatise of the Supervisor and Guardian of the Cinnamon Sea* (12th c.). *Treatise on Bamboo* (5th c.). *Treatise on Bamboo Shoots* (10th c.). *Tried and Proven Good Recipes* (Yuan era). *Tried and Proven Good Recipes of Shao, the Perfected one* (15th c.). *Tried and Proven Later Recipes* (Song era). *Tried and Proven Recipes* (different authors, different times). *Tried and Proven Recipes from the Hall of Preserving Long Life* (16th c.). *Tried and Proven Recipes of Tang Yao* (unclear).

Uncertain Words (16th c.). *Unofficial Histories* (different texts, different times).

Vitality in Heaven and Earth (15th c.).

Wang Anshi (1021 – 1086). Wang Bing (8th c.). Wang Guan (Tang era). Wang Gun (Song era). Wang Haicang (13th c.). Wang Ji (1463 – 1539; et al.). Wang Qiu (12th c.). Wang Shuhe (3rd c.). Wang Wei (701 – 761). Wang Ying (16th c.). Wang Zhen (13th c.). Wang Zhizhong (12th c.). Wei Zhi (16th c.). *What one should know about pregnancy and birth* (Yuan to Ming era). *Wings to the Examples of Refined Usage* (Song era). *Writings on Awakening to the Truth* (10th/11th c.). Wu Min (16th c.).

Xia Ziyi (Song era). Xiao Bing (Tang era). Xu Kai (920 – 974). Xu Shen (58 – 147). Xu Shenweng (12th/13th c.). Xu Shuwei (1079 – 1154). Xu Xueshi (see Xu Shuwei). Xu Zhicai (died 572). Xuan fu (alias Confucius). Xuan zong (8th c.). *Xuan's Canon* (Han era or earlier). Xue Yongruo (9th c.). Xun Bozi (5th c.).

Yan Shigu (Tang era). Yan Zili (Song era). Yang Qi (16th c.). Yang Qingsou (Yuan era). Yang Renzhai (13th c.). Yang Shen (1488 – 1559). Yang Shiying (13th c.). Yang Yi (974 – 1020). Ye Mengde (1077 – 1148). Ye Shilin (see Ye Mengde). Yu gong (uncertain, BCE). *Yu pian* (6th c.). Yu Yan (1258 – 1314). Yuan Zhen (779 – 831). Zan Ning (919 – 1001).

Zan Yin (9th c.). Zhang Bo (3rd c.). Zhang Congzheng (1158 – 1228). Zhang Ding (8th c.). Zhang Gao (Tang era). Zhang Hua (Western Jin era). Zhang Ji (see Zhang Zhongjing; also: 767 – 830). Zhang Jiegu (12th c.). Zhang Rui (12th c.). Zhang Shizheng (11th c.). Zhang Wenzhong (7th/8th c.). Zhang Yi (3rd c.). Zhang Yuansu (see Zhang Jiegu). Zhang Zhongjing (2nd c.). Zhang Zihe (see Zhang Congzheng). Zhao Jin (13th c.). Zhao Xihu (Song era). Zhen Quan (541 - 643). Zheng Kangcheng (see Zheng Xuan). Zheng Xiao (1499 – 1566). Zheng Xuan (127 – 200). Zhong Jun (died 113 BCE). Zhou Caochuang (s. Zhou Mi). Zhou Chu (c. 236 – 297). Zhou Mi (1232 – c. 1298). Zhou Xian wang (1379 – 1439). Zhu Duanzhang (12th c.). Zhu Gong (Song era). Zhu Zhenheng (1281 – 1358).

Glossary

Aggregation-illness. Painful lumps emerging from time to time in both flanks. BCGM Dict I, 371.

An infant's headrest. Identical with an infant's-headrest pain. A condition following delivery with swelling and lumps caused by stagnant blood (the "infant's headrest") in the abdominal region, accompanied by pain. BCGM Dict I, 147.

An infant's-headrest pain. A condition following delivery with swelling and lumps caused by stagnant blood (the "infant's headrest") in the abdominal region, accompanied by pain. BCGM Dict I, 147.

Archer's poison. An ancient notion of bugs that live in waters and shoot their poison at humans, causing disease. BCGM Dict I, 432.

Attachment-illness, influx-illnesss. A notion of a foreign pathogenic agent, originally of demonic nature, having attached itself to the human organism. BCGM Dict I, 688-695.

Bedroom exhaustion. An etiological agent of excessive or inappropriate sexual intercourse. BCGM Dict I, 152.

Collapsing center. Excessive vaginal bleeding outside of a menstruation period. BCGM Dict I, 58

Concretion-illness and conglomeration-illness. The two terms are often used interchangeably and do not signify two distinctly different conditions. Concretion-illness and conglomeration-illness result from a disharmony of cold and warmth resulting in a failure to transform beverages and food. Nodes form when the clash with the qi of the long-term depots. BCGM Dict I, 677

Corpse [bugs/worms] throat. A condition of a disease affecting the throat with pain and itching and loss of voice. BCGM Dict I, 458.

Depot dryness. A condition of women whose spirit is depressed and who feel sad and begin to weep for no apparent reason. BCGM Dict I, 662.

Doubled danger. A reference to the meaning of the 29th hexagram of the *Yi jing*.

Doubled tongue. A condition with the growth underneath the tongue, mostly in children, of what appears like a second tongue. BCGM Dict I, 92.

Effusion of the back. A condition of obstruction-illnesses and impediment-illnesses developing on one's back. As it was believed that the transporter holes of the five depots and six palaces are located on the back, conditions of obstruction-illnesses and impediment-illnesses there, often apparent as abscesses, were considered threatening. BCGM Dict I, 148.

Elevation-illness, elevation illness-qi. A group of conditions characterized by violent abdominal pain, in some cases associated with constipation and anuria. Also notion of a foreign item that has entered the scrotum, causes pain, and may ascend and descend. BCGM Dict I, 417, 419.

Female *dan*-illness. Identical with *dan*-illness resulting from exhaustion with women. A condition of resulting from excessive sexual intercourse. BCGM Dict I, 361, 262.

Fetal poison. A heat poison transferred from a mother's body to a fetus during pregnancy, resulting in a child's predisposition for developing smallpox and other diseases. BCGM Dict I, 485.

Flowery *xuan*-illness. Identical with *xuan*-illness. Conditions of dermal lesions with initially erythema, papules, and itching gradually slightly elevated with small papules, blisters, and/or scales and scraps. The central lesion may appear to heal spontaneously, and it may reappear. Also, a designation of local lesions with itching, release of liquid, and shedding of scabs. BCGM Dict I, 222, 591.

Gu 蠱 is an ancient conceptualization of diseases traced to a magic pathogenic agent. Originally it was assumed to be a most poisonous bug, the only creature in a closed jar surviving competition with hundreds of other poisonous bugs. This bug was believed to be instrumentalized by greedy persons to appropriate the belongings of others. The resulting disease was termed *gu* poison(ing). See BCGM Dict I, 191.

Impediment-illness. An obstruction of vessels or other ducts inside the body. Qi rushing against the impediment may cause a local swelling and eventually break through the surface to cause an abscess. BCGM Dict I, 277.

Influx. 1.) A pathological mechanism of evil qi moving around in, and erratically entering, various parts of the human body. 2.) A condition of sores with pus in deep-lying regions of the human body. BCGM Dict I, 323.

Influx pain. An illness sign of pain erratically changing its location. BCGM Dict I, 694.

Innocence. An illness accompanied by scrofula affecting the head and neck. BCGM Dict I, 537.

Intestinal wind. A condition of bloody stools with the blood being fresh and red. BCGM Dict I, 79.

Jie-**illness**. Vaguely identifiable skin ailment. BCGM Dict I, 249.

Leaking fetus. A condition of vaginal bleeding during pregnancy. BCGM Dict I, 327.

Leg qi. Painful, weak, swollen legs. BCGM Dict I, 248.

Marriage pain. An injury inflicted on a woman's outer genital parts following crude and violent sexual intercourse. BCGM Dict I, 244.

Massive wind. May refer to sores caused by a massive intrusion of wind evil and also to conditions of leprosy. BCGM Dict I, III.

Melting with thirst. Most likely including cases of diabetes. BCGM Dict Vol I, 567.

Mouse fistula. Identical to scrofula pervasion-illness.

Nine mansions diagram. An ancient astronomical projection on a square divided into nine subsquares, so called "mansions," onto the sky to identify the position of celestial bodies and their movement in the course of a year.

Nipple moth. Most likely including cases of acute tonsillitis. BCGM Dict I, 410.

Obstruction-illness. An obstruction of vessels or other ducts inside the body. Qi rushing against the obstruction may cause a local swelling and eventually break through the surface to cause an abscess. BCGM Dict I, 641.

Obstruction-illness and impediment-illness. Two vaguely distinguished obstructions/impediments of vessels or other ducts inside the body. Qi rushing against the obstruction may cause a local swelling and eventually break through the surface to cause an abscess. BCGM Dict I, 642.

Old blood. Identical with residual blood, a condition of stagnant blood forming long-term accumulations in the body that are difficult to dissolve and may in turn cause further diseases. BCGM Dict I, 480.

Palpitating qi. A condition with fright, fear, and heart palpitation. BCGM Dict I, 240.

Pervading joints wind. A condition of pain wind, characterized by spontaneous sweating, shortness of qi/breath, aching joints, and difficulties in bending and stretching. BCGM Dict I, 314.

Pin-illness. A deep-reaching and festering hardness in a tissue, eventually rising above the skin like a pinhead. BCGM Dict I, 127-129.

Red bayberry poison sores. Most likely including cases of syphilis. BCGM Dict I, 293, 294.

Repudiation-illness, including cases of leprosy. BCGM Dict I, 293.

Roaming wind. A condition of roaming and sudden pain and itching brought about by wind evil. BCGM Dict I, 645.

Robber sweating. 1.) An illness sign of a profuse sweating during sleep that ends when one wakes up. 2.) A pathological condition with robber sweating as major sign. BCGM Dict I, 122.

Robber wind. A condition caused by qi that appear in a season they do not belong to. More at BCGM Dict I, 667.

Scrofula pervasion-illness. When two or more connected swellings of the size of plum or date kernels appear either on the neck or in the armpits, or somewhere else on the body. BCGM Dict I. 329.

String-illness. A condition of acute pain located in the abdomen to the left and right of the umbilicus. BCGM Dict I, 591.

Suspended obstruction-illness. A condition of **obstruction-illness** developing either in the perineum or in the bend between the jaws and pharynx. BCGM Dict I, 593, 641.

Suspended rheum. A disease brought forth by rheum flowing into the region below the flanks with cough and vomiting causing pain. BCGM Dict I, 59.

The Three Peng. The the three corpse spirits Peng Ju, Peng Zhi, and Peng Jiao residing in the human body in the head, the heart, and the abdomen and aiming to bring about premature death.

Thundering head wind. A condition of head wind characterized by headache together with lumps rising in the face and/or sounds in the head. BCGM Dict I, 303.

To poke life. The mixing of food or beverages with poison, and *gu*-poisoning, i.e. the insertion of a poisonous bug into a human's food, are two crimes that are believed to be primarily committed in the South.

Visitor heat. An etiological agent identified as heat evil intruding into the human organism from outside. BCGM Dict I, 282.

Well splendor water. The first water drawn from a well in the morning. BCGM Vol. II, 05-15-01.

White overflow. A condition of white mucus excreted from one's urinary tract/genital region as a result of excessive sexual intercourse or unfulfilled desires. BCGM Dict I, 49.

Yellow *dan*-illness. Most likely including cases of jaundice. BCGM Dict I, 225.

Yin (and yang) exchange. A condition of a communicable disease acquired by males through sexual intercourse with a female who had just been cured of harm caused by cold. BCGM Dict I, 639.

Yin poison. A condition a.) of harm caused by cold, resulting in a flourishing of only yang qi and a diminution of yin qi, with cold extremities and a greenish facial complexion, pain in the abdomen and affecting the entire body, as well as a deep-lying and fine movement in the vessels, and b.) poison qi with a cold quality. BCGM Dict I, 633.

Founded in 1893,
UNIVERSITY OF CALIFORNIA PRESS
publishes bold, progressive books and journals
on topics in the arts, humanities, social sciences,
and natural sciences—with a focus on social
justice issues—that inspire thought and action
among readers worldwide.

The UC PRESS FOUNDATION
raises funds to uphold the press's vital role
as an independent, nonprofit publisher, and
receives philanthropic support from a wide
range of individuals and institutions—and from
committed readers like you. To learn more, visit
ucpress.edu/supportus.